P9-CKT-186

DYSLEXIA

Theory & Practice of Instruction

Third Edition

JOANNA KELLOGG UHRY

DIANA BREWSTER CLARK

WITHDRAWN

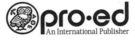pro·ed
An International Publisher
8700 Shoal Creek Boulevard
Austin, Texas 78757-6897
800/897-3202   Fax 800/397-7633
www.proedinc.com

████████████████████████
████████████████████████
████████████████████████

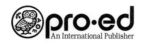

© 2004 by PRO-ED, Inc.
8700 Shoal Creek Boulevard
Austin, Texas 78757-6897
800/897-3202   Fax 800/397-7633
www.proedinc.com

All rights reserved. No part of the material protected by this
copyright notice may be reproduced or used in any form or by
any means, electronic or mechanical, including photocopying,
recording, or by any information storage and retrieval system,
without prior written permission of the copyright owner.

Printed in the United States of America

1 2 3 4 5   10 09 08 07 06

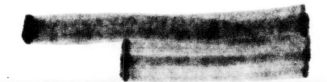

Table of Contents

Preface to the Third Edition

The first edition of this book was written by Diana Brewster Clark and published in 1988. Diana, my colleague and friend from our days studying at Teachers College Columbia University, died early in 1993 as she was beginning to plan a second edition. I eventually wrote the second edition, which was published in 1995. This third edition provides a systematic update of research and programs since that time. It includes new chapters and a somewhat different structure. The purpose of the book, however, remains the same: to provide an overview of the research literature on the nature of dyslexia and how children with dyslexia can be taught most effectively. The book is written for teachers and the final chapters are practical in nature.

In her preface to the first edition, Dr. Clark stated that there were several important realizations about dyslexia that prompted her to write this book, one of which follows:

> [T]he separation of reading education, special education, and remedial reading education into three ostensibly autonomous domains of instruction—the first two residing in schools, the third for the most part in the private sectors—has been extremely detrimental to dyslexic students, causing unnecessary confusion over their identification and treatment. Sharing and integrating ideas between these three, now separate, disciplines is essential if dyslexic students are ever to be served effectively.

In 1988, classroom teachers were provided with little training in special education or specialized remedial reading instruction, and were not expected to provide reading instruction in the classroom for children with reading difficulties. Reading specialists and special educators served as pull-out specialists. They pulled children out of the classroom for blocks of specialized instruction, or, in some cases, provided instruction all day long in special classes. Neither of these specialties involved training in the remediation of dyslexia. Three trends, representing changes in the field, have helped break down this compartmentalization since 1988.

CHANGES IN THE FIELD
BALANCED READING INSTRUCTION IN THE CLASSROOM

Since the second edition of this book, two major analyses of the research literature on learning to read have been published. Both have played a role in the current trend away from the dichotomy of the reading wars (i.e., skills versus meaning) and toward instruction that balances skills—especially phonics skills—with meaning-based instructional approaches that developed out of the whole-language movement.

The first of these two analyses of the research literature was carried out by a committee of the National Academy of Science at the joint request of the U. S. Department of Education and the U. S. Department of Health and Human Services. Catherine Snow served as committee chair for the report, Preventing Reading Difficulties in Young Children (Snow, Burns, and Griffin 1998). The second analysis was the National Reading Panel Report (2000; Ehri et al. 2001), a meta-analysis and summary of what the team called "scientific research" on reading instruction. Linnea Ehri served as Chair of the Alphabetics subgroup, which analyzed phonemic awareness and phonics data. These reports came at a time when Congress was urging more evidence that federal money was supporting well-researched, effective programs.

TREND TOWARD INCLUSION CLASSROOMS

When the first edition of this book was published, it was assumed that teachers working with children with dyslexia would be reading specialists, but this notion is changing. Many children with reading difficulties are being taught in inclusion classrooms, classrooms with a mix of children, some of whom have individualized education plans (IEPs), assessment-based instructional plans generated after establishing the need for special services. The best inclusion classes involve collaboration between a special educator and a regular educator working together in the same classroom. In less ideal cases, especially in high-need, under-resourced schools, classroom teachers may be solely responsible for children with reading disabilities for part or all of the day. This means that classroom teachers need to increase their knowledge and skills in a wide array of teaching strategies. They need enormous amounts of self-confidence, and they need to believe that all children can learn to read.

Primary-grade teachers need to know how to identify and teach to minimize the early symptoms of dyslexia. They need the tools to spot the early signs and to provide immediate and effective instruction. Teachers in the upper elementary grades need to know how to plan effective remediation. Both lower and upper grade teachers need extraordinary organizational skills in order to group students for instruction at various levels and to modify instruction to meet the needs of all.

TREND TOWARD MORE TEACHER PREPARATION IN READING

In its most recent standards for teacher preparation, the International Reading Association (IRA) recommends that initial elementary teacher education programs include five literacy courses in the curriculum. Most colleges and universities do not meet this standard, but there certainly is a movement toward more emphasis on reading in the curriculum and in later professional development.

Louisa Moats' work on classroom teacher training (1994b) found that many teachers do not, themselves, have strong phonemic awareness. Phonemic awareness and other linguistic knowledge and skills have been a neglected area in teacher education programs. Teachers who are well prepared to teach these aspects of language can make an enormous impact. As Moats says,

> Most reading problems can be greatly ameliorated through appropriate instruction. According to the convergent findings of numerous studies from the 1990s, classroom teaching is the best antidote for reading difficulty (Moats 2000).

The current edition is written at a time when educational accountability has become a national agenda. Given enough background in reading methods and in the linguistic processes underlying early reading acquisition, teachers should feel confident that they can be accountable for teaching all children to read.

ORGANIZATION OF THE THIRD EDITION

As with previous editions, the book is divided into three parts. Part I continues to outline the underlying psychological and cognitive processes that support both beginning reading and mature, skilled reading, and to address issues of assessment for dyslexia. Additional material has been added to the assessment chapter regarding the increasingly important role of the classroom teacher in using assessment to identify early difficulties and to modify instruction.

Part II addresses general principles of instruction for students with dyslexia such as systematic, direct instruction, and assessment-based planning. The chapters in Part II continue to be structured around application of these principles within the various components of a language arts program such as phonemic awareness, phonics, fluency, vocabulary, comprehension, spelling, handwriting, and written composition. Two changes have been made in the organization of Part II. First, the chapter on *The Reading-Writing Relationship* has been moved to the spot after *Phonemic Awareness* and before *Phonics Instruction*, and it has been rewritten and renamed *Spelling to Read* (see Chapter 6). This acknowledges the strong role that invented spelling can play in the transition from phonemic processing to written language. The other change involves a new chapter on *Vocabulary* (Chapter 9), with information that was embedded in the *Comprehension* chapter in the first two editions.

Part III, as before, is devoted to descriptions of particular programs for students with reading difficulties. The chapter on IBM's *Writing to Read* has been removed. IBM no longer produces educational software. In many schools, the computers once used in Writing to Read centers have been moved into classrooms for general computer use and most schools no longer employ Writing to Read specialists. The chapter on Robert Calfee's Project READ has also been removed from this edition because it is not being used in schools and the training is no longer available to teachers. Not to be confused with Enfield and Greene's Project Read, Calfee's program (e.g., Calfee and Henry 1985) served as the literacy component of Stanford University's Accelerated Schools program. It was distinguished by its integration of direct skills and meaning-based instruction. In his introduction to a new book by his colleague Marcia Henry, he described Projct READ as an early balanced literacy program. Materials for teaching word reading were developed for Project READ by Henry whose subsequent work integrates reading, spelling, and morphological patterns for meaning for both beginning readers (Henry 2003) and older readers (Henry 1990), and is designed for typically developing as well as disabled readers.

Two new chapters have been added to Part III, one reviewing several early intervention programs, and one on *Success for All*. The sequence of the chapters in Part III has been reorganized, proceeding from early intervention to school-wide interventions that constitute a form of universal design or instructional plan that is so direct and intensive that it will benefit all readers, to specialized remedial programs, usually administered through tutoring and designed specifically for students with dyslexia.

The most important change in this edition is the name of the book. The word remediation no longer appears in the title. When the book was first written, remediation was really the only option for a child with dyslexia. Few children with this word-level reading difficulty received help until they were found to be several years below grade level. Today, we know a great deal about early identification and intervention. Appropriate instruction can begin very early and it can begin in the classroom. Thus, the book covers a range of instructional options including, but not limited to, remediation.

Classroom teachers are an audience for this edition of the book as well as reading specialists, special educators, and dyslexia specialists. There are two reasons for this. First, in a time of dramatic school budget cuts, the classroom teacher may need to accept responsibility for inclusion students with dyslexia. Second, on a more hopeful note, if the classroom teacher of very young children does his or her job with expertise, many students with dyslexia will not need outside referrals.

Acknowledgments

I am grateful to Diana Clark for beginning this project, and I continue to look to her work for guidance and inspiration. I am grateful, as always, to Margaret Jo Shepherd, whose short talk about Uta Frith's model of spelling and dyslexia in a doctoral seminar many years ago led to an interest that became the focus of much of my subsequent work, including this book. Linnea Ehri has informed my understanding of the beginning reading process since I first read her work, and she has continued to do so in conversations, in our work together, and through her work on the National Reading Panel. I am grateful to Judith Birsh for conversations about phonemic awareness and early interventions, and to Eileen Marzola and Virginia Pepe for conversations about assessment.

This edition was written during the period of a grant to Fordham University from the Hello Friend/Ennis William Cosby Foundation. The grant provides funding for 18 credits of professional development for K–2 classroom teachers. The goal of this professional development has been to develop a model for early identification and appropriate instruction of children with dyslexia right from the start. I am grateful to the Foundation and to its Education Director, Carolyn Olivier, for this opportunity to study teachers and their children during the learning-to-read process. I am grateful to Linnea Ehri and Margaret Jo Shepherd for serving on the Board of Advisors and for their many helpful insights into the program and the process of teaching children at risk. And I am especially grateful to the Cosby scholars. Many of these teachers critiqued the second edition, helping to make this third edition more readable. Even more important, they shared their teaching lives and their understandings of the children they teach. Their help has been invaluable.

Fordham has hosted three summer institutes in collaboration with the Hello Friend/Ennis William Cosby Foundation. We are grateful to the following speakers for informing our practice: Richard Allington, Isabel Beck, Judith Birsh, Vinita Chabbra, Jonathan Cohen, Linnea Ehri, Virginia Goatley, Phyllis Hunter, Prisca Martens, Eileen Marzola, Reid Lyon, Anne McGill-Franzen, Darrell Morris, Eileen Perlman, Michael Pressley, Kenneth R. Pugh, Cathy M. Roller, Hyla Rubin, Charlena and Harry Seymour, Sally and Bennett Shaywitz, Margaret Jo Shepherd, Lydia Soiffer, Dorothy S. Strickland, Darlene M. Tangel, and Barbara Wilson. And thank you to institute participants Bryan Collier, Emily McCully, and Faith Ringgold for reminding us through their brilliant children's books why learning to read is so important.

Valerie Rowe, Beatrice Samson, LaVern Lariosa, and Laura Salvatierra provided enormously helpful information and advice about the new chapter on Success for All.

And thank you, of course, to Elinor Hartwig.

Dedication

To Alfred, and to our parents, our children, and our grandchildren Alene, Jim, and Maddie who are readers now, and Grace, Jane, and Max who are still listeners, but especially to Phoebe and Eleanor who learned to read during this revision

—JKU

To Elise, Ashley, and Brewster

—DBC

I

Reading and Dyslexia

1

Perspectives on Reading and Learning to Read

In kindergarten, Nora and Katie were in the same print-rich classroom with a loving and lively teacher who provided extensive time each day for stimulating emergent reading and writing activities. Both of these bright, healthy children came to kindergarten with experiences listening to books at home and in preschool. Both had attentive, supportive, college-educated parents who were professionally involved with books and literacy. By the end of kindergarten, Nora could finger-point read familiar text (i.e., touch each word as she said sentences from memory), could sound out, as she put it, "any word with three letters and *a* in the middle," and she could read a few words without having to sound them out. She enjoyed writing stories and she did this well enough for her teacher to be able to read what she wrote. Katie, on the other hand, didn't like to write, and when she did, neither she nor her teacher could read it. She still struggled to remember the names of some letters and could not sound out any words. Her teacher was surprised because she had a huge vocabulary and was precocious in math. By mid-first grade, Nora seemed to learn sight vocabulary almost by magic and new words were sounded out successfully. She eagerly picked out books to take home each night and begged to stay up late to read one more book at bedtime. Katie, on the other hand, either made up text from the pictures or from her own experiences or struggled to sound out words, but wasn't very good at the letter sounds. She needed reminding to take books home and resisted taking them out of her backpack to read with her mother, because, "Reading is boring." By third grade Nora read for pleasure, had polished off every series she could find, and was writing her first novel. Katie almost never read for pleasure, was embarrassed by not being able to read what her friends read and pretended to be reading the latest *Harry Potter*. Her spelling was weak and her stories short and repetitive. Reading was still "boring" and she "hated" writing. Katie is dyslexic.

It is the intent of this book to provide an overview of the nature of dyslexia and of how children and adults with this reading disorder can be helped to be better readers. In order to understand what goes wrong with reading acquisition in individuals with dyslexia, the development of skilled reading in normally achieving children needs to be examined. What processes are involved in mature skilled reading? And how do these processes develop? These two questions are crucial to the understanding of dyslexia.

The psychology of reading has been under investigation since the beginning of this century. Combined efforts of reading educators and researchers from related disciplines (e.g., psychology, neurology, linguistics) have led to new theoretical perspectives on the acts of reading and of learning to read, several of which have contributed substantially to the understanding of reading disability. One such perspective views reading as an *information processing system*. It attempts to identify the psychological processes involved in the act of skilled reading and to determine how they are coordinated. A second perspective focuses on reading as a *developing process*. Understanding how normal reading is acquired is crucial to the understanding of what goes wrong during the development of reading in children with dyslexia.

READING AS INFORMATION PROCESSING

Comprehension is the purpose of reading. We read to gain information or to enjoy a story. How does comprehension happen? How do skilled readers look at a page filled with letters and understand a message written by someone else in another time and place, a process involving movement from sensory input to higher level thought?

One model for analyzing such interactions is called *information processing*. It draws parallels between the human mind and a computer. The mind is viewed as a system for taking in information at the sensory level, organizing and interpreting it, keeping it temporarily in short-term memory or storing it in categories for later retrieval. Executive control processes or monitoring mechanisms, which are affected by prior experiences both with life and with print, help in guiding this process. For example, expectations about what will come next in a story affect the way incoming information is perceived and organized.

Viewing reading as information processing provokes questions about what subprocesses are involved, the order in which they occur, and the relative contribution of the various available information sources. One extremely important query, for example, concerns the extent to which reading might be guided by print, the small pieces of information that enter the system at the sensory level, or by meaning and context, which are influenced by prior experiences. Any and all of these processes could conceivably guide the self-monitoring process. Reading theorists have developed models, or theoretical representations of the reading process, to explain their points of view on these issues. Three distinctly different positions on the reading process are discussed below.

TOP-DOWN THEORY

Proponents of the *top-down* theory of reading, led by Kenneth Goodman and Frank Smith, take a strong meaning-based position. They maintain that reading is primarily dependent upon the reader's purpose for reading a text. According to these theorists, rather than reading every letter in every word, good readers sample only the essential print information for meeting this purpose (Goodman 1967; Smith 2004). Such readers rely heavily on their acquired knowledge of the world and of conventional graphemic, syntactic, and semantic structures to hypothesize or predict the words to come and to confirm the sense of what they have read. Only when they find that the text does not make sense do they go back and focus on individual words or examine letters in words. In this model their perception of sensory input—what they think they see—is guided by metacognitive monitoring.

Goodman calls reading a *psycholinguistic guessing game* (Goodman 1967), implying that the reader makes an informed guess that is consistent with what is known so far from the text in regard to both parts of speech and meaning. Both Goodman and Smith describe reading as a *top-down* procedure that moves from higher order (cognitive) to lower order (sensory and perceptual) mental processes. One argument used to support this model is that skilled reading is so rapid and automatic that it could not possibly involve a close look at every letter in every word.

The implication suggested by the top down model involves reading instruction that is aimed from the beginning at the meaning level, and that limits instruction at the letter and word level to situations within the context of a meaningful passage of text. Classrooms adhering to this model have commonly been referred to as *whole language* classrooms. Teachers adhering to a *whole language* philosophy consider beginning reading to be an extension of oral language development. In these classrooms, a teacher reads aloud to emerging readers who then build print knowledge from an oral-language meaning base. Goodman argues that skilled readers read in this way and that beginners use the same process, but are simply not very skilled at it yet. Beginning reading is practiced by matching oral language, memorized from several readings, with written language. Teachers support this through *Shared Reading* (Holdaway 1979), a school version of the sort of book experiences parents provide for their children when they share a text as they read aloud. In school, oversized or big books are read aloud by the teacher with print held up facing the children. The teacher models how she learns and how she knows what she knows (e.g., " I wonder what this word is. I think I'll go back to the beginning of the sentence and see if I can think of a word that makes sense here.") This sharing or modeling is considered a form of Vygotskian scaffolding or support by an expert who helps the new reader acquire strategies that eventually will be used independently. The teacher encourages the children to join in and she chooses texts in which words can be predicted from illustrations, rhyme, or repetition as in "'Oh lovely mud,' said the cow. 'Oh, lovely mud,' said the sheep,' from Joy Cowley's (1990) *Mrs. Wishy-Washy*. Eventually text is read to the point of at least partial memorization, which enables constant joining in.

Shared reading is highly motivating and encourages playful engagement in pretend reading of smaller versions of the big books. Pretending to read by saying the memorized text aloud and turning the pages becomes real reading, little by little, as a match is made between spoken words and written words.

This transition from pretend reading is called *concept of word in print* (Morris, 1983, 1993; Morris et al. 2003) or *finger-point reading* (Ehri and Sweet 1991; Uhry 1999, 2002a). These researchers have provided strong evidence that finger-point reading is facilitated by *phonemic awareness* (ability to identify small speech sounds or phonemes in spoken words). The other important component is letter knowledge. Knowing the name of the letter *m* (which sounds like the initial phoneme sound /m/ in the spoken word *mud*) allows a child to point to the printed letters *mud* at the right time while reciting "Oh, lovely mud," in the memorized text. Eventually, the match between words in speech and words in text is memorized and the child acquires sight words. See Chapter 6 for an elaboration of the role that phonemic awareness and invented spelling play in finger-point reading.

Guided reading is the next step in learning to read in whole language classrooms (e.g., Fountas and Pinnell 1996). Again, the teacher scaffolds learning, but here the children know enough words to read on their own. Using texts at what is called *instructional reading level*, with most but not all words read by sight, the teacher reinforces strategies such as predicting what will happen next based on previous text, and at using personal experiences to make self-to-text connections. She assists in figuring out new words through encouraging children to skip over unknown words while trying to figure them out from pictures or from syntactic or semantic context. The idea is that meaning is paramount in figuring out new words.

The whole language idea of skipping over words rather than using letters to figure them out is highly controversial. Goodman and Smith's *top-down model* has been called into question by studies that demonstrate that proficient readers do not skip over letters, words, and phrases, nor do they rely only on context to gain information. Instead, they fixate on almost all letters in text. Researchers are able to document individual eye fixations, as well as saccades (i.e., rapid movements to the next fixations), and regressions (i.e., returns to earlier words during reading). Their findings indicate that even though skilled adult readers often read as many as 200 to 300 words a minute, they do process every letter (e.g., Just and Carpenter 1980; Rayner 1985, 1992, 1993). Keep in mind that when you read a word with a complex orthographic pattern, as in the word *bright*, you visually process every letter in the pattern. This doesn't mean that you sound the word out one letter at a time, but doesn't seeing *bight* or *briht* slow you down? Research also indicates that fluent readers are less reliant on context in processing textual information than poor readers because they are more adept at quickly processing letters and words within text (Stanovich 1986b). Thus accurate and automatic word recognition appears to be an essential component of proficient reading.

BOTTOM-UP THEORY

Diametrically opposed to the Goodman-Smith perspective on reading is the *bottom-up* perspective. This model describes reading as a hierarchical procedure that moves from processing the smallest bits of graphemic information, individual letters, to ever-larger chunks of information and only attaches semantic meaning after words have been identified (LaBerge and Samuels 1974). In this model a series of associations must be built between low-level pieces of information, such as sounds and letters, before they can be interpreted and associated with specific meanings.

An important contribution of the bottom-up model is its emphasis on the subprocesses of the reading act and its contention that many of these subprocesses, such as letter and word identification, must become automatic in order for readers to be fluent. David LaBerge and

S. Jay Samuels (1974), who were among the first investigators to focus on the attentional demands of reading, hypothesize a *limited capacity mechanism* in human information processing that controls the distribution of attentional resources. As they explain it, during execution of a complex skill such as reading, many component processes must be coordinated within a very short time; if none of these processes is carried out automatically, there will not be enough attention available to execute the reading act successfully.

The implication for instruction here involves teaching letter sounds before words, words before sentences, and sentences before passages. Only then can passages be read and understood. Carrying the theory into practice would imply teaching decoding in isolation and mastering decoding before teaching reading comprehension. There are few classroom examples of this theory in pure form, but several Orton-Gillingham remedial reading programs follow this model (e.g., see Chapter 21, *Alphabetic Phonics*). However, there are numerous examples of classrooms using basal reading series that outline a program of activities including workbook exercises for teaching letter-sounds in isolation and for pre-teaching sight words in isolation before they are encountered in a reading passage. While comprehension instruction is not absent in such programs, it is not a major focus in the early grades. One criticism of bottom-up programs is that the language in phonics-controlled readers (also called *decodable text*) is not natural language, which makes it difficult to use a full range of predicting strategies. The argument against these readers is that the stories are often contrived and the content can be dull and unmotivating. There really is not any research indicating whether or not decodable text is effective, but if children are taught using a phonics-decoding method, words at their reading levels are bound to be words that can be decoded using the alphabetic strategy.

INTERACTIVE THEORY

Top-down and *bottom-up* models represent extreme theoretical perspectives on the act of reading. Both describe reading as a series of sequentially ordered processes and are therefore referred to as *serial processing models*. In both models, control over the reading process runs in only one direction. Each processing event triggers another processing event, either one step up or one step down in a hierarchy. In contrast, another view of reading holds that many of the component processes occur at the same time or in parallel.

David Rumelhart (1977), who originally proposed this less extreme theory, contends that readers simultaneously initiate word identification and predict meaning, and he maintains that these are reciprocal events. He cites several sources of knowledge that the good reader has available to help extract the message in the text: knowledge of the graphophonemic system, knowledge of particular sight words in the lexicon, knowledge of the syntactic and semantic aspects of language, background knowledge, and metacognitive knowledge of how to self-monitor during reading. Note that the first knowledge source involves print and its relationship with the phonological aspects of spoken language, whereas the remaining sources refer to oral language alone. Rumelhart believes that these knowledge sources can be activated concurrently and that they operate reciprocally; he refers to his theory as an *interactive* model of the reading process.

Rumelhart's colleague Mark Seidenberg, in collaboration with James McClelland, developed what they call a *connectionist* model, which is similar to the *interactive model*. Their reasoning is that reading involves a series of associations or connections resulting in accumulated lexical knowledge. The model involves connections in both directions between context and meaning, and then additional two-way connections between meaning, orthography, and phonology (i.e., meaning-orthography, orthography-phonology, and phonology-meaning). The term phonology refers to the sounds in spoken language and the term *orthography* refers to the letter patterns in written words. In other words, connections or associations between any two processors can trigger other associations in any direction and contribute to the overall reading process. Seidenberg and McClelland have used computational simulations of word learning to provide evidence of the interactive nature of the relationship between phonology and orthography. Theoretical *hidden units*, to which Seidenberg and McClelland assign statistical weights, mediate these connections (1989).

Skilled reading involves rapid decoding; an often cited study by Rayner and Pollatsek (1987) puts the rate at more than five words every second. As described by Seidenberg and McClelland, rapid word reading triggers associations with several other processors. Pronunciations and word meanings are generated by visual word recognition, as are hypotheses about possible syntactic patterns. All of this contributes to comprehension, so that "text and discourse are interpreted essentially as the signal is perceived" (Seidenberg and McClelland 1989, p. 523). The point here is that these connections are made all at once rather than in a linear, hierarchical fashion (i.e., either top-down or bottom-up). As Marilyn Adams puts it:

> In order for the connections, and even the connected parts, themselves, to develop properly, they must be linked together in the very course of acquisition. And, importantly, this dependency works in both directions. One cannot properly develop the higher-order processes without due attention to the lower. Nor can one focus on the lower-order processes without constantly clarifying and exercising their connections to the higher-order ones (Adams 1990, p. 6).

Instruction following from applications of this theory involves not just introducing all the processors or cue systems at the same time rather than in a hierarchical sequence, but actively helping children connect each cue system with the others. Questions such as, "What does a cow say?" and, "What letter would you expect to see if the word is *moo*?" encourage the child to use the entire system of processors.

Sylvia Farnham-Diggory describes an idealized model for reading instruction that she attributes to ancient Greece and Rome and that is consistent with the interactive model. First order skills (enciphering and deciphering) and second order skills (comprehension and composition) are taught together. She describes a teaching/learning model that resembles *whole language* instruction in combination with systematic direct instruction designed to highlight the rule-based nature of what she calls the *orthographic cipher* or letter-sound system of English. Both first- and second-order skills are taught in a way that emphasizes the reciprocal relationship between reading and writing and both are taught within the context of meaningful projects (Farnham-Diggory 1990). Her teaching model is consistent with the one proposed by Adams (1990) in which meaning-based and code-based strategies are taught together.

WHAT HAPPENS WHEN ONE OF THE SYSTEMS DOESN'T WORK WELL?
Gough's Simple View of Reading

Philip Gough and William Tunmer present a model of skilled reading comprehension that is dependent on two components: (a) the ability to look at print and recode it into spoken language, and (b) the ability to understand spoken language (Gough and Tunmer 1986). In order to function effectively in regard to reading comprehension, the reader must be good at both components. Gough and Tunmer concede that the model is an oversimplification and that reading, in reality, is a highly complex task, rather than a simple one. However, the model provides a very clear view of what might go wrong in skilled reading. To refer back to the connectionist model, if the processors that are involved in turning print to speech, or if the processors that are involved in prior knowledge, understanding of words, or comprehension of complex oral syntax are not working efficiently, then the connections between them will break down. Without all systems working well, text cannot be understood. According to Gough and Tunmer, in skilled reading both word reading and listening comprehension must work well to facilitate proficient reading comprehension.

Stanovich's Compensatory Model

The term *compensate* means "to make up for." A crutch is used to support the body while a broken leg heals. The question in reading instruction is whether to work on the weak area and, metaphorically, heal the leg, or learn to use the crutch on an on-going basis. Should we keep working on handwriting and spelling indefinitely with a dyslexic sixth grader or should we teach him to use ViaVoice, a computer program for composing by dictating? The bigger question is how does the brain compensate when some processes critical to reading do not work well?

Stanovich (1981, 1984) emphasizes the potentially compensatory nature of interacting processes and calls his own view of reading an interactive-compensatory model. The finding that readers with poor word recognition are more reliant on context than good readers is one example of such compensation. Stanovich's interactive-compensatory model illustrates the trade-offs that can occur among the component subskills of reading, and helps to explain individual differences in reading ability. Therefore it has considerable appeal for those of us concerned with disabled readers. There is much similarity between this theory and Perfetti's verbal efficiency theory.

DEVELOPMENTAL PERSPECTIVES ON READING

CHALL'S DEVELOPMENTAL MODEL

Reading at proficient levels and reading as a developing skill are quite different behaviors. Reading is learned over many years, and for most people important changes in reading behavior occur over this span of time.

Jeanne Chall (1983b), who was a leading researcher in reading education in this country, developed a stage theory of reading development, which she preferred to call a scheme or model. She hypothesized six qualitatively different stages from readiness to maturity. She maintained that most people progress through these stages in the same order, through not necessarily at the same rate and despite the fact that many people do not reach the higher stages, or expert levels, of reading ability. She believed that rate and success in learning to read are determined by the interaction between learner and environment. Borrowing from Jean Piaget's stage theory of cognitive development (Inhelder and Piaget 1958; Piaget 1970), Chall described reading as "a form of problem solving in which readers adapt to their environment through the processes of assimilation and accommodation" (1983b). Assimilation referred to the learner's application of previously acquired skills to a particular task or problem. Accommodation referred to the learner's ability to adopt new skills or new ways of thinking in performing an unfamiliar task or solving a new problem. Chall provided ages and grade levels at which the average student could be expected to reach each of the six stages, but urged that they be considered only approximations.

Stage 0: The Prereading Stage

The first stage in Chall's model is Stage 0, the prereading stage. It lasts from birth to around age six and comprises a greater number of developmental changes than any other stage. This period goes from the very beginnings of an individual's language awareness to the ability to recognize and name letters of the alphabet and even to read some names on signs or a few words in familiar books. Chall talked of readiness concepts—which we call *emergent literacy* today—such as understanding the purpose of reading, understanding the relationship between pictures and print, and understanding the relationship between written and spoken words.

Stage 1: Decoding

Stage 1, the initial or decoding stage, is attained by most children between the ages of six and seven while in first and second grade. The major accomplishment of this period is grasping the *alphabetic principle*—the principle that tiny units of sound in spoken language map onto letters in written language—and learning the letter-sound correspondences, or the alphabetic code. Children increasingly attend to graphic elements in words rather than treating words as wholes. Chall explains the successful transition from Stage 0 to Stage 1 as a process of accommodation: Children apply their newly acquired readiness concepts and skills, which include the ability to analyze parts within wholes, to the challenge of reading unfamiliar words. However, if these readiness skills are lacking, children approach new challenges through assimilation, continuing to use the strategies learned in the previous stage: viewing all words holistically and relying on contextual cues such as pictures and memory for stories.

Stage 2: Confirmation

Stage 2 involves confirming what has been learned in the previous stage and gaining fluency. Although phonics knowledge continues to develop during this period and even later, it is confirmation of old knowledge that is the focus here. Children gain confidence in "their decoding knowledge, the redundancies of the language, and the redundancies of the stories" (Chall 1983b, p. 19). They begin to develop speed as well as accuracy in word recognition. At this point, the learner should be attending to both meaning and print and using cues from these information sources interactively. Stage 2 is a particularly critical period for the developing reader. If progress breaks down, the individual can remain "glued to print," as Chall expresses it. Many factors may contribute to this arrest, among them unstable phonics knowledge, limited experience with language and ideas, and lack of reading practice.

Stages 3–5: Reading to Learn

Stage 3, which commences around fourth grade at roughly nine years of age, is primarily distinguished from the previous stage by a change in motivation for reading. At this point, the individual begins to read in order to learn new information. Where Stages 1 and 2 are referred to as "learning to read," Stages 3 through 5 are called "reading to learn." Reading in content area subjects (science and social studies) is introduced in school. Vocabulary enlargement and expansion of world knowledge become increasingly important. For the most part, the material encountered during this stage presents only one point of view. However, in the second half of Stage 3 (grades seven through eight or nine), which covers junior high, as students begin to read newspapers, magazines, and more adult reading materials, they are exposed to differing points of view and they begin to read critically.

The ability to deal with multiple viewpoints is more fully developed in Stage 4 (roughly ages fourteen through eighteen), which covers the high school years. This ability is acquired mainly through formal education.

Readers who attain the highest level of reading development, Stage 5, have learned to read selectively and are able to develop their own opinions and make their own judgments about what they read. As Chall expresses it, the reading process at this stage is "essentially constructive;" readers construct their own knowledge from that of others. Stage 5 is not usually reached until college age or later and may, in fact, be reserved for individuals who have an intellectual bent; Chall points out that four years of college does not ensure its attainment. It has not yet been determined what proportion of the general population become expert readers.

Each stage builds on the skills acquired in previous stages, and success in meeting the challenges confronted at each stage is to a large extent dependent upon mastery of those skills normally acquired in earlier stages, according to Chall. Readers become increasingly flexible in their reading style, able to adjust the pace and the distribution of attention as the complexity of the material and the purpose for reading warrants.

DECODING STAGES WITHIN CHALL'S STAGES

Even within Chall's stages, growth in reading acquisition represents qualitative changes. A number of reading researchers have used observations and research findings to construct stage models for the acquisition of decoding. These models usually involve four phases in which four strategies develop, each dependent on those that come before.

Phase 1: The Logographic Phase

British reading theorist Uta Frith calls the earliest reading phase *logographic* (Frith 1985, 1986). When using this strategy, young children are highly dependent on the look of a word within a particular context. Some researchers claim that a few words are recognized instantly at this stage through memorization of the exact shape of the word. Others say that the word needs to be linked to context-dependent cues. For instance, the word "McDonald's" might be recognized under the golden arches but not on its own. "Xepsi" on a soda can logo might be read as "Pepsi" (Masonheimer, Drum and Ehri 1984). Letters can be used in a limited way at this stage but attending to letter order is not a characteristic of the logographic strategy (Frith 1985, 1986; Marsh et al. 1981). For many years both researchers and teachers believed that children needed to acquire a sight vocabulary of roughly 40 memorized words before they could take advantage of letter cues. The lexicon of sight words was believed to provide insight into the letter-sound relationship and to provide a base for the next strategy.

Linnea Ehri has questioned the size of this pre-phonics lexicon through an experiment that demonstrated that even readers who knew only a few words could use letter cues to learn new words (e.g., GRF for *giraffe* and LFT for *elephant*), and that the use of letter-sound cues was a more efficient strategy for them than the use of visually distinctive letter patterns (Ehri and Wilce 1985). Letter-sound associations are built on letter-name knowledge. For instance, the name of the letter G provides a clue to its sound and helps children remember how to read a particular word. In other words, this initial visual-cue or logographic phase may last only a very short time. Some researchers doubt that the stage exists at all. Rebecca Treiman's work with spelling supports the usefulness of letter names prior to formal acquisition of letter sounds (1994).

Phase 2: The Partial-cue Phase

Linnea Ehri has called the next phase the *phonetic-cue* (Ehri and Wilce 1987a, 1987b) or *rudimentary phonetic* (Ehri 1995) or *partial-cue* phase (Ehri and McCormick 1998). Here letters play a more important role, but children still do not use every letter in a word. Associations are made between salient letters, such as the initial *j* and final *l* in the printed word *jail* and a stored memory of the word *jail* (Ehri and Wilce 1987b). When phonetic-cue readers see the *j* and *l* together in a word they scan their lexicon for a match that sometimes involves the correct word and sometimes a look-alike word. The phonetic-cue strategy helps children remember particular words but it does not help them sound out new words.

Phase 3: The Cipher or Alphabetic Phase

The *cipher* phase (Gough and Hillinger 1980) is also called the *alphabetic* phase (Frith 1985, 1986). This strategy takes full advantage of the alphabetic system upon which our writing system is based. Letters are sounded out, one at a time, from left to right, and then the sounds are blended together into words. To do this a child needs to have knowledge of letter-sound associations, some of which are learned intuitively through knowing letter names (e.g., *j* and *m*), and some of which need to be taught more explicitly (e.g., *y* and *w*). The beginning cipher reader also needs metacognitive knowledge about units of sound in speech, a knowledge which is called *phonological awareness*, and of how these speech-sound units, once segmented, can be mapped onto letters in print, which is called the *alphabetic principle*. Only at this phase of strategy development can the beginning reader actually read a word that has not been memorized. A reader at this phase should be able to read accurately using letter-sound associations.

Phase 4: The Orthographic Strategy.

The term *orthography* comes from Greek roots, which can be translated as *perfect writing*. In the context of reading stage theory the term refers to spelling patterns, or units of letters commonly occurring together. The *orthographic* (Frith 1985, 1986) or *analogy* strategy (Goswami 1986) involves recognizing a unit of letters that forms a spelling pattern that represents a sound. Both Goswami, and Rebecca Treiman (1985) provide evidence that the natural break-point in a word for young readers is after the initial consonant or consonants (e.g., *c-* or *cl-*), which is called an *onset*, and before the vowel-consonant or vowel-consonants units (e.g., *-at* or *-ink*), which is called a *rime*. Being able to read *cat* allows a child to recognize the *at* portion of *sat*. Capitalizing on this phenomenon is a method of instruction called *word families* in which same-spelling-pattern words are taught together. According to a version of the four-phase model proposed by Marsh and his colleagues (Marsh et al. 1981) analogies can be made at the *morphological* level as well. This involves groups of letters that are units of meaning, or *morphs*, such as the unit *know* in *knowledge*. Note that here the unit of letters actually differs in sound from word to word while the meaning remains constant.

While the analogy strategy is considered the most sophisticated form of decoding according to the four-phase model, British researcher Usha Goswami has carried out experiments demonstrating that even very young children can read unknown words through analogy to a known word (e.g., Goswami 1986, 1988). Goswami chose analogous words with similar endings using the argument that end-analogies or *rimes* (e.g., *beak, peak*) are easier to learn than beginning-analogies (e.g., *beak, bean*) because the break between *onset* (i.e., initial letter or letter cluster) and *rime* (i.e., vowel unit and final consonant unit) is an easier form of segmentation for young children. In Goswami's training studies, a target word was taught and then embedded in a word list of unknown words that included a few rimes of the target word. More of the rime words were read successfully than were other unfamiliar words (Goswami 1986, 1988). Practitioners have used these experiments as evidence that children should be taught using a word-families approach right from the start.

Linnea Ehri later carried out an experiment that confirmed Goswami's finding that very young readers can read by analogy, but she found that those subjects who knew how to use a cipher strategy were better at using the analogy strategy than were the children who were still using a phonetic-cue strategy. The phonetic-cue readers, who read using associations between partial letter cues and a stored lexicon could not figure out new words from old words, whereas the cipher readers could (Ehri and Robbins 1992). Goswami, too, has found evidence that skill in phonological awareness, a crucial factor in cipher reading, contributes to analogy reading (Goswami and Mead 1992).

Word families, then, may play two roles in decoding. In the early stages of reading, they support emergent readers' success in "reading" rhyming words by reading the onset (e.g., cat, sat, fat, rat) but there is not evidence that this helps children learn to read other letters in these words or to read these words in other contexts. Later, after learning to read letters in all positions in words, word families help young readers *chunk*, or read quickly, letters that they already know how to read slowly and accurately. For teachers, instructional decisions about word families ought to be based on knowing about a child's reading stage.

EHRI'S STAGE THEORY

Through her research, Linnea Ehri has done much to clarify the role of reading strategies at each of these four phases, as noted above. She has produced much of the evidence that demonstrates just what processing demands are associated with each phase. Her subjects are carefully screened so that she is able to document differences between children she considers nonreaders, novices, and beginning readers.

Early Links between Letters and Sounds

One of Ehri's important contributions to the field of early read-ing is the role of letters in teaching phonemic awareness. She has carried out research indicating that learning to spell facilitates learning to read (1989; Ehri and Wilce 1987b). She argues that this helps children listen for the sounds in words (phonemic awareness) and also helps them link these sounds with letters (phonics). She has also found that phonemic awareness is easier to learn when sounds are represented by letters (Hohn and Ehri 1983).

Alphabetic Reading as a Foundation for Sight Word Reading

Another important contribution made by Ehri (1992) is in regard to the relationship between word attack skills, used to decode or decipher unfamiliar words based on letter-sound relationships, and the acquisition of *sight words*, which have been memorized and can be recognized instantly. It is part of both historical theory and school lore that instruction involves either one approach or the other. For example, teachers talk of using either a *sight approach* or a *phonics approach* to teaching reading. Often they try to fit a particular approach to a particular child depending on whether they view the child as a *visual learner* or an *auditory learner*. The term *dual route* is used to express these alternate routes to meaning. According to the dual route theory, there are two avenues to meaning. The first of these hypothesized routes involves sounding out a word, or turning print into speech, in order to trigger a connection with its meaning in a *lexicon* or stored bank of vocabulary words. The second depends on a rote-learned arbitrary connection between print and meaning without the intermediate step of recoding the letters to a phonological system.

Ehri's model of the relationship between what she calls *recoding* (or moving from print to speech through the use of letter-sound associations) and sight word acquisition casts doubt on this dichotomy. Ehri is critical of the connectionist notion that arbitrary associations can be made between a printed word and its meaning. She notes that the research literature does not support either a *phonological route* or a *visual-semantic route*. Ehri suggests a third route, which she calls the *visual-phonological route*. According to her theory, a series of complex connections are made on several levels. Letters are connected with phonemes. In Ehri's example, the letter *l* in *belt* is connected with the sound /l/. Units of letters are connected with parts of spoken words (e.g., the letter unit *elt* is connected with the sound /elt/). The whole printed word is connected with the whole spoken word (e.g., *belt*). In addition, the printed word *belt* is connected with its meaning. Ehri uses the term *cipher sight word reading* when words are recognized quickly as a result of connections made through the cipher strategy. In other words, the cipher strategy facilitates decoding until a word has been read enough times to be recognized rapidly through what Ehri calls "a complete network of visual-phonological connections in lexical memory" (Ehri 1992, p. 138).

The implication of Ehri's theory in terms of word reading stage theory is that at each phase in strategy acquisition (e.g., logographic, phonetic–cue, cipher, orthographic) the connections between print and oral language become more elaborated and the lexicon of sight words is more easily built and more automatically retrieved. She suggests that instruction can facilitate sight word learning most effectively if phonics instruction is linked to acquisition of a few highly practiced, phonetically regular words at any one time. That is, when short *a* is taught in phonics instruction, sight word instruction should involve short *a* words (Ehri 1992).

FRITH'S CONTRIBUTIONS TO READING STAGE THEORY

British researcher Uta Frith presents a model of decoding acquisition, cited in descriptions of the phases outlined above (1985, 1986). Note that her model skips the phonetic–cue phase and moves directly from *logographic* to *alphabetic* reading. Frith's model is insightful in two regards. Her first contribution to stage theory is her notion that there are two steps at each of her three phases, one involving the acquisition of the strategy for reading and the other for spelling. At each of her three phases these skills develop, one behind the other, but not always in the same order. Reading develops first, before spelling, at the *logographic phase*. That is, children become aware of letters and written words through exposure to environmental print, on cereal boxes and traffic signs for example, before they learn to write letters or words.

Spelling to Read

At the *alphabetic phase*, the order is reversed. Children can spell using an alphabetic, left-to-right, letter-by-letter strategy before they can read alphabetically. That is, they continue to use a *logographic* strategy to recognize a few memorized words while spelling *alphabetically*. Often they can spell phonetically regular words that they cannot read. The notion of using alphabetic spelling instruction as a way of leading young children into using the alphabetic strategy for reading appears to be quite sound. Linnea Ehri and Lee Wilce (1987b) found that kindergarten children trained in listening carefully to the sounds in words and then in representing these sounds with letters were able to read words composed of these letters more accurately than children trained in letter-sound associations alone. Ehri presents evidence, however, that these kindergarten children were using a *phonetic-cue strategy* (the strategy omitted by Frith's theory) rather than the full *cipher* or *alphabetic* strategy.

At the *orthographic phase*, again, the order of spelling and reading acquisition is reversed. Exposure to print in books helps children recognize units of letters in order to read by analogy while they are still producing phonetic rather than orthographically conventional spellings. Using memorized units to spell appears to be the last strategy to develop.

Dyslexia as Failure at the Alphabetic Phase

Frith's second contribution to stage theory is the notion that it is at the *alphabetic phase* that children with dyslexia begin to fail in reading. In other words, they are able to memorize a few words using logographic strategies, but are unable to use the alphabetic principle to invent spellings or to decode new words they have not seen before (1985, 1986). This is consistent with detailed descriptions of individuals with dyslexia from the research literature presented in Chapter 2 of this book. Phonemic awareness is an important facilitator at the alphabetic phase and deficits in phonemic awareness are characteristic of dyslexia (see Chapter 5). Support for acquisition of the alphabetic principle is the basis for most of the programs currently in use for remediation of dyslexia, as outlined in Part III of this book.

EDUCATIONAL IMPLICATIONS OF DIFFERING PERSPECTIVES OF READING

Not all reading authorities agree that a strong focus on the alphabetic code is essential for learning to read. Perspectives on this issue have important implications for reading instruction. Theorists who espouse a strong meaning-based or top-down view of reading tend to minimize the importance of learning phonics and advocate an indirect or incidental learning approach to letter-sound knowledge. Kenneth Goodman, for instance, is critical of the use of phonics instruction in the early stages of reading (1993). He argues that English phonics rules are arbitrary and unreliable, and are not helpful out of context. What Jeanne Chall called the *great debate* in reading instruction goes back long before the advent of whole language philosophy (Chall 1983a). In the 1930s, for instance, advocates of John Dewey's philosophy recommended teaching whole words, rather than letter-sounds, because words put children directly in touch with meaning right from the start. During the late 1960s and early 1970s advocates of open classrooms suggested teaching reading using meaningful materials, such as the children's own writing, as well as *language experience* text generated by groups of children and written down by teachers. Historically, periods in which naturalistic, child-centered approaches to reading instruction dominate have alternated with periods characterized by a swing toward an emphasis on skills.

In 1967, Jeanne Chall published a massive review of the literature on reading instruction that she updated in 1983. After examining
the relevant research studies, Chall concluded that early intensive phonics instruction produced greater gains in reading by third grade in comparison with other approaches. She made the point that because
English is an alphabetic language, all children who learn to read will
learn some phonics, either by figuring it out themselves from exposure
to words, or through *direct instruction*. Chall presents convincing evidence that direct, systematic phonics instruction is significantly more
effective than the alternative, often called *indirect* or *intrinsic* learning.
Chall did not intend to limit instruction to phonics at the early stages.
Keep in mind the importance of comprehension in her reading stage
model, both in terms of oral language in the pre-reading stage and as
the major focus of reading once decoding has been acquired. However,
Chall served, for many years, as a central focus of criticism from the
anti-phonics movement that has been part of a political debate revolv-
ing around reading instruction.

Like Chall, Marilyn Adams (1990) carried out an extensive
review of the literature on learning to read. However, Adams was much
more explicit than Chall in outlining the importance of connections
between meaning processors and letter-sound processors. She concluded that to be effective, phonics instruction must be linked with
language-based reading instruction. She provided a detailed description
of this in discussing *Reading Recovery*, an individual reading program for
beginning readers who are behind their peers in Grade 1 classrooms
(see Chapter 15). In this reading model, children are explicitly
instructed in how to coordinate the use of various cue systems.

Two new research reviews have been carried out since the 1995
edition of this book. The first, *Preventing Reading Difficulties in Young
Children* (Snow, Burns, and Griffin 1998) was written by the
Committee on the Prevention of Reading Difficulties in Young
Children under the auspices of the National Research Council. The
goal was to construct a team of researchers from diverse traditions and
to review and synthesize research from these traditions. The focus was
on beginning reading instruction, especially for young children at risk.
The team, lead by Catherine Snow, recommended instruction using
the alphabetic principle to acquire fluent alphabetic reading, as well as
motivating children to read for meaning and pleasure. Their curriculum recommendations for Grades K-3 included direct instruction in
phonological awareness, phonics, sounding out words, sight word
acquisition, text-reading fluency, and writing. In addition to direct
instruction, they recommended time and resources for both guided literacy activities and independent reading and writing for all children,
and supplemental support for children lagging in the developmental

components of oral language or literacy. Materials for both teachers and parents were generated as part of this project. One publication, *Starting Out Right* (Burns, Griffin, and Snow 1999) is organized with a section on early language and reading aloud for preschoolers, as well as sections for parents and teachers working with grades K-3.

The second new review was written by a panel charged by congress with assessing the state of research-based knowledge of reading instruction. The National Reading Panel Report, titled *Teaching children to read: An evidence-based assessment of the scientific research literature on reading and its implications for reading instruction* was published in 2000 by the National Institute of Child Health and Human Development. Instead of reviewing and synthesizing research as in Snow's (1998) report, the panel carried out a series of meta-analyses. First, they identified areas for analysis (phonemic awareness, phonics, fluency, vocabulary, comprehension, teacher education, and technology in reading instruction). Each of these areas was assigned a subcommittee of the Panel to construct a report. Each subcommittee selected research studies that met criteria for scientific methods. The meta-analysis involved using a statistical technique that allowed the subcommittee to compare studies in terms of the effectiveness of instruction for reading outcomes. Briefly, the findings were consistent with Chall (1983a), Adams (1990), and Snow et al. (1998) in that direct, systematic instruction in phonemic awareness and phonics was more effective in teaching word reading, especially with young children and children at risk, than other forms of early reading instruction without this direct instruction. More detailed findings are included in later chapters on instruction.

SUMMARY

Reading acquisition involves a series of developmental stages in which more and more features of printed words are used to recode print as oral language. Direct instruction in phonemic awareness and phonics facilitates this development. As the processing of print becomes more and more automatic, more and more processing space is available for comprehension. Skilled reading involves rapid connections between processing systems for almost instantaneous print-to-meaning operations. What goes wrong in this process for children with dyslexia? Why are some children, like Nora, able to master skilled reading so easily, while others, like Katie, are not?

2

The Nature of Dyslexia

It is believed that roughly 10 million children in the United States are affected by reading disabilities (Lyon 1995). Like Katie in Chapter 1, children with dyslexia have difficulty learning letter sounds and learning to read and spell words. Special instruction has been developed to minimize these negative outcomes. Without this special instruction, children with dyslexia struggle learning to read words. Later they have difficulty reading automatically and fluently, and have little processing space left to think about meaning as text becomes more and more complex in the late elementary grades. Reading is not pleasurable and they do not read very much and do not pick up oral vocabulary or background knowledge from books. Without special instruction, many adolescents with dyslexia drop out of school. Without special instruction, many adults with dyslexia have difficulty holding jobs. Some learn to compensate, and, with great effort, learn to read, but not fluently, and learn to write, but with continuing difficulty with spelling. There is evidence from the field of neurology that individuals with dyslexia have normally developed brains, but that without special instruction, their brains do not function, during reading, in the same way as the brains of typically developing readers. These differences in the functioning of the brains of dyslexics are now known to involve the processing of phonological information during reading. Scientists have known for well over 100 years that some otherwise high-functioning individuals have unexpected difficulty with learning to read, but a scientifically precise explanation has taken a long time to develop. This chapter will present a short history of the evolution of knowledge about the nature of dyslexia, and it will lay the groundwork for later chapters on identification, early intervention, and remediation.

DEFINING DYSLEXIA

The term *dyslexia* is derived from the Greek *dys* (difficult) and *lexicos* (pertaining to words) and was first used by Berlin in 1887 to describe extreme difficulty reading and spelling words. The World Federation of Neurology has defined dyslexia as follows:

> *Specific developmental dyslexia* is a disorder manifested by difficulty learning to read despite conventional instruction, adequate intelligence, and adequate sociocultural opportunity. It is dependent upon fundamental cognitive disabilities that are frequently of constitutional origin (1968; cited in Critchley 1970).

The qualifier *developmental* refers to a disorder of suspected congenital or hereditary origin, in contrast to acquired dyslexia, a disorder resulting from brain injury after the onset of reading (Frith 1986). It is important to state that the word *developmental* does not mean that the disorder will disappear with maturity. A distinguishing characteristic of dyslexia is, in fact, its persistence, although appropriate remedial treatment and the development of compensatory strategies may moderate its effects.

The qualifier *specific* is intended to connote a disorder limited specifically to reading rather than involving a general learning problem. As Keith Stanovich describes this notion,

> Simply put, it is the idea that a dyslexic child has a brain/cognitive deficit that is reasonably specific to the reading task. That is, the concept of a specific reading disability requires that the deficit displayed by the disabled reader not extend too far into other domains of cognitive functioning (Stanovich 1988a, p. 155).

Stanovich (1988b) refers to poor readers who are poor in cognitive ability as well as in all academic areas as *garden variety poor readers*. Reading is not discrepant from IQ in these children as it sometimes is in children with dyslexia. The weak reading of garden variety poor readers is not unexpected as it is in dyslexics.

There is even evidence that dyslexia is limited not just to reading, but to very specific aspects of reading. Philip Gough's theoretical *simple view of reading* holds that there are two contributors necessary to skilled reading comprehension: (a) listening comprehension and (b) decoding (Gough and Tunmer 1986). That is, children with reading problems could be having difficulty at either the word reading level or with understanding what they have read once they have decoded or deciphered written words into spoken words. Wesley Hoover has tested

Gough's model using data from 900 children on the Iowa Test of Basic Skills. He analyzed subtest results for listening comprehension, decoding, and reading comprehension to confirm Gough's two independent contributors to reading comprehension; he found that each is necessary but not sufficient for reading success (Hoover 1994). Dyslexia is conceptualized as difficulty at the word-reading level. Reading comprehension is affected, but it is decoding, and not listening comprehension, that causes the difficulty.

Dyslexia is considered a learning disability in the Federal Register under Public Law 94-142 (see Kavanagh and Truss 1988). As with other learning disabilities covered under this law, dyslexia involves what is called an *exclusionary* diagnosis. That is, in this definition, instead of describing characteristics directly, the definition describes all the conditions that must be ruled out (e.g., low IQ, physical handicaps, environmental factors, etc.) before making a diagnosis.

The term *learning disabilities* is actually a political label coined by Samuel Kirk (see Farnham-Diggory 1992). The term was adapted to secure special services for students with mild learning handicaps. Some of these children did not qualify for placement in established special education categories (i.e., mentally handicapped, emotionally handicapped, physically handicapped). Others' parents did not want their children classified with these more severely handicapped students. Although the majority of students who are classified as *learning disabled* have reading difficulties, in many cases these difficulties can be attributed to mild handicapping factors or conditions other than dyslexia, such as low average intelligence. These children, in terms of Gough's *simple view of reading* are poor at both decoding and listening comprehension. They are considered *garden variety poor readers*. Much of the research on reading disorders has been muddied by failure to distinguish between children who are dyslexic and those who are classified for school instruction as learning disabled, with poor reading as part of a more extensive set of difficulties (e.g., borderline IQ, poor mathematics skills, poor listening).

Stanovich and Gough base their models on a very specific language deficit in the area of phonological processing, a deficit that will be discussed later on in this chapter in more detail. The idea of a specific deficit distinguishes dyslexia from other, less specific learning disabilities. The following definition was the result of the Dyslexia Consensus Project[1], a collaboration between the International Dyslexia

---

[1]The goal of the Definition Consensus Project was "to provide a foundation for meaningful research, diagnosis, and intervention in order to maximize the potential of individuals with learning disabilities and dyslexia to lead independent and productive adult lives" (IDA, 2002, p.9). The ten participants who met in August of 2002 included G. Reid Lyon, Chief of the Child Development and Behavior Branch of NICHD and Harley Tomey , President of IDA, as well as Susan Brady, Hugh Catts, Emerson Dickman, Guinevere Eden, Jack Fletcher, Jeff Gilger, and Bennett and Sally Shaywitz.

Association (IDA) and the National Institute of Child Health and Human Development (NICHD). It was first published in the winter, 2002 edition of the International Dyslexia Association (IDA) publication *Perspectives*, and in the 2003 edition of its journal, *Annals of Dyslexia*:

> Dyslexia is a specific learning disability that is neurobiological in origin. It is characterized by difficulties with accurate and/or fluent word recognition and by poor spelling and decoding abilities. These difficulties typically result from a deficit in the phonological component of language that is often unexpected in relation to other cognitive abilities and the provision of effective classroom instruction. Secondary consequences may include problems in reading comprehension and reduced reading experience that can impede growth of vocabulary and background knowledge (Lyon, Shaywitz, and Shaywitz, 2003, p. 1).

In the article in which the definition appears, Lyon, Shaywitz, and Shaywitz elaborate on the key points in the definition. Dyslexia is unexpected given cognitive functioning. It is specific to weak word reading and spelling and a consequence of phonological deficits. It is neurological in origin. Difficulties in other areas such as comprehension, vocabulary development, and background information are a secondary consequence rather than an organic part of the primary disability.

HISTORICAL AND CURRENT VIEWS ON ETIOLOGY

Although the term *dyslexia* has been used consistently since 1887 to indicate difficulty at the word-reading level, theories about the exact etiology or causes of dyslexia have changed over time. Much of the very early thinking about possible causes grew out of work with brain injured adults who had lost the ability to read. James Hinshelwood, an ophthalmologist practicing in Scotland at the turn of the Century, was one of the first scientists to describe clinical studies of children who failed to read (e.g., 1896; 1917). He surmised that his patients with reading disorder, which he called *congenital word blindness*, must have had either birth injuries to the brain or brain defects. Hinshelwood believed that these defects were in the left hemisphere of the brain in areas related to the storage of visual memory because these children seemed to have difficulty remembering the names of letters and words.

Samuel Orton, an American neurologist, also published theoretical work in which visual processes were implicated. According to Orton, reading reversals (e.g., *b* for *d* and *saw* for *was*) were caused by problems with cerebral dominance in the early stages of reading. He theorized that both right and left visual fields received visual input and relayed this as mirror images to the visual cortices. While in most people one side of the brain becomes dominant over the other and suppresses the image from the non-dominant hemisphere, he believed that dominance was poorly established in people with dyslexia and that the backwards image was often perceived rather than inhibited or suppressed, resulting in what he called *strephosymbolia*, or twisted symbols (1928). Thus, children with dyslexia would see the word *saw* but perceive its mirror image, the word *was*. Orton's model is often misinterpreted, however, as a deficit at the sensory input level involving actually seeing mirror images. This was never his intention.

Orton was also one of the first to associate dyslexia with language disorders (Geschwind 1982), and this constituted the major thrust of his work. Orton's work on language formed a basis for many of the remedial programs that are currently in use. However, it is his visually-based mirror-image explanation that caught on in the popular literature and that continues to be a widely held misconception.

VISUAL EXPLANATIONS OF DYSLEXIA
The Visual-Perceptual Deficit Hypothesis

Orton's mirror-image theory was discredited by the 1970s on several grounds, one being that reversal and sequencing errors did not appear to account for a greater proportion of the total reading errors made by readers with dyslexia than those made by normal readers (Stanovich 1986a). In other words, although children with dyslexia may make more oral reading errors than do children who are good readers, the ratio of reversal errors to other errors is the same. Most readers make occasional reversals, especially in the beginning stages of acquiring reading. If they do not receive appropriate early instruction, children with dyslexia continue to make decoding errors typical of early readers.

Another reason to question the visual-perceptual deficit hypothesis is that readers with dyslexia have not been found to differ from average readers in their performance on nonlinguistic tasks, such as the ability to distinguish visual designs or faces (Liberman and Shankweiler 1979). In studies performed by Frank Vellutino and his colleagues, poor readers had no more difficulty than good readers in copying or recognizing letters or words from a novel alphabet, which were essentially nonverbal stimuli (Vellutino et al. 1975; Vellutino, Steger, and Kandel 1972). Furthermore, Vellutino (1978, 1983) demonstrates that poor readers are almost as adept as good readers at copying visually confusable letters and words from memory, although they are significantly less good at naming or pronouncing these items on second exposure. He attributes the naming problems of poor readers to less well established verbal codes for letter or word forms rather than to visual-perception deficits. Vellutino (1987) suggests that the mirror writing exhibited by some dyslexics (as well as some normally developing readers) reflects their incomplete grasp of letter-sound relationships rather than a visual-perception deficit. That is, it is not the case that they confuse the look of the letters; rather, they cannot remember which name goes with which letter.

In a review of the literature, however, Dale Willows and Megan Terepocki suggest that there is some evidence for non-linguistic directional confusions in children with reading disorder. While the look-alike and sound-alike properties of *b* and *d* could indeed result in a naming-based reversal problem consistent with Vellutino's model, we need to continue to refine research methods for examining directional confusions in children with reading disorder (Willows and Terepocki 1993).

Probably the most compelling arguments against attempting to correct dyslexia through correcting visual-perception come from studies carried out in the 1970s indicating that visual-perception training is generally ineffective in improving reading skills in individuals with dyslexia (Bateman 1979; Bryant 1979). This training was once quite popular. For example, during the 1960s Marianne Frostig developed a test for visual perception and a remedial training program involving tracing, and copying shapes and patterns (Frostig 1967; Frostig, Lefever and Whittlesey 1964). Although Frostig apparently meant these materials to supplement rather than replace reading training, many training programs were based, misguidedly, on her materials alone. There simply were no studies from that period indicating that this training had any positive effect on reading ability.

Optometric training for visual-perception deficits is another historical trend. As Larry Silver has pointed out, optometric training programs that proliferated in the 1960s and 1970s have been both controversial and generally unsuccessful in promoting reading acquisition (Keogh and Pelland 1985; Metzger and Werner 1984). Optometric training alone is not sufficient to improve reading. This point of view grows out of a compelling body of research in the mid- to late-1970s suggesting that *diagnostic-prescriptive teaching* or *process training* (remediation of weak processes, usually visual-perception processes) did not produce gains in reading (e.g., Arter and Jenkins 1979). Close to 20 years ago, Larry Silver argued that the most effective remedial therapy for children with reading problems involves direct instruction in reading (Silver 1987) and this conclusion continues to represent best practice for individuals with dyslexia.

Erratic Eye Movements

The above research has centered on misperception or failure to integrate stationary visual forms. Other work has focused on the temporal aspects of vision. One such line of research involves questions about eye movements. According to Alexander Pollatsek (1993) when the eyes view letters and words, or any other stationary visual stimuli, they fixate briefly (for roughly 200 to 300 ms) while constructing an image to be perceived by the brain before performing a *saccade* or eye movement (for roughly 10 to 40 ms) to the next fixation. Visual information from the saccade is suppressed. This *saccadic suppression* insures a series of discrete rather than overlapping images. In reading, most movements are from left-to-right but there are also right-to-left movements when we go back to confirm a letter or word.

Because erratic eye-movement patterns have been observed in children who are poor readers, it has been hypothesized that this is a cause of dyslexia (Pavlidis 1985; Punnet and Steinhauer 1984). However, it seems likely that erratic eye movement is the result rather than the cause of reading problems; in most cases it is not observed when poor readers are reading at their independent reading levels, but rather when they read text that is too hard for them. Consistent with this explanation, Richard Olson and his colleagues compared younger good readers with older poor readers in a reading-age-match study (Olson, Conners and Rack 1991) and found similar eye movement for the two groups during the reading of similar text.

At the same time, some researchers continue to suggest that there may be a small percentage of children who are dyslexic and whose abnormal fixation patterns reflect a primary visual-spatial disorder (Benton 1985; Eden et al. 1995; Keogh and Pelland 1985; Rayner 1985). For example, there is recent research suggesting that both language and visual skills contribute to reading ability and that this is true for good as well as poor readers. Guinevere Eden (Eden et al. 1995) administered visuospatial and oculomotor measures to subjects who were already participants in a longitudinal study of reading disability conducted by Frank Wood and his colleagues at Bowman Gray Medical School (see below). These children were discrepantly poor readers, with IQs significantly stronger than reading ability, and with deficits in phonological skills. In comparison with normal readers of comparable IQ they were poor at several visuospatial skills (i.e., vertical tracking and fixation stability with the left eye, which is ordinarily used as the lead eye during movement). Note that they were no poorer at these visual tasks than a third group of *garden variety poor readers*. Eden states that her results are consistent with the sort of visual deficits in poor readers reported by Lovegrove and his colleagues (see below).

Deficits in Timing in the Visual Pathways.

Another, more complex visual explanation for reading disorder in some children emerged during the early 1990s. In this model there is a deficit in regard to *saccadic suppression* (see above) involving one of the two systems that transmit information from the eye to the brain. The sustained or *parvocellular* system operates during fixations and the transient or *magnocellular* system operates during saccades or movements to the next fixation. Keep in mind that it is information from the fixation rather than the saccade that is perceived. During the saccade, in normal readers the image from the first fixation is suppressed before the next fixation.

There is some research suggesting that the transient system operates somewhat sluggishly in some poor readers in comparison with normal readers (e.g., Livingstone 1993; Lovegrove 1992; Lovegrove and Williams 1993), and fails to suppress the initial fixation as efficiently as is the case for good readers. Note that this body of research is based on tasks designed to measure identification of images under both quickly and slowly changing conditions, but that the tasks are not reading tasks. However, it has been hypothesized that during reading, failure of the transient system to suppress one fixation before moving on to the next would result in perception of two overlapping sets of letters, which would gradually fade to a single set. Children with *saccadic-suppression deficits* should be able to read words in lists more easily than in connected text (Breitmeyer 1993; Lovegrove and Williams 1993). However, as Charles Hulme points out, this is not the case (Hulme 1988).

If Livingston and Lovegrove are correct, some forms of dyslexia may involve a neural deficit which cannot be corrected and which causes a perceptual deficit (Breitmeyer 1993). The implications for instruction have not been addressed fully, but Breitmeyer and others suggest that reading may be improved by using colored lenses (i.e., Irlen lenses) or transparent colored overlays to cover text. This has been a highly controversial treatment for reading problems (e.g., Blaskey et al. 1990; O'Connor et al. 1990; Robinson and Conway 1990; Solan 1990). Up until this point there has been no theoretical model or research to explain why some individuals report increased ease in reading with these lenses. Breitmeyer (1993) suggests that while certain complex properties of red light would exacerbate the deficit, blue lenses could actually help to counteract the effects of the sluggish transient system. Note that there is insubstantial evidence to draw conclusions about either the model or the treatment.

Visuoconstructive Ability and Dyslexia

A number of highly respected researchers continue to carry out studies exploring the possible influence of non-linguistic factors in dyslexia. For example, Guinevere Eden and her colleagues recently published a study with evidence that some weak readers, while drawing clocks, exhibit symptoms similar to brain damaged patients with right hemispheric damage. They under-use the left side of a clock while representing the clock's face (Eden, Wood, and Stein, 2003).

Keith Rayner (1993) points out that with the publication of Frank Vellutino's *Dyslexia* in 1979, the field began to shift away from a notion of dyslexia as a visual problem and toward the unitary view that dyslexia was caused by a language deficit involving phonological processing. Rayner suggests that we need to be careful not to assume that dyslexia has a unitary cause. He advocates continuing examination of the most current models of skilled reading (e.g., Seidenberg and McClelland 1989) with attention to the various points at which reading might break down. At this time, though, there is no persuasive and comprehensive body of research pointing to a visual-deficit explanation for dyslexia in English speaking children.

AUDITORY-VISUAL HYPOTHESIS

INTERSENSORY DEFICIT HYPOTHESIS

Another hypothesized explanation for dyslexia has involved difficulty integrating information that must be processed simultaneously in two or more modalities. This theory seemed logical when first introduced, for in reading, both auditory and visual systems are involved. Herbert Birch, who first proposed the intersensory deficit hypothesis, developed a test of auditory-visual integration that requires children to match rhythmic patterns with dot patterns, and found that some poor readers were markedly less proficient than good readers at this task (Birch and Belmont 1964). However, other researchers, such as Naomi Zigmond (1966), found that some disabled readers were inferior to readers of normal ability when processing in a single modality, as on auditory tasks; therefore, their inferior performance on intersensory tasks can be expected. In a further challenge to the intersensory or cross-modal deficit hypothesis, Frank Vellutino and his colleagues (Vellutino, Steger, and Pruzek 1973) found no significant differences between poor and adequate readers on nonverbal paired-associate matching tasks that measure both within and between modality functioning (visual-visual; auditory-auditory; visual-auditory). By contrast, similar studies carried out with verbal stimuli, such as words and letters, reveal notable differences for poor and adequate readers. These investigators conclude that verbal, rather than intersensory, deficits distinguish dyslexics from normal readers.

Subtypes or Unitary Disorder?

With so many possible explanations, a question that has provoked specialists and researchers for some time is whether dyslexia is a unique syndrome or whether it comprises a number of identifiable subcategories. The question has led to studies aimed at classifying dyslexia into discrete subtypes based on patterns of symptoms.

Some researchers have identified subtypes based on spelling errors. Elena Boder (1971), for example, claimed to find three distinct spelling patterns among dyslexics. She terms these error patterns *dysphonetic* (reflecting deficits in sound–symbol association), *dyseidetic* (representing difficulty remembering visual aspects of words with non-phonetic spellings), and *dysphonetic-dyseidetic* (a combination of both problems). Attempts to validate Boder's subtypes, however, have not been successful (Carpenter 1983; Moats 1983; Nockleby and Galbraith 1984). In a recent study, Dale Willows and Gillian Jackson found Boder's categorization measures to be unreliable in terms of consistency between examiners (Willows and Jackson 1992).

Rebecca Treiman and Jonathan Baron (1983) examined spelling behaviors in dyslexia from the perspective of rule application. They found evidence of individuals with dyslexia who were overly reliant on spelling-sound rules, and whom they labeled *Phoenicians*, and another group who depended on word-specific associations, whom they called *Chinese*. These investigators allege that the Phoenician type of dyslexic is able to spell nonsense words but tends to over-generalize phonics rules to exception words.

Another approach to the subtyping of dyslexia involves a dichotomy between what is called *surface dyslexia*, or failure on an orthographic level to move directly from print to meaning, and *deep dyslexia*, or failure in using phonological processes to decode unfamiliar words. This dichotomy is consistent with the dual route theory of processing in which either the direct lexical route or the phonological route is used. The terminology comes from studies of adults who were once normal readers and who lost either one ability or the other following brain damage (Patterson, Marshall, and Coltheart 1985). When used with children these terms are altered to *developmental surface dyslexia* and *developmental deep dyslexia*.

In a review of the literature on nonword reading, John Rack, Maggie Snowling, and Richard Olson make the point that while studies using large numbers of subjects generally fail to distribute all subjects into distinct subtypes, not all individuals with dyslexia have the same profiles (Rack, Snowling, and Olson 1992). Snowling and her colleagues have documented a number of case histories of children with average or higher IQ's and extraordinary difficulty with word reading and these profiles fall into two types, children with phonological deficits and those with visual memory deficits (Goulandris and Snowling 1991; Snowling, Goulandris, and Stackhouse 1994; Snowling and Hulme 1989).

At this point there is no single subtype classification system that is supported by a comprehensive body of research or that is useful in choosing remedial programs for English-speaking children with dyslexia. Thirty-five years ago practitioners tried to match children with instruction depending on whether they were *auditory learners* or *visual learners*, but there is no research base to support this dichotomy. While not supported by research, and thus, misguided, this idea is appealing and lingers on in educational folklore. The best practice involves teaching children to coordinate phonology and print because both are crucial to skilled reading.

DYSLEXIA AS A LANGUAGE-BASED DEFICIT

For the past 30 years the prevalent view has been that dyslexia is a language-based problem (e.g., Catts 1986, 1989; Elkonin, 1973; Liberman 1973, 1984; Shaywitz 2003; Stanovich 1986a; Vellutino 1979). Language is a highly complex function with multiple dimensions. Language *form* involves phonology (units of sound), morphology (units of meaning), and syntax. *Semantics* involves overall meaning. *Pragmatics* involves usage or purpose. Each of these three aspects involves both receptive and expressive language. It is fairly universally agreed that oral language is a precursor to reading. The question is, how is each of these areas related to reading and which causes dyslexia?

Early Language Difficulties and Reading

Research substantiates a strong relationship between early oral language problems and later reading problems. Follow-up studies of children diagnosed with early specific language impairment (SLI) have shown the incidence of later reading disability to be 90 percent or greater (e.g., Stark et al. 1984; Strominger and Bashir 1977). That is, most children who struggle to learn to listen and talk also struggle to learn to read and write.

Although the incidence of later reading difficulties for children with early language impairment is very high, the reverse is not always the case. Not all children with dyslexia have histories involving early language disorder. For example, in a prediction study, Natalie Badian used a screening including a number of language measures with four-year-olds to predict sixth-grade reading (Badian 1988). Almost all of the four-year-olds with low screening scores developed later reading problems, but only a little more than half of the children with later reading problems had scored below the screening cut-off as four-year-olds. We really have two groups of children here, those whose global language impairment causes later reading impairment, and those whose dyslexia affects more specific areas of language development (see Catts 1989).

Children with global language difficulties often babble late as infants and speak late as toddlers. Some have difficulty with receptive language. Some understand what they hear, but have marked expressive language problems with vocabulary or syntax. Children with autism fail to make eye contact as infants and have difficulty developing and using language for communication. Children with these severe language problems are typically referred for speech/language assessment and remediation prior to entering school.

Although all of the above dimensions of oral language can have an impact on written language development, not all aspects of language are implicated as primary causes in developmental dyslexia. Dyslexia tends to be associated with milder and subtler linguistic differences that often go unnoticed in the preschool years.

Specific Deficits in Phonological Processing and Dyslexia

These subtle differences tend to involve the phonological aspects of oral language. One explanation of dyslexia is failure to construct complete inner models of the sound structure of words. The classic example is scrambling sounds in long words, such as saying "aminal" for *animal*, long after age peers have corrected this typical early mispronunciation. Another difficulty is substituting words that sound alike. An adult I know referred to the "wind chill factor" as the "windshield factor" and another adult, with an oil leak in her car, talked of her "Cadillac converter." A 10-year old, after hearing the name Judy Blume on a list of authors on his summer reading list, commented, "Isn't that kind of young for me? And I didn't know Judy Blume was an author. Isn't she a character in a book? You know, *Judy Blume, Toothless Wonder.*" I realized that he was confusing this author with the title character in his younger sister's book, *Junie B. Jones, Toothless Wonder.* We all make these malapropisms now and then, but the verbal world of individuals with dyslexia is overwhelmingly full of phonological confusion.

Keith Stanovich has suggested that the entire range of difficulties often attributed to dyslexia may stem from what he calls the *phonological core deficit*. He argues that failure to learn to decode words because of phonological processing problems causes subsequent deficits in reading comprehension, vocabulary development, and even IQ, through lack of access to print experiences. Stanovich calls this the *Matthew effect* from Bible verses in which the rich get richer and the poor get poorer. There is evidence that this phonological core deficit is of organic origin. There is also evidence that its symptoms are responsive to remediation. What is the range of phonological processing abilities?

Phonological Awareness. The term *phonological awareness* refers to the metacognitive ability to focus on the form of a word rather than the meaning, and to understand that spoken language is made up of a series of sounds that occupy a particular sequential order. Keep in mind that this is quite different from skills in phonics knowledge, a low-level, paired–associate form of learning that relates letters and sounds on an automatic or rote level.

Phonological awareness is the most intensively researched of the phonological processing abilities, and the one with the clearest relationship to dyslexia. The earliest work on phonological awareness in the United States was carried out by Isabelle Liberman together with her students at the University of Connecticut and her colleagues at Haskins Laboratories (Liberman, 1973; Liberman et al. 1974; Liberman et al. 1977). Liberman asked children to use a wooden dowel to tap the number of sounds or phonemes in words. Virtually none of the children could represent phonemes accurately at age four, a few at age five, and most by age six. Liberman's work also suggested that this skill was poorly developed in children with reading problems.

Several British researchers have provided evidence of a link between deficits in phonological awareness and deficits in reading. In a series of often cited case histories, Maggie Snowling and her colleagues have documented the pervasive phonological deficits of children with dyslexia seen over a period of time in a clinical setting (e.g., Snowling and Hulme 1989). While it has been argued that phonological awareness may be an effect of mature reading rather than its cause (Morais et al. 1979), it has also been demonstrated that the degree to which phonological awareness is developed prior to reading instruction plays a powerful role in determining reading outcomes. In a reading–age match study, Snowling (1980) found that older poor readers matched on reading level with normal younger readers were much poorer at phonological tasks. This suggests that the deficit has a cause beyond lack of exposure to reading. It is likely that the relationship is reciprocal; phonological awareness drives reading in the early stages and then exposure to print increases phonological awareness once reading catches on. Two components of a large-scale, longitudinal study carried out in England by Lynette Bradley and Peter Bryant (1983) have confirmed the causal role of early phonological awareness in later reading. They followed hundreds of young children over a period of time and found that the young prereaders who were good at phonological awareness became the later good readers. In the second component of this study, they trained prereaders in phonological awareness and found that they had a later advantage over controls in reading and spelling. The findings from these early studies have been confirmed over and over through a body of research carried out during the late 1980s and 1990s through funding from the National Institute of Child Health and Human Development (NICHD) and other sources. See Chapter 5 for more information on phonemic awareness.

Speech Perception Deficits. Ability to perceive sound is a prerequisite for phonological awareness, but does not appear to be the key issue in dyslexia. During the 1980s, a recurring question in the field was whether or not difficulty with the phonological aspects of reading was caused by difficulty with auditory perception. Findings from research from that time indicated that there were no differences between children with and without dyslexia in perception of nonverbal environmental sounds (Brady, Shankweiler, and Mann 1983; Godfrey et al. 1981). Differences did appear to occur related to speech sounds, however, and were especially marked when speech sounds occurred in the presence of background noise. Susan Brady and her colleagues at Haskins Laboratories carried out a series of experiments comparing good and poor readers in ability to listen to words and repeat them back. In an early study, there were no differences except when stimuli were presented under conditions of background noise (Brady, Shankweiler, and Mann 1983). In this study, the words were all a single syllable in length. In a later study, differences were found in listening and repeating back nonsense words and multisyllable words even in the absence of background noise. Brady hypothesizes that the difficulty is not at the perceptual level but at the level of phonological representation. This results in poor ability to encode phonological information. That is, under less than optimal conditions (unfamiliar words, long words, and under noisy conditions), children with this reading-related deficit have difficulty remembering sounds and encoding them into spoken reproductions (Brady, Poggie, and Rapala 1989).

Paula Tallal and her colleagues (e.g., 1980; Tallal, Miller, Jenkins, and Merzenich 1997; Tallal and Stark 1982; Tallal et al. 1996) have proposed a model of language learning impairment (LLI) characterized by difficulty in perceiving and analyzing rapidly presented speech sounds (i.e., tens of milliseconds). For example, some consonant sounds are of very short duration. The "stop" consonants /b/ and /d/ are almost impossible to pronounce without saying /buh/ and /duh/, whereas /s/ is of longer duration and easier to perceive and pronounce. Tallal believes that for some children, the short duration of stop consonants interferes with the ability to detect fine distinctions between phonemes in words and, consequently, with the ability to make connections between graphemes and phonemes in attempting to read. She and her colleagues have trained children to perceive these sounds by increasing their temporal processing thresholds through modifications to acoustically slowed speech over a four-week period (Tallal et al. 1996). Tallal and her colleagues have used Fast ForWord, a program with a computer game format, to increase this threshold (Merzenich et al. 1996). This approach is still new and somewhat controversial. Although Tallal's team has reported growth in phonemic awareness and reading attributable to Fast ForWord, other researchers have reported greater benefits for the Orton-Gillingham approach when the two methods were compared (Hook, Macaruso, and Jones 2001).

Verbal Short-term Memory.   The ability to listen, remember, and repeat back speech sounds involves being able to build a phonological model of the sounds in a word or word string in inner speech. This is one of the characteristic phonological processing difficulties reported in a review of the literature on the relation between phonology and reading by Wagner and Torgesen (1987). Their term for verbal short-term memory is *phonetic recoding to maintain information in working memory.* Memory for words appears to depend on their sounds. Three common measures of verbal short-term memory involve repeating back longer and longer sentences, or strings of digits, or strings of unrelated words.

Individuals with dyslexia have been found to perform less well than age-matched typically developing readers on tasks requiring them to repeat back information verbatim (e.g., Mann, Liberman, and Shankweiler 1980). A number of studies comparing children of equivalent IQ but of both high and low reading ability report deficits on the Digit Span subtest of the Wechsler Intelligence Scales for Children (WISC-R) for the poor readers (see Jorm 1983). The idea here is that verbal information is held in memory more efficiently when it is stored in a phonological code. Individuals with impaired phonological processing have difficulty doing this. Holding meaningless material in short-term memory involves heavier demands on phonological coding than does memory for materials that are meaningful. For example, in a group of six- and seven-year-olds referred for reading disorder, there was a significant discrepancy between ability to repeat back sentences, the easier task for this group, and unrelated word strings, which was more difficult (Shepherd and Uhry 1993).

As Peter Bryant and Lynette Bradley (1985) have pointed out, verbal short-term memory is another area in which one can question the causal role in reading. Does the pre-reading level of facility in remembering oral linguistic material drive later reading ability? Or is verbal short-term memory exercised during reading through needing to remember strings of words until the end of a sentence is reached? Bryant and Bradley make a strong case for this practice effect, and thus for the effect of reading on verbal memory. To test their hypothesis, they measured memory in 368 children over a period of four years. They found that verbal short-term memory at age 4 was not a very good predictor of reading at age 6, but that reading at age 6 was a good predictor of verbal short-term memory at age 8. Virginia Mann and Isabelle Liberman (1984) reported contradictory evidence when they found that memory for word strings in kindergarten predicted some of the variance in first-grade reading.

Speech Articulation Rate.   It can be argued that at least some of the variance in verbal short-term memory tasks may be accounted for by motoric elements affecting articulation rate. That is, as a child prepares to repeat back lists or sentences, they are retained in an *articulatory loop* in which material is sub-vocally rehearsed in order to retain it in short-term memory. Slowness in vocalization can cause the phonological impression to deteriorate and can interfere with accuracy of reproduction. This could be caused by speech–motor deficits. Peter Wolff and his colleagues at the Children's Hospital in Boston have reported evidence that both children and adults with dyslexia are slow and dysrhythmic when asked to repeat the same sequence of syllables (e.g., *pa-ta-ka*) over and over to the rhythm of a metronome. Furthermore, these speech motor deficits are correlated with deficits in reading (Wolff, Michel, and Ovrut 1990b). Hugh Catts has reported similar findings. He found children with reading disorder to be significantly slower in repeating multisyllabic words when compared to normal readers (Catts 1986).

Rapid Naming. Inability to retrieve the names of objects previously known is symptomatic of adult acquired aphasia. Early studies of children with anomia or word-finding problems have grown out of the literature on adult aphasia. There are two forms of rapid naming, *discrete trial* or *confrontational* naming in which objects are presented for naming one at a time, and rapid serial naming, which involves stimuli (e.g., letters, numerals) presented in linear format, and named in a series, one after the other. The first, discrete trial naming-finding problems are typical of individuals with SLI and can be associated with comprehension issues, but are not typical of dyslexia. Rapid serial naming, the second form of rapid word retrieval difficulty appears to be unequivocally linked with dyslexia. Martha Denckla and Rita Rudel have carried out seminal work using an instrument they designed to measure this dyslexia-related naming problem. Called the Rapid Automatized Naming Test (RAN; Denckla and Rudel 1974, 1976a, 1976b), the instrument uses 10 x 5 grids of the same five colors (and then numerals, pictured objects, and letters) repeated over and over in random serial order. Denckla and Rudel found that the length of time it took to name these stimuli varied with age; older children were quicker than younger children. It also varied with reading ability; good readers were quicker than poor readers at any given age (Denckla and Rudel 1974). This has been confirmed through more recent studies (e.g., Wolf 1999; Wolff, Michel, and Ovrut 1990a).

This task is very similar to the act of reading. In both cases a child looks at a visual stimulus and speaks a response. It could be argued that good readers, in effect, practice for the RAN test when they practice reading, whereas poor readers, who read far fewer words in a day or a week, practice less and thus are slower on the RAN. The Oxford psychologist Peter Bryant and his research colleague Lynette Bradley have made the point that only through reading-age-match studies can rapid automatized naming be linked specifically with dyslexia, rather than with the early stages of reading. That is, slow naming is associated with slow reading, but the direction of causality is not clear.

Wagner and Torgesen (1987) consider rapid serial naming a form of phonological processing. They call it *phonological recoding in lexical access* because the child moves from a visual code to an auditory code in naming letters or digits. Other researchers consider rapid serial naming a measure of orthographic processing speed. Patricia Bowers and Marianne Wolf (1993; Bowers, 1995; Bowers and Swanson, 1991; Bowers, Sunseth, and Golden, 1999; Wolf, 1991; 1999) have presented a model in which this task taps non-phonological functions, such as precise timing mechanisms for orthographic processing. They use the term *double deficit* for readers who are weak in phonemic awareness as well as in speed of naming.

Where deficits in phonological awareness are associated with later deficits in word-reading accuracy, deficits in rapid serial naming appear to be related to word-reading fluency. See Chapter 8 for information on instruction to improve rate and fluency in reading.

NEUROLOGICAL AND BIOLOGICAL CORRELATES
Hemispheric Specialization

Historically, overt neurological problems have been difficult to identify among children with dyslexia (Rutter 1978). Therefore, investigative efforts to understand the neurological underpinnings of dyslexia were focused on behavioral differences, which were thought to indicate neurological differences, with much of the exploration in the area of differences in hemispheric specialization. The basic assumption behind this research has been that language processing in dyslexics may not be controlled by the same areas of the brain as in individuals without dyslexia. For the majority of the population, these areas lie in the left cerebral hemisphere. Much of this research examined *laterality differences*, which were presumed to reflect *lateralization differences*. By *laterality* we mean the choice of hand, eye, or foot in performing everyday activities. *Lateralization* refers to "the involuntary brain functioning of the left and/or right cerebral hemispheres" (Obrzut and Boliek 1986), otherwise called hemispheric specialization.

The relationship between left-handedness and reading disability has received considerable attention. Within the general population, the incidence of left-handedness has been estimated to be 8 to 10 percent (Kinsbourne and Hiscock 1981); lateralization indices are not as easily determined. Drake Duane, a neurologist, reported that 98 percent of right-handed people and 70 percent of left-handed people have language lateralized in the left hemisphere (Duane 1983). An interesting finding from one study (Hardyck and Petrinovich 1977) is that left-handers with a family history of left-handedness appear to have less hemispheric specialization than right-handers, whereas left-handers with no family history of left-handedness seem to process language in the left hemisphere like most right-handers. Confounding the issue is the possibility that some cases of left-handedness may be the result of early brain injury (Satz, Saslow, and Henry 1985). Clinical investigations of reading disorder may involve such *pathological left-handers* and cognitive deficits in such cases would more likely be due to cerebral insult than to deviant cerebral lateralization (Hiscock and Kinsbourne 1982). Any data pertaining to the connection between left-handedness and dyslexia, therefore, would be falsely skewed.

Finding left-handedness to be more common in males than females, the late Norman Geschwind, a neurologist who pioneered research on the etiology of dyslexia, proposed a theory based on epidemiological research that links male sex hormones, left-handedness, and autoimmune diseases to dyslexia (Geschwind 1983; Geschwind and Behan 1982). Further exploration of this hypothesized association has been carried out by Geschwind's colleagues at Beth Israel Hospital in Boston, principally Albert Galaburda (Galaburda 1985). Among educators, psychologists, and neuropsychologists, opinions on the theorized association between handedness patterns and reading disability varied considerably in the 1980s.

Other Measures of Lateralization

Several measures of central language processing have been devised that are now considered to be better indices of cerebral lateralization than handedness. One of these measures is dichotic listening, where paired stimuli are presented simultaneously to each ear and the subject's response pattern, favoring one or the other ear, is thought to indicate the dominant hemisphere for that particular stimulus type: a right-ear advantage (REA) reflecting left-hemispheric processing and vice versa. Another measure, visual half-field (VHF) technique, involves presenting verbal or nonverbal stimuli tachistoscopically to either the left or right visual fields, or to both fields simultaneously in bilateral presentations. Response performance comparisons are considered to reflect degree of lateralization to one or the other hemisphere.

Brain Structure Differences

During the late 1970s and 1980s, a few postmortem anatomical studies were conducted on the brains of persons previously diagnosed as dyslexic (Galaburda 1983, 1985; Galaburda and Kemper 1979) to see if the brains of dyslexics were different from the brains of typical readers.

Although biological anomalies were indicated, the number of cases was not sufficient to draw any definitive conclusions about the occurrence of cerebral abnormalities in dyslexics (Geschwind 1986). However, in the opinion of the investigators, one finding was considered important. Whereas in most individuals the left hemisphere is larger than the right, the dyslexic brains examined by Albert Galaburda (1985) appeared relatively symmetrical due to a larger-than-normal right hemisphere in the brains of individuals with dyslexia. This finding led Galaburda to postulate that the etiology of dyslexia lies in abnormal migration of neural cells during fetal development (Galaburda, Rosen, and Sherman 1989).

Early efforts to look for possible cerebral abnormalities in dyslexic individuals involved a number of noninvasive techniques, such as *electroencephalography* (EEG), an electrical scanning procedure, and *computerized tomography* (CT), a radiological scanning technique. Neither of these brain scanning methods has been effective in providing a clear image of the working brain (Connors 1978; Denckla 1978; Denckla, LeMay, and Chapman 1985; Duane 1983).

Until the early 1990s, studies of blood flow in the brain involved the radioactive isotopes used in *positron emission tomography* (PET) scans, which limited experimental use with children. However, experiments with *magnetic resonance imaging* (MRI) are far less invasive and provide the sort of detailed picture available prior to MRI only through postmortem studies. Work with MRI indicates that there are physiological differences between individuals who read normally and those who are dyslexic. For example, Lubs and his colleagues found differences in patterns of asymmetry in the two hemispheres; whereas normal readers tend to be asymmetrical in the angular gyrus area of the parietal lobe, with left side larger than right, the pattern is reversed with individuals who are dyslexic (Lubs et al. 1991). In another example of imaging techniques, Frank Wood and his colleagues at Bowman Gray Medical Center have carried out studies indicating that blood flow differences involving Wernicke's area of the left hemisphere are present in adults diagnosed with dyslexia as children, in comparison with those without a history of reading disorder. These studies were carried out during performance of an auditory-to-orthography task; subjects were asked to indicate whether a word they heard had four letters (Flowers 1993; Wood et al. 1991).

Brain Function Differences

Functional Magnetic Resonance Imaging (fMRI) has had an enormous impact on research on dyslexia. For example, a group of neurologists, psychologists, and linguists are currently using fMRI to explore the neurobiological basis of dyslexia through a collaboration between Haskins Laboratories and the Yale School of Medicine. This technique provides a picture of how various cortical areas are activated during different reading tasks. Sally and Bennett Shaywitz and Kenneth Pugh are part of this collaboration. Sally Shaywitz's new book *Overcoming Dyslexia* (2003) is written for parents and provides a clear description of the tasks used in fMRI imaging, and of the findings of her group's studies using this technology.

Two findings are particularly relevant to dyslexia. First, there are different pathways used for sounding out words in the early stages of reading and for quickly recognizing words later during skilled reading. Second, this quick system is implicated in dyslexia. According to Pugh and the Shaywitzes (e.g., Pugh et al. 2000, 2001), two left-hemisphere posterior systems are activated during reading. The first is the left hemisphere *temporo-parietal*, or *dorsal* circuit, which is activated during phonological tasks such as reading new words. This system is activated in response to the reading of low frequency words and nonwords. It works slowly, connecting speech sounds to print in unfamiliar words, and connecting these units to information from other language systems such as the morphological and semantic systems. In teacher terminology, this system could be related to the accurate sounding out of words so that they can be recognized and understood. This is the system that needs to work well during Chall's alphabetic or decoding stage of reading.

Once these connections have become integrated, words are recognized and understood through activation of a second left hemisphere posterior circuit, the *occipito-temporal* or *ventral* system. One characteristic of this system is its rapid response time (i.e., 150-180 ms). The ventral system appears to process orthographic information, that is, to recognize visual patterns and to connect them to patterns stored in memory. This system develops later in the reading process and appears to benefit from the "highly integrated representations" formed by the earlier developing dorsal system (Pugh et al. 2001, p. 483). Again, in teacher terminology, this system relates to automaticity and fluency. In this model, then, the dorsal system processes the sounding out of words and the building of what Ehri calls amalgamations or connections with other lexical elements. Once these connections are firm, the ventral system recognizes words almost instantly during fluent reading. These two systems need to work together, using what Pugh and his colleagues call "functional connectivity" (p. 485).

These patterns of cortical activation are found to be different in readers with dyslexia. The team at Haskins Laboratories and the Yale School of Medicine have carried out neuroimaging studies indicating that the functioning of both the dorsal and ventral anterior systems appears to be disrupted in both adults and children with dyslexia. In contrast with nonimpaired readers, there was little activation of the dorsal system in response to phonological recoding tasks by adults and children with dyslexia. Likewise, readers with dyslexia did not show the characteristic quick response in the ventral area in response to print. Moreover, functional connectivity is disrupted (Shaywitz et al. 1998). In addition to evidence of disruption of these left hemisphere posterior systems, there is also evidence that readers with dyslexia compensate through activation of anterior regions when processing phonological information (Pugh et al. 2000; Shaywitz et al. 1998). That is, they compensate by misusing parts of the brain that are poorly suited to the task of rapidly recognizing words. These findings are consistent with studies from the fields of reading and educational psychology in terms of disruption of phonological processing in dyslexia.

The value of this recent ability to form an image of the brain of a living person engaged in a specific linguistic task lies not so much in diagnostic benefit for individuals, as in its ability to confirm that dyslexia is an organic disorder. A second benefit lies in its ability to document effective instruction. There is encouraging news from a recent study carried out by a team including an instructional specialist and neuroscientists in which progress in reading was documented as being causal to changes in brain functioning (Shaywitz et al. 2004). Benita Blachman provided systematic, direct, phonologically based reading instruction to second and third grade children with low ability in phonological processing. See Blachman et al. (2003) for a more detailed description of the treatment. At the end of the intervention, their phonological awareness and reading ability were superior to that of controls. Before and after the year-long intervention, the children were flown from upstate New York to New Haven, Connecticut for fMRIs. At pre-test, their cortical functioning was similar to that of the children with dyslexia previously tested by Pugh and the Shaywitzes. At post-test, functioning was similar to that of children without dyslexia, while untreated controls with low phonological processing skills continued to show the left hemisphere posterior cortical anomalies typical of children with dyslexia. That is, appropriate instruction not only taught these children to use phonological processes for reading, it changed the way their brains functioned during reading. Sally Shaywitz describes this as being able to "rewire or 'normalize' the brain." Additional reading on the neurobiological implications of dyslexia can be found in Bennett Shaywitz's article in the third edition of the *Handbook of Reading Research* (Shaywitz et al. 2000) and in Sally Shaywitz's book *Overcoming Dyslexia* (2003).

Ironically, while fMRI confirms the role of phonemic processing deficits in beginning reading with physical evidence, fMRIs have also provided evidence that dyslexia is not univerally associated with phonemic processing difficulties. In a recent study using evidence from fMRIs for eight Chinese children with reading disorder and eight typically developing readers, brain activation differences occurred but differed from those found in fMRI studies of English-speaking readers (Siok et al. 2004). Activation was similar for the two Chinese groups in the left temporoparietal cortex. However, the children with reading disorder demonstrated less activation than typically developing children in the left middle frontal gyrus. This area is described as helping to associate shapes and meaning, a task more typical of reading in Chinese orthography than in English. Pilcher (2004) quotes Guinevere Eden as saying, "The study shows that the neural basis of reading is complex and differs depending on the nature of the writing system," in response to the study. This study raises the point that dyslexia as a phonological processing deficit may be more characteristic of individuals learning to read in English and other alphabetic languages than of those reading languages utilizing logographic characters.

Gender

The stereotype of the male dyslexic grew out of statistical descriptions based on children referred to clinics and to special school placements. Using these samples, it looked as though there were roughly four times as many boys as girls with dyslexia or severe reading disorder (Vogel 1990). Re-evaluation of these ratios has been carried out in projects involving, for example, the Connecticut Longitudinal Studies (Shaywitz et al. 1990), Bowman Gray Medical Center (Wood et al. 1991), and the Colorado Reading Project (DeFries et al. 1991). Instead of figuring ratios of boys to girls in samples of referred children, these studies tested large numbers of children within school districts. When tallies were kept of the number of children whose reading was lower than expectations based on IQ, there were close to as many girls as boys with reading deficits. One possible explanation of the discrepancy is that boys are referred more often than girls because they are more apt to have attentional and behavioral problems (Vogel 1990) and thus their reading problems are more visible than those of girls.

Attention Deficit Hyperactivity Disorder and Dyslexia

Up until fairly recently the distinction between children with dyslexia, and those classified as *learning disabled* who read poorly and also had behavior problems, was not made clear in much of the research literature. One important recent step has involved isolating *attention deficit disorder* with and without *hyperactivity disorder* (ADHD)[2] as distinct from other learning disorders.

---

[2] Historically, several terms have been used in different editions of the *Diagnostic and Statistical Manual of Mental Disorders* (e.g., attention deficit disorder with and without hyperactivity). For the sake of simplicity, the current term ADHD is used throughout this discussion for ADDH and ADD.

During the 1960s and 1970s, the term *minimal brain dysfunction* (MBD) was used to describe children assumed to have subtle neurological problems causing both learning and behavior problems. Neurological *soft signs* such as reflexes or borderline performance on the EEG were used diagnostically by the medical community. These children were often assumed to have suffered birth injuries resulting in erratic behavior and learning problems. They most likely shared symptoms with the brain injured children described earlier by Werner and Strauss (1940; or see Farnham-Diggory 1992). There was never clear agreement in the educational and medical communities on either diagnostic procedures or a clinical profile for MBD and the concept lost favor by the 1980s. We now believe that many of these children may have suffered from ADHD among other conditions.

Research by Sally and Bennett Shaywitz of the Yale University School of Medicine, and others in the field, have helped us to identify ADHD more easily and to differentiate it from learning disabilities. The Shaywitzes have developed what they call the Yale Children's Inventory (YCI), which includes a parent questionnaire about behavior (Shaywitz et al. 1988). The YCI examines academic, language, and fine motor development as well as behaviors such as attention, activity, and negative affect. Portions of this questionnaire are reprinted in a book edited by the Shaywitzes that summarizes some of the recent work on ADHD (Shaywitz and Shaywitz 1992). The YCI was used with 445 children who participated in the Connecticut Longitudinal Study. Data including the YCI as well as school-based testing were collected on all of the kindergarten children from 12 Connecticut towns at the beginning of the 1983-84 school year and again during the spring of their second- and fourth-grade years. Results from this study have helped clarify the relationship between ADHD and reading and other academic problems. Based on findings from this nonreferred population, as well as from other sources, the Shaywitzes report that somewhere between 10 and 20 percent of children have ADHD (Shaywitz and Shaywitz 1991).

The relationship between reading disorder and ADHD is complex. There is evidence that the two syndromes represent independent factors. That is, either syndrome can exist with or without the other. In a clinic-referred population of 192 children studied at the University of Arkansas Child Study Center, roughly 50 percent of those who met criteria for ADHD from the *Diagnostic and Statistical Manual of Mental Disorders* (*DSM III*) also had specific reading problems using the criteria of reading scores that were significantly lower than Verbal scale IQ. That is, not all children with ADHD have specific reading difficulty (Dykman and Ackerman 1991). The degree of overlap between these syndromes tends to depend on whether or not subjects are studied by researchers through a school system or through a referred clinic population. As many as 80 percent of clinic-referred children with academic disorders were found to have ADHD in very early studies, whereas only about 30 percent of the children with reading disorder in the Connecticut Longitudinal Study had concomitant ADHD.

In looking at the ADHD-reading relationship Frank Wood and Rebecca Felton report three longitudinal studies carried out through the Bowman Gray Medical Center with both children and adults. These studies indicated that while ADHD certainly predicts academic success in general, it does not predict specific success or failure at the word-reading level (Wood and Felton 1994). In one of these studies, 485 children were followed from first to fifth grade. Specific linguistic factors related to phonological processing were far better at predicting later word-level reading ability than were measures of ADHD (Felton and Wood 1989). In other words, while ADHD and dyslexia can be *comorbid*, or both present in the same child, they are separate factors and ADHD does not appear to affect the acquisition of word-level decoding skills in a specific way.

Erik Willcutt and Bruce Pennington studied hundred of twins, with and without reading disability in order to examine the relationship between ADHD and reading disability (RD). They found that students with RD were significantly more apt to have signs of ADHD than those with typically developing reading skills and that attentional difficulties were more prevalent in the weak readers than were signs of hyperactivity. Interestingly, far more boys than girls showed signs of hyperactivity. This finding sheds light on gender issues described above. These researchers state,

> This difference may provide a partial explanation for the discrepancy between the gender ratio obtained in referred (approximately 4 boys to 1 girl) and non-referred (1.2 to 1.5 boys to 1 girl) samples of individuals with RD. Specifically, the hyperactive and impulsive behaviors exhibited by boys with RD may be more disruptive than the inattentive behaviors exhibited by girls and may therefore precipitate more frequent referrals for clinical attention (Willcutt and Pennington 2000).

Willcutt and Pennington's study is consistent with work on comprehension carried out by the Shaywitzes, who have reported evidence that silent reading comprehension difficulties may be associated with ADHD (Shaywitz 1993). This may be because ADHD involves a generalized inability to attend during complex tasks that need a high degree of self-monitoring, rather than a difficulty specific to reading.

Heritability

Clinicians have long been convinced that dyslexia runs in families. They often find a parent or sibling with dyslexia when collecting date on family history in the initial phase of an evaluation or preparation for tutoring a referred child.

Research carried out as part of the Colorado Twin Study has provided convincing evidence that relatives of dyslexics are more predisposed to dyslexia than individuals in families of good readers. With the genetic etiology of dyslexia in mind, John DeFries and his colleagues carried out the Twin Study. This involved collecting data on pairs of twins, both identical (*monozygotic* or MZ) and nonidentical or fraternal (*dizygotic* or DZ) twins, from 27 Colorado school districts. Initial data was used to screen for any set of twins in which there was at least one member with a history of school reading problems. Extensive testing of IQ, reading level, phonological awareness, and eye movements was carried out, as well as tests to confirm *zygosity* (the twin relationship). Ninety-nine identical pairs were identified, as well as 73 same-sex and 39 different-sex pairs of fraternal twins. If dyslexia were primarily of environmental influence one would expect roughly the same number of co-occurring instances of dyslexia in fraternal as in identical twins. That is, what the researchers call the *concordance* rate should be the same in the two sets of twins. However, this was not the case. In 70 percent of the identical pairs, when one twin had a reading disorder, the other did as well, while in the fraternal twins the concordance rate was only 48 percent (DeFries et al. 1991). These rates confirm findings from earlier, smaller studies from other researchers, in suggesting the heritability of dyslexia.

An interesting additional finding from the Twin Study involved analysis of phonological processing data. Although there was a strong genetic influence on phonological skills, this was not the case with orthographic skills. That is, when subjects were poor at reading and this was associated with weak phonological processing, there was a genetic link, but this was not so when orthographic processing was considered. This is consistent with findings from a British twin study in which the genetic component of spelling disorder appears to influence phonology but not orthography (Stevenson 1991).

Using a different model but asking a similar question, Herbert Lubs and his colleagues also find a familial predisposition to dyslexia. Eleven families with dyslexic members were traced for three generations in an attempt to locate a gene leading to dyslexia. The pattern of inheritance that emerges from this and other studies is called *autosomal dominant inheritance* (Lubs et al. 1993). Some unaffected members appear to carry the gene, but remain asymptomatic, while others appear to have recovered or compensated. The latter are more apt to be women than men.

A number of recent studies have tried to identify a gene for dyslexia. For example, Shelley Smith and her colleagues have worked on gene localization using a technique called *sib pairs*, in which DNA samples are analyzed in pairs of siblings. The argument for this technique is that pairs of siblings who are both dyslexic will have similar DNA in regard to the dyslexia gene, while this will not be the case in disconcordant pairs. Smith found encouraging results for both chromosome 6 and chromosome 15 (Smith, Kimberling, and Pennington 1991). A more recent study favors chromosome 6 (Cardon et al. 1994). This work is in the very early stages and caution should be exercised in interpreting results.

While there is much still to be learned about the genetic characteristics of dyslexia, it does seem clear at this time that it can be inherited. Bruce Pennington, one of the principal researchers in the Colorado Reading Study, cites evidence that dyslexia is both *"familial* (about 35%-40% of first degree relatives are affected)," and *"heritable* (with a transmission rate of about 50%)" (Pennington 1991, p. 48).

SUMMARY OF CURRENT VIEWS OF DYSLEXIA

Much of the scientific evidence for the current definition of dyslexia comes from a series of NICHD-funded studies in the late 1980s and early 1990s. This funding encouraged clearer definitions of research populations, use of well-normed tests, and communication across disciplines. Major findings from this research and other research teams are incorporated into the history above and are summarized as follows.

Dyslexia is a Difficulty with Learning to Read and Spell Words

Individuals with dyslexia struggle inordinately with word reading. The definition of dyslexia from the NICHD and the IDA describes, "difficulties with accurate and/or fluent word recognition and . . . poor spelling and decoding abilities."

Dyslexia Involves Deficits in Phonological Processing

Phonemic awareness, rapid, automatic naming, and verbal short-term memory tend to be areas of deficit in individuals with dyslexia. This makes it very difficult to learn to read words. Direct and systematic instruction in phonemic awareness and phonics helps children with dyslexia make progress in word reading. The NICHD definition states, "These difficulties typically result from a deficit in the phonological component of language that is often unexpected in relation to other cognitive abilities and the provision of effective classroom instruction."

Dyslexia is Genetic

Dyslexia tends to run in families. Family members of individuals with dyslexia have roughly a 50% chance of being dyslexic. Being the child or sibling of an individual with dyslexia places one at risk.

Dyslexia is Not Gender Specific

Girls are just as likely to be dyslexic as boys. More boys with reading disability are referred to special education than girls, but this may be because of behavior.

Dyslexia is Not a Developmental Lag

Dyslexia can be overcome to some degree through appropriate instruction, but it is not merely a developmental lag. Time will not take care of the deficit. The term *developmental dyslexia* means that the deficit is innate to the developing child and not the result of trauma such as head injury, which is called *acquired dyslexia*.

Dyslexia Involves Differences in Brain Functioning

Brain fMRI's look different for children and adults with dyslexia in comparison with typically developing readers. These differences show up in what is believed to be compensatory overuse of frontal areas of the brain that become more pronounced over time, and underuse of the back of the left hemisphere areas that are typically activated in good readers. Evidence from fMRI's helps to confirm the nature of dyslexia as organic rather than environmental.

Individuals with Dyslexia Can be Taught to Read

Despite the organic nature of dyslexia, there is evidence that appropriate reading instruction can make important contributions to improvement in reading outcomes for individuals with dyslexia, and that this instruction is more effective when it begins very early in the reading acquisition process. Lack of good instruction cannot cause dyslexia, but it can exacerbate the symptoms. Good instruction can ameliorate or overcome the symptoms.

ACADEMIC MANIFESTATION OF DYSLEXIA

Dyslexia is generally perceived first and foremost as a word-reading disorder. At the time of the first edition of this book there was fairly general agreement in the field that along with this word-reading level disorder there might be a wide range of other disorders including persistent difficulty in spelling, phonological processing, reading rate, comprehension, expressive writing, and handwriting. The picture has shifted toward primary deficits in phonologically driven word-level reading as the area of deficit in dyslexia as NICHD studies have provided better control in terms of careful description of the samples of children examined.

Oral Reading
Word Attack Skills

The most pronounced among the reading difficulties that individuals with dyslexia experience is the inability to decode unfamiliar words (e.g., Olson et al. 1985; Shaywitz 2003; Siegel 1985; Vellutino 1983). This problem appears to be the common denominator in all cases of dyslexia (Gough and Tunmer 1986). The basis for the decoding deficiencies among dyslexic readers is a deficit in phonological processing that affects ability to make use of letter-sound associations (i.e., phonics knowledge), possibly related to rapid retrieval problems. Deficits in understanding the sound structure of speech (phonological awareness) confound mastery of the relationship between sounds in speech and letters in words. In short, children with dyslexia have extraordinary difficulty in using word attack skills to read new words as well as trouble committing decoded words to memory. These children have trouble breaking down spoken words in order to identify their component parts when they spell, and in blending together these parts into words when they read. Sound sequencing errors (articulating letter sounds in the wrong order), as well as letter-sound confusions (producing the wrong sound for a given letter or letters), are often observed in their oral reading. Word attack skills have proven to be the most sensitive identifier of disabled readers (Read and Ruyter 1985; Richardson, DiBenedetto, and Adler 1982; Ryan, Miller, and Witt 1984; Siegel 1985).

Nonwords are widely used to measure ability to use word attack skills to read unfamiliar words. Studies documenting the nonword-reading deficit are often carried out through matching dyslexic and normal readers by word recognition level. The question here is, do the older dyslexics, matched on real-word reading level with younger normal readers, have more difficulty in reading nonwords? Maggie Snowling provided early documentation of the nonword reading deficit in a *reading-age-match* (RAM) comparison in which children were asked to respond to words using pairs of modalities (visual-visual, auditory-auditory, visual-auditory) and say whether the words were the same or not. Children with dyslexia were as competent as normal readers in making same-different judgments of pairs such as *torp* and *trop* in the visual-visual and auditory-auditory modes. Only when they needed to see one word in print and listen to the other did they have substantially more difficulty than normal readers (Snowling 1980).

In another often-cited study, Richard Olson and his colleagues made a similar comparison of 15-year-olds with dyslexia and 10-year-old normal readers. They were asked which of a pair of written words (e.g., *caik-dake*) sounded like a real word. The older readers were poorer than the younger normal readers, despite the match in real word reading level (Olson et al. 1985). In a more recent study with much larger numbers of students, including twin pairs from the Colorado Twin Study, this phonological coding deficit was confirmed, as was its heritability (Olson et al. 1989).

Word Recognition

If individuals with dyslexia are not facile at decoding unfamiliar words, how do they read? One argument is that they compensate using an area of strength to make up for their phonological weakness and that this strength involves visual memory for letter strings, which is considered an orthographic skill. Richard Olson tested this theory in an experiment using the same 15-year-old-dyslexic and 10-year-old-normal readers tested for phonological ability above. This time he asked them to choose between two phonologically similar written words, one real and the other its pseudohomophone (e.g., *street-streat*). The task here is essentially a proof reading task. Which word looks right? Here the two groups did not differ. Keep in mind, however, that the dyslexic children were five years older than the normal readers. These children's strength in orthography is a relative one in comparison with their weakness in phonological skills. Compared to typically developing readers of their own age, they read far fewer words (Olson et al. 1989).

Dyslexia is most evident when words are presented in isolation (Perfetti 1984; Stanovich 1980). This is logical because children with dyslexia are relatively strong in comprehension. Understanding a paragraph can help in understanding an unknown word. Once enough words have been learned to enable at least some degree of comprehension, then comprehension enables decoding of unfamiliar words.

Linnea Ehri has challenged the belief that there are dual routes to word reading, one using phonological processing and the other using an instant word-unit-to-meaning recognition (1992; Ehri and Saltmarsh 1995). She argues that letter-sound knowledge is used even in what is commonly called *sight word* reading, and that even the most irregular word has some phonetically regular letters. She has found evidence that beginning readers without phonemic deficits are better at learning new sight words than older readers with disabilities.

Reading Rate

Word recognition skills improve with remediation, and there is even evidence that word attack skills can be improved through intensive training in phonological awareness, but individuals with dyslexia continue to read more slowly than typically developing readers. That is, accuracy can be remediated more effectively than rate. Much of the recent research on reading rate has been carried out through the Colorado Reading Project in the laboratories of Richard Olson. He and his colleagues have found significant differences between dyslexic and normal readers in vocal response latencies—the time between presentation of a stimulus and a subject's response—when single words are presented on a computer screen.

Another way of looking at rate is to time entire passages of text. P. G. Aaron and Scott Phillips examined the academic skills of college students with dyslexia and found their reading comprehension scores to be well above these students' own scores for reading rate (Aaron and Phillips 1986).

SPELLING PROBLEMS

For individuals with dyslexia, spelling presents even greater challenges than reading. Although reading is remediable, sometimes to a high degree, spelling deficits appear to persist through adulthood (Aaron and Phillips 1986; Cone et al. 1985; Ganschow 1984; Rutter 1978).

Roderick Barron (1980) observed that poor readers are more likely to use a visual-orthographic strategy in reading and to apply a phonological strategy to spelling. Lynette Bradley and Peter Bryant find this same strategy differential in young normal readers (Bradley 1985; Bradley and Bryant 1979). They believe that the independence of reading and spelling behaviors is a natural developmental phenomenon; young children who have not yet learned to read often spell words on the basis of sound. Are children with dyslexia simply behind on a developmental continuum, or do they spell differently from children without dyslexia?

In analysis of the spelling errors of children who are dyslexic but have received intensive remediation, Mary Kibel and T. R. Miles found persistent difficulty with a type of errors not found in spelling-age matched controls. The errors involved both cluster reduction (e.g., spelling *blend* as "bend") and substitution of phonologically confusable pairs (e.g., *e/a*, *b/d*, *r/l*). An analysis by Louisa Moats produced similar evidence of cluster reductions and unstressed syllable reductions in the spelling errors of third and fifth grade children with dyslexia, again in comparison with spelling-age matched controls (Moats 1993). Maggie Bruck and Rebecca Treiman have also found consonant clusters to be particularly troublesome for spellers with dyslexia (Bruck and Treiman 1990). These studies are more sophisticated than earlier ones that attempted to categorize errors as either phonological or orthographic, in that highly specific phonological processing deficits are the focus here, rather than a wider array of phonetic errors.

The unanswered question here is why individuals with dyslexia appear better able to compensate for phonological processing deficits in reading than in spelling. If orthographic spelling develops over time through exposure to print, this should fall into place eventually, after remediation of reading. It may be that orthographic processing in spelling is particularly dependent on successful phonological processing and subsequent representations of the sound structure of words.

READING COMPREHENSION

Children with dyslexia have been found to be poorer at reading comprehension than good readers, which is consistent with Philip Gough and William Tunmer's *simple view of reading* (1986). If decoding is poor, even in the presence of well-developed listening comprehension, then reading comprehension will be poor. This is also consistent with Keith Stanovich's *Matthew effect* (1986b). Reading comprehension is a skill that needs development over time; it is difficult to practice comprehension if decoding is undeveloped.

Lack of reading accuracy and automatic recognition at the word level appear to place limitations on the comprehension of text, as well as on reading fluency (Stanovich, Cunningham, and Feeman 1984). David LaBerge and S. Jay Samuels (1974) attempted to explain this apparent trade off in attentional resources by hypothesizing a limited capacity mechanism in working memory. In the same vein, Charles Perfetti (1984, 1985b) proposes a verbal efficiency mechanism to account for the strong relationship between speed and accuracy of word identification and reading comprehension shown in correlational studies.

Tests of the *simple view of reading* indicate that reading comprehension cannot surpass its two components, word decoding and listening comprehension (Hoover 1994). However, this data comes from very large numbers of readers drawn from the general population of school children. In examining the relationship between decoding and comprehension in readers with dyslexia in the Colorado Twin Study, Richard Olson and his colleagues provide a different story. When children with dyslexia were matched with controls in regard to timed word recognition ability, their comprehension levels were significantly higher on several measures. Keep several things in mind. The match was on *timed* word reading. Had accuracy been the matching criterion, the match would have been with higher functioning controls. Also, the children with dyslexia were older and thus had an intellectual advantage.

Maggie Bruck reports data from a study of college-age students with dyslexia. Some of these subjects comprehended very well despite poor decoding skills. Bruck proposes the possibility of what she calls a "minimum threshold level" for word recognition, saying, "Once critical levels of word-recognition skill have been achieved, variation in comprehension levels may be best accounted for by higher level component processes" (Bruck 1990, p. 450). That is, bright individuals with dyslexia use their oral language strengths (e.g., vocabulary, general knowledge, interpretation of context) to compensate for weak decoding skills.

LISTENING COMPREHENSION

Dyslexia is "characterized by difficulties with accurate and/or fluent word recognition and by poor spelling and decoding abilities" (NICHD/IDA 2002). According to this definition, listening comprehension should not be an area of deficit. As definitions of dyslexia have become more and more specific, and more driven by the NICHD's insistence on careful descriptions of research participants, listening comprehension presents as a skill that should be average to strong in individuals with dyslexia. However, there are a number of individual differences across the dyslexic population and evidence of listening problems for some of these individuals.

Keith Stanovich has been an advocate of limiting the term *dyslexia* to individuals with a discrepancy between listening and reading comprehension (Stanovich 1988a, 1988b), which makes it strictly a reading problem. However, one explanation of weak listening skills in older students with dyslexia is linked to his *Matthew effect*. Because of their general lack of reading experience some dyslexic individuals may fail to develop a strong vocabulary and knowledge base, which limits their ability to comprehend. This can be considered a second-order comprehension problem.

Maggie Bruck, on the other hand, has not found diminished levels of either listening comprehension or verbal IQ in adults with dyslexia (1990). Her data suggest a hierarchy of skills in both high- and average-IQ adults with dyslexia, in which low-level, phonologically driven skills such as nonsense-word reading are less developed than high-level skills such as reading and listening comprehension. Whether or not listening has been diminished by phonological processing deficits, there is agreement that decoding is poorer than reading comprehension, which, in turn, is poorer than oral language skills.

Hugh Catts (1989) calls dyslexia a language problem but limits it to those aspects of language that are phonological. Catts' model is consistent with that of Isabelle Liberman and her colleagues, who have led this line of research. Liberman maintained that as we read or listen we must hold incoming linguistic information in working memory in phonological form while we process sentences (e.g., Liberman and Shankweiler 1985; Mann, Shankweiler, and Smith 1984). Thus, the deficit that affects word reading could also affect listening. Support for this view can be found in a recent study carried out in Australia by Gail

Gillon and Barbara Dodd. They tested 8- to 10-year-old poor readers matched on reading level with younger good readers, using a number of measures of phonological processing as well as measures of syntax and semantics. While the poor readers were weaker than reading-age-match controls in all oral language areas, they were particularly poor in phonological processing (Gillon and Dodd 1994).

Athough the International Dyslexia Association adapted the phonologically oriented NICHD definition of dyslexia for research purposes in 1994, it continued to use a second, broader definition in order to be able to procure special dyslexia-oriented services for children with a range of more global deficits in expressive and receptive language. This is a common- sense approach in terms of thinking about remedial instruction. The treatment for word reading problems is the same, with or without listening problems, and if a child has vocabulary and comprehension issues as well, then these areas need extra instruction, too.

EXPRESSIVE WRITING PROBLEMS

When we consider the three potential areas of writing difficulties for individuals with dyslexia—composition, spelling, and handwriting (Cicci 1983)—spelling stands out as by far the most prevalent area of deficit (Ganschow 1984; Poplin et al. 1980). Other types of deficiencies can also be found in the writing samples of dyslexic students—for example, poor punctuation, word omissions, lack of subject/predicate number agreement, and lower percentages of compound and/or complex sentences—but there is little consistent documentation of their prevalence. In a study in which students with learning disabilities were asked to dictate stories to an examiner and then to write stories by hand or on a word processor, the dictated stories were significantly longer, of better quality, and contained fewer grammatical errors. These findings suggest that ". . . mechanical and conventional demands of producing text appear to interfere with the fluency and quality of written expression" (MacArthur and Graham 1988). It can be argued that deficits in spelling absorb so much energy and attention that all other aspects of writing are diminished in quality (Uhry and Shepherd 1993b). Perhaps the most serious writing problem among individuals who are dyslexic is a general resistance to writing. Diana King (1985), who works with adolescents, affirms that without remedial intervention this resistance tends to build throughout the school years.

OVERCOMING DYSLEXIA THROUGH INSTRUCTION

Historically, dyslexia has appeared to be pervasive throughout the lives of individuals. Frank Wood and his colleague Lynn Flowers have examined adults first diagnosed by neurologist Samuel Orton. It was after Samuel Orton that The Orton Dyslexia Society (now renamed the IDA) was named. Many of these individuals with dyslexia were tutored as children by Orton's wife, June Lyday Orton. Brain differences in regard to blood flow were found in these individuals as adults even in cases where reading had been successfully remediated during childhood (Flowers 1993; Wood 1993). When these same adults were examined for neuropsychological and academic residue of dyslexia, they were found to have deficits in nonword reading, phonological awareness and rapid automatized naming (Felton, Naylor, and Wood 1990). Of the three symptoms, rapid automatized naming seems to be the most pervasive and to determine the degree to which recovery from dyslexia is possible (Wood and Felton 1994). There is evidence, by contrast, that phonological awareness and nonword reading are remediable to some degree (e.g., Alexander et al. 1991; Kibel and Miles 1994; Shaywitz 2003; Shepherd and Uhry 1993; Uhry 1997; Uhry and Shepherd 1997; Wise et al. 1989). Put in terms of word reading, accuracy can be improved over time, but reading rate remains slow.

Recovery rate research has been hard to interpret because of inconsistent documentation of the characteristics of participants and instruction across studies. Are there some symptoms of dyslexia that are easier to remediate than others? Is it important to begin early? What instructional methods work best? Since the last edition of this book, several large-scale longitudinal treatment studies have been completed by research teams in Florida (Torgesen 1995) and Texas (Foorman, Francis, and Fletcher 1995). In addition, the National Reading Panel (2000) has carried out a meta-analysis of these and other treatment studies. Specific recommendations are included in the chapters in Parts II and III of this book.

No two individuals with dyslexia need exactly the same instruction. What we know from scientifically designed treatment studies is what works best for most children. Most of these programs have some features in common, but what is exactly right for a particular individual can only be determined through assessment of the individual's strengths and weaknesses in a number of areas. The following chapter presents a conceptual plan and practical suggestions for the educational assessment of individuals with dyslexia.

3

Assessment for Dyslexia

There is much overlap between the terms *assessment* and *evaluation* in an educational context. Both terms involve the gathering and interpretation of data for planning instruction and making other educational decisions about a student. I use the term *assessment* here to mean the general process of on-going inquiry, both formal and informal, used to answer questions—in this case, questions about an individual's struggle to learn. I use the term *educational evaluation* to characterize an event—the formal process of gathering information on background and on response to classroom instruction, formulating hypotheses, choosing and administering measures to test hypotheses, and writing up a report with a logical presentation of conclusions. In many ways the two terms refer to the same process, but assessment tends to be ongoing, whereas an educational evaluation takes place at a specific time and involves larger questions.

The IDA/NICHD definition of dyslexia (see Chapter 2) carries two important ideas. The first, as is the case with all learning disabilities, is a discrepancy between cognitive functioning and achievement. The second idea, which is specific to dyslexia, is the presence of a deficit in phonemic processing.

The traditional method of testing for any learning disability has been to compare IQ to academic achievement. In the case of dyslexia, the comparison would be between IQ and reading achievement. A number of highly respected researchers have pointed out that the discrepancy model is problematic for a number of reasons (e.g., Fletcher et al. 1998). First, there is little agreement about the discrepancy formula. Is the discrepancy valid if the two tests are not normed on the same population? How large should the discrepancy be? Can a straight comparison be used, or should discrepancy be defined by a regression formula that adjusts for the upper and lower ends of IQ? Using a straight comparison of standard scores, a 30-point discrepancy might qualify a child as dyslexic but with a reading score of 112 and an IQ of 137, does a child qualify for remedial reading services? What about a child with an IQ of 98 and a reading score of 86? Should this child need to wait until the discrepancy is larger to get help? In addition to these quandaries, there is little evidence that children classified as dyslexic have different reading profiles or different instructional needs than children with very low reading scores but without this discrepancy.

One alternative to the discrepancy model suggests that the presence of phonological processing deficits be used as a marker of reading disability and the need for intensive instruction in this area. Fletcher et al. (1998) point out that this model could entitle children to special services based on an early screening. In this model there is no need to wait until a child is reading several years below grade level. There is support for this model from other researchers. For example, Torgesen and Wagner suggest that diagnosis should be based on "specific linguistic-cognitive markers." In their model, early assessment in phonological awareness, verbal short-term memory, and rapid automatic naming would identify those children who will benefit from early, direct, and intensive instructive in phonological processing (Torgesen and Wagner 1998). As Torgesen points out,

> Children who are delayed in the development of phonemic awareness have a very difficult time making sense out of "phonics" instruction, and they certainly have little chance to notice the phonemic patterns in written words on their own (Torgesen 2002).

This is true for children with IQ-reading discrepancies and those without this discrepancy. For both groups of children, it is the phonological core deficit that prevents successful response to instruction, and appropriate instruction is effective for both.

Another diagnostic alternative to the discrepancy model involves a student's response to instruction. Douglas and Lynn Fuchs suggest a model in which the diagnosis of learning disability is reconceptualized. In this model, the need for special services is established through documentation of failure to progress in reading in a situation in which other children are learning well. They point out that when an entire class or school is failing to thrive, then the system needs changing, but that when a child is struggling in the presence of instruction that seems appropriate for others, then that child needs additional educational services (Fuchs and Fuchs 1998; Fuchs 2003).

This chapter provides information about both informal and formal steps in assessment for dyslexia in terms of both early screening and later evaluation. It also presents several case studies of the assessment of struggling readers in light of the models outlined here.

STEPS IN ASSESSMENT FOR DYSLEXIA

The following guidelines for assessing children who may be dyslexic draw on three sources of knowledge. The first is research. During the 1990s substantial federal funding culminated in clearer descriptions of dyslexia. Many of the references in this chapter are taken from the record of an April 1992 National Institute of Child Health and Human Development (NICHD) conference on learning disabilities assessment organized and later edited into a book by Reid Lyon (1994). The second source involves practical experience at the Teachers College Columbia University Child Study Center[3] during the five years that I taught teachers how to carry out educational evaluations. We worked with children referred because of struggles with reading that had not been resolved by their schools. The third source is a series of case studies written by my Fordham students in the Ennis William Cosby Graduate Certificate Program. These classroom teachers are committed to using assessment in planning instruction and as an effort to insure that at least most children will not need to be referred out of their classrooms for special help.

SCREENING FOR EARLY IDENTIFICATION AND INTERVENTION

In the best of all possible worlds, all teachers would screen for dyslexia early in the kindergarten year, and continue with informal assessment during this year to keep track of all children's response to instruction. Research tells us that the best kindergarten predictors of later word-level reading are letter name knowledge and phonemic awareness (Wagner and Torgesen 1987). Thus early screening can double as assessment for classroom planning.

---

[3]The Child Study Center was a site within the Department of Special Education at Teachers College Columbia University designed for the practical training of graduate students in the diagnosis and remediation of children with special needs. The first author served as Director for five years. The pronoun we, used throughout this chapter, refers to the group of faculty, clinicians, and students who collaborated at the Child Study Center during the early 1990s on what we called *the dyslexia project*. This was an exploration of the clinical description of dyslexia and of effective strategies for its remediation (Shepherd and Uhry 1993; Uhry 1997; Uhry and Shepherd 1997). Notes on the assessment of KM come from several formal evaluations conducted by Margaret Jo Shepherd and from notes from her tutors and her school, and from ongoing, research-based assessment by Joanna Uhry.

One informal assessment that is useful to kindergarten teachers is a survey of letter name recognition. This pinpoints instruction and can be updated every few months. Another informal, curriculum-based observation involves invented spellings. Invented spelling requires both letter knowledge and phonemic awareness. Can the child stretch out words and represent the initial sound with a written letter? By the end of kindergarten, typically developing readers can usually spell the beginnings and ends of words in their stories or on a short list of words. Children come to kindergarten with a range of skills. It is progress that we are looking for here. Children who come to school without ability to write any letters for sounds in words, but make good progress, will most likely be able to benefit from first grade reading instruction as well. Children who struggle to learn letters and still cannot stretch out words after kindergarten instruction in phonemic awareness may be dyslexic.

More systematic but still relatively informal assessment could involve Darrell Morris's invented spelling test (1999). This 12-word, dictated list can be used with a whole class of children every few months. The test is developmentally scored and the words are chosen to reveal specific linguistic patterns over time. Invented spelling has been shown to be an excellent predictor of later reading skills (e.g., Morris and Perney 1984). Two other tests assess ability to blend, and ability to segment and manipulate phonemes. The Roswell-Chall Auditory Blending Test (Chall, Roswell, and Blumenthal 1963; Roswell and Chall 1997) involves saying phonemes and asking the child to blend them (e.g., /u/-/p/, /b/-/oat/,/s/-/a/-/d/). Jerome Rosner's (1974, 1975, 1999) *deletion* or *elision* task asks children to listen to words and then repeat them with phonemes removed (e.g., Say *meat* without the /m/). It tests a child's concept of the sound structure of spoken words. The blending and deletion tasks are purely auditory; letters are not used. In combination these three measures are enormously helpful in planning phonemic awareness instruction as an intervention for individuals or small groups.

Each of these measures takes around 10 minutes for a teacher to administer. Indications that a child is below age norms in invented spelling, blending, or segmenting indicates the probable usefulness of more direct small-group classroom work in these areas. There is evidence that by combining several of these tasks and looking at them together with early word recognition skills, in an instrument called the Early Reading Screening (Uhry 1993a), children at risk for dyslexia can be identified quite accurately in kindergarten. Tests of blending, invented spelling and phoneme manipulation are short and straightforward. A teacher who is skilled in pronouncing and hearing phonemes accurately can use these tests in the classroom. They are widely used in both diagnostic work and in research. This testing can confirm a teacher's hunch that phonological processing is an issue. Testing, together with careful observation, can help in fine-tuning instruction.

Intense and direct PA instruction from a skilled kindergarten or first grade teacher can make a world of difference to all children but especially to those with dyslexia. Many programs provide extra instruction for the lowest readers in a class. For example, see the section on *Fundations* in Chapter 14 This K-2 program can be used for a whole class and includes supplemental instruction for children needing extra help. If a teacher is still worried about lack of progress in the presence of direct and refined instruction, the next step is to involve the child's parents. They will most likely have ideas and want to play a role in shaping instruction. Many times, this process is reversed and it is a parent who first voices concerns to the teacher. Without suggesting a formal evaluation yet, consult with the school's reading or learning specialist and collaborate on a more intensive classroom intervention. Ask the specialist to observe and make suggestions.

If, after ongoing informal assessment and intensive classroom instruction, the child does not seem to be making progress, a more formal screening should be carried out. Wagner, Torgesen, and Rashotte's Comprehensive Test of Phonological Processing (CTOPP; 1999) is a standardized test of phonological processing skills with several subtests: (a) Elision, (b) Rapid Color Naming, (c) Blending Words, (d) Sound Matching, (e) Rapid Object Naming, (f) Memory for Digits, and (g) Nonword Repetition. Standard scores are provided for each subtest, and for three composite scores: Phonological Awareness, Phonological Memory, and Rapid Naming. This test is usually administered by a professional with more time and standardized testing expertise than a classroom teacher has.

Early identification and intervention works. This is confirmed by large scale, longitudinal studies reported by the National Reading Panel (2000; Ehri et al. 2001). Many local school districts construct their own version of early identification and intervention. Hyla Rubin has worked with a Connecticut school district to screen kindergarten children using invented spellings. In a controlled study, 478 kindergarten children were trained in a three-part sequence: (a) rhyme and syllable analysis, (b) analysis of spoken words into phonemes, and (c) transfer activities such as invented spelling. By the end of the kindergarten year, children performing at the mean for this group could represent all sounds (e.g., medial vowels as well as initial and final consonants) in invented spellings. Performance on all tasks was significantly better than controls. The finding of greatest importance to this discussion is that referrals to special first grade instruction were substantially reduced in comparison to earlier years (Rubin and Eberhardt 1996). This study is not unique. Early screening followed by intervention can reduce the severity of dyslexia and increase potential for successful reading. Not all children are lucky enough to be in schools that provide early screening and intervention. Unfortunately, many children are not assessed and do not receive appropriate instruction until after they have failed to read.

CLASSROOM ASSESSMENT AND INTERVENTION

Where assessment used to begin with a teacher's passing along a reading concern to a specialist (e.g., a child not keeping up with group instruction), today's teachers have much more research-based instructional and assessment knowledge available to them to use in the classroom. Assessment should begin in the classroom with ongoing, day-to-day informal curriculum-based assessment for all children. Kenneth and Yetta Goodman call this "kid watching." In a book called *Fragile Evidence* that criticizes the use of standardized tests in the assessment of reading, Jane Hansen states, "Evaluation is all day, noticing what is happening," (1998, p. 105). While I think the book overstates its case, I do agree that classroom observation is the best place to start assessment and should be used in planning programs for all readers including those who are struggling.

Classroom assessment should focus on response to the curriculum, with an eye toward immediate small adjustments to instruction. Can the student read words and books that others at this grade level can read? If not, at what level can the student experience success? What strategies does the student use to read unfamiliar words? What strategies might be taught next? As with younger children, spellings provide a rich source of data. Can the student segment sounds in order to represent them with letters? If not, does more direct instruction in segmenting help? Does the student know what letters go with those sounds? If not, teach the letter sounds directly and systematically, little by little, with much review to automaticity. Do spellings capture a sense of the sound structure of words even if they are not conventional? Can he understand what he reads? If not, teach comprehension strategies directly. Is comprehension better when the student listens? What about handwriting? Following careful analysis of these detailed curriculum-based observational notes and adjustments to instruction, teachers should continue assessing and adjusting instruction.

PREPARATION FOR FORMAL EVALUATION

Eventually, if short-term classroom interventions do not result in progress, either the teacher or parents may suggest that a formal evaluation for dyslexia be carried out by an educational evaluator with special reading expertise, in consultation with a psychologist. The role of the psychologist is to provide IQ testing in order to explore cognitive functioning, as well as personality testing, which can provide insight into emotional issues that might be factors in school difficulty. This can take place in a school setting or with an outside team. Although many researchers find fault with the discrepancy model of assessment, it is still common practice and is still usually necessary as a venue for qualifying for special services.

The purpose for the evaluation should be clarified at the onset. Is the purpose to come up with a remedial plan including teaching materials and methods? Is classification for special school services the goal? Is a new school or tutor the issue? Will an older student want to use the evaluation report to qualify for untimed school tests or college entry exams? Does the student wish to be exempt from studying a second language? Both family and student should have a voice concerning the purpose of the evaluation and should understand possible benefits. Both should be involved in feedback sessions.

A formal educational evaluation should begin with a thorough family history of possible reading difficulty. The Colorado Twin Study indicates that dyslexia is familial (DeFries et al. 1991; Olson et al. 1989; Olson et al. 1990). Another question is whether there have been prolonged school absences during critical periods in learning to read. What reading methods are used in school? Weakness in phonics can be exacerbated by lack of instruction. Virginia Berninger and Robert Abbott make the point that we ought to be looking at failure to respond to appropriate instruction over time as an indicator of disability (Berninger and Abbott 1994).

The actual process of testing for dyslexia can be conceptualized as having three phases. Results from the first establish a diagnosis of dyslexia using a discrepancy model, often a necessary step for services. The second phase provides a second source of evidence to confirm this diagnosis through checking for the phonological processing deficits often associated with dyslexia[4]. The third provides an inventory of which reading and writing skills and strategies are solid and which ones remain to be taught. This third step provides a baseline for later measurement of progress, and serves as a guide in planning intervention or remediation. In reading the following, keep in mind that it is a framework for testing many possible hypotheses. All of the following would be too much for any one child.

---

[4]Results from large-scale longitudinal NICHD studies in the 1990s indicate that instruction including direct instruction in phonics and phonological awareness is effective for children both with and without dyslexia. This evaluation phase should be carried out for struggling readers even without a finding of discrepancy scores.

PHASE I: EVALUATION FOR DISCREPANCIES

The objective of a discrepancy phase is to establish that the individual's reading is weak in the presence of other academic or cognitive strengths. This involves the use of standardized test scores to establish average or higher IQ (i.e., an IQ above 85) and a discrepancy between word-reading and other verbal abilities. The discrepancy model is built on an assumption of the word-reading difficulty being specific, rather than symptomatic of more far-reaching difficulties. Each of the following ways of testing for discrepancy is based on the hypothesis of phonological processing difficulties that cause word reading and spelling to be weaker than expected, given an individual's relative strengths or even gifts in other areas of academic or cognitive development. Use of assessment for phonological processing is not necessarily part of school-based assessment.

IQ/READING COMPREHENSION DISCREPANCY

The Reading Comprehension subtest from the Wechsler Individual Achievement Tests[5] (WIAT; Wechsler 1992) provides an ideal way to look for a discrepancy because the WIAT is normed on the same population sample as the Wechsler Intelligence Scales for Children (WISC-III; Wechsler 1991[6]). The WIAT manual provides tables of score differences that can be considered significantly discrepant. Linda Siegel (1989) made the point that the relationship between achievement and IQ is most likely bidirectional and others since then have concurred. That is, once children reach the middle elementary grades, IQ is dependent on vocabulary and background information acquired in reading. In support of this point, in our clinical practice we have seen IQ's fall over time when children are not reading. With older, reading-deprived and thus vocabulary- and knowledge-deprived children, an experienced clinician needs to weigh data from a number of tests to make a diagnosis.

LISTENING COMPREHENSION/READING COMPREHENSION DISCREPANCY

Keith Stanovich (1991) suggests comparing listening comprehension and reading comprehension to avoid the use of IQ tests. It is important to choose two tests from the same battery; the two tests are thus normed on the same sample. It is common practice in reading assessment to compare comprehension of a passage a child reads aloud

---

[5]A newer edition, the WIAT-II, was published in 2002.
[6]The WISC-IV was published in 2003.

with comprehension of a parallel passage read to the child by the examiner. Keep in mind that any conclusion needs to consider idiosyncratic background knowledge; does this child really understand better when he listens or does he just know a lot more about baseball than about the topic of the parallel passage he read himself? In contrast, scores on standardized tests tend to reflect performance over a number of passages. Use of the WIAT, for example, provides a standardized comparison between multiple reading passages and multiple listening passages. The listening versus reading comprehension comparison, interpreted in the light of Philip Gough's simple view of reading (Gough and Tunmer 1986), implies a deficit in word reading in the child who understands spoken text better than text she must read herself.

Word reading should also be a focus in exploring discrepancies. By definition, dyslexia involves weak reading at the word level. A number of contrasts provide support for this hypothesis, and may help to qualify a child for special services in cases where the IQ-reading discrepancy is not large enough.

STRONG LISTENING OR READING COMPREHENSION WITH WEAK WORD READING

This is a discrepancy that will be apparent to parents and teachers as well as to a trained evaluator. It will seem surprising that a child who is bright and responsive while listening to books has so much trouble learning words. Use of the word reading and listening comprehension subtests from the same battery can confirm what parents and teachers already know. Keep in mind that listening is always stronger than word reading in six-year-olds; many more words can be understood than can be read. What is being compared here are standardized scores. Compared to the six-year-olds in a norming sample of hundreds of six-year-old students a child with dyslexia might have a standard score of 107 on listening and a standard score of 82 on word reading.

Another way to look for dyslexia involves looking at discrepancies between decoding and comprehension. In our clinical practice, we have worked with older, remediated children with dyslexia who can comprehend at reading levels close to those commensurate with age, IQ, listening ability, and school experiences, but who continue to decode somewhat inaccurately and extremely slowly. While this is counter-intuitive, given Gough and Tunmer's *simple view of reading*, in some individuals who are very bright, compensatory mechanisms allow the acquisition of a large enough sight vocabulary to comprehend beyond what might be expected. A discrepancy here makes a powerful argument for a specific decoding disorder. Keep in mind that even though a bright child may have acquired a near-adequate sight vocabulary through this compensation, more appropriate instruction will make this process easier in the future, leaving more processing space for even stronger comprehension.

ACCURACY VERSUS RATE

This contrast is complicated because both can be weak in children with dyslexia. Word reading accuracy is associated with phonemic awareness and letter-sound knowledge, which support the development of sounding out and eventually, of sight word acquisition. Accuracy can improve dramatically in response to good instruction (see Chapters 5 and 6 on Phonemic Awareness and Phonics Instruction). Word-reading rate is typically predicted by early rapid serial letter naming rate. Rate is dependent on accuracy, but also on automaticity. Rate is harder to remediate than accuracy (see Chapter 8). Although phonemic awareness and reading accuracy can be remediated to some degree, individuals with dyslexia rarely become rapid readers.

Word lists for measuring word reading accuracy are plentiful. Some lists are grade specific, such as those supplied in informal reading inventories. Others are what we call "basal-ceiling tests[7]," which are long lists of words progressing in difficulty from kindergarten to adult levels, with standardized scores provided for whatever portion of the list is read accurately. Note that the number of words provided on these K through 12 basal-ceiling tests varies a great deal from test to test. There are 44 words listed on the Woodcock-Johnson Tests of Achievement (Woodcock and Mather 1989b), 55 on the WIAT, 66 on the Peabody Individual Achievement Test (PIAT-R; Markwardt 1989), and 106 on the Woodcock Reading Mastery Test (WRMT-R; Woodcock 1987). The higher the number of items, the more reliable a test will be; a single missed word has more influence on the total score if there are not many items at the child's reading level, and this diminishes the reliability of the results.

Word reading rate for words in lists can be measured using Joseph Torgesen's standardized *Test of Word Reading Efficiency* (TOWRE; Torgesen, Wagner, and Rashotte 1999). The Sight Word Efficiency subtest includes a progressively more difficult word list that a student is asked to read as quickly as possible, skipping unfamiliar words, for a score of how many words can be read accurately in 45 seconds. A sec-

---

[7] These tests have three hypothetical sections for every reader. Words in the middle section comprise the test and credit is given for all of these words that are read correctly. Credit is also given for "too easy" words that appear before a *basal* of roughly 5-6 correct words in a row, because it is assumed that these words can be read. No credit is given beyond the *ceiling* of roughly 5-6 missed words in a row, because it is assumed that these words cannot be read. The norming for basal-ceiling tests must be extensive in order to make statistical assumptions like these.

ond subtest, Phonetic Decoding Efficiency, is similar in format but uses nonwords. The TOWRE tests both accuracy and fluency and is quick and easy to administer. The Gray Oral Reading Test (GORT-4; Wiederholt and Bryant 2001) is structured like an informal reading inventory, with graded oral reading passages and comprehension questions. However, it provides standardized scores for word reading accuracy and rate, as well as for comprehension.

CONTEXTUALIZED VERSUS DECONTEXTUALIZED WORD READING

Readers with dyslexia are more reliant on context than proficient readers, who tend to use letters efficiently to get at words. This does not mean that strong readers do not use context; their reading is so automatic that they use context to comprehend. Young readers with dyslexia continue using pictures, their own experiences, and the context of the story to predict unknown words and even whole stories, much as preschoolers do during "pretend" reading. While all cue systems are important in reading, children with dyslexia tend to underutilize letters and over-rely on other sources of story information. As is the case with many beginning readers, older individuals with dyslexia often can read words in books that they cannot read in lists. Their standardized scores on reading words in passages (e.g., GORT) tend to be higher than their scores on reading words in lists (e.g., Word Identification subtest of the WRMT). Use of word-list tests does not suggest that children should be counting on letters alone when they read, but it does give us useful information about their progress with sounding out. It is, after all, weakness in phonological processing (i.e., phonetic decoding) that is the earmark of dyslexia.

REAL VERSUS NONWORD[8] READING

Another method of measuring discrepantly weak sounding-out strategies involves the use of nonwords. To read a nonword is to use phonics skill to sound out an unfamiliar word, either letter-sound by letter-sound (e.g., by blending /f/-/a/-/m/ into *fam*) or through analogy to a known word (e.g., *fam* is like *am*). Critics of this sort of testing protest the high degree of decontextualization, but it can be argued that many, many non-words are syllables in real words (e.g., *fam* in *family*, *lan* in *Atlantic*). One good test of nonword reading is the Word Attack (WA) subtest of the WRMT, with its Word Identification (WId) subtest providing the contrast. We used to think that individuals

---

[8]Note that *nonwords* are also called *nonsense words* or *pseudowords* in the literature. They are constructed of phonetically regular combinations of sounds and letters but are not real words, e.g., *zim, clab, firtual.*

with dyslexia maintained a discrepancy (i.e., WId > WA) into adulthood, but current thinking, supported by research, indicates that effective phonics-based instruction can remediate a nonword or new-word reading problem (e.g., Alexander et al. 1991; Uhry and Shepherd 1997). However, as with real-word reading, rate of nonword reading is apt to be affected by dyslexia, particularly in individuals who also have slow serial naming skills (i.e., the "double deficit"). Torgesen's *Test of Word Reading Efficiency* provides lists of words to be read in a minute (see above) and, in addition, nonwords to be read in a minute, providing an opportunity to compare real-word versus nonword reading rate.

DISCREPANCIES ACROSS DOMAINS

Spelling tends to be poor in young children with dyslexia, and to remain poor even after decoding improves. Louisa Moats (1994a) suggests choosing a spelling measure that has high reliability and that samples a broad domain of orthographic and morphological patterns. By contrast, Patricia Lindamood (1994) advocates looking at spelling without using letters at all, through the use of her Lindamood Auditory Conceptualization Test (LAC; Lindamood and Lindamood 2004). In our clinic, we used the WIAT Spelling test for three reasons. First, it has a balance of word types (phonetically regular words, high frequency words which are less regular, and words that are homonyms). Second, it is reliable, and third, spelling can be compared with word reading, reading comprehension, and listening comprehension on the same measure. It makes sense to use the LAC as a follow up to a weak spelling score but not instead of a spelling test.

A discrepancy between reading and math can also be used to support the hypothesis of a specific rather than general learning disability. Some children with dyslexia are strong in math and weak in reading, and some are even strong in math concepts, but weak in computation. Lack of automaticity in retrieval can cause difficulties in both decoding and in computation. Batteries such as the WIAT, the PIAT-R, or the Kaufman Test of Educational Achievement provide an opportunity for some or all of these comparisons. Keep in mind that a comparison must use tests normed on the same sample, and that each test or subtest needs to have high reliability, preferably close to .90 or higher (Hill 1981; Jensen 1980).

In interpreting these comparisons, the important thing to remember, as in all uses of standardized scores, is that we should be looking for multiple sources of information. Just as a single score never tells the complete story, we need to look beyond a single discrepancy. Once standardized testing of some of the above discrepancies has been completed, it is helpful to arrange the scores into a pattern. We developed the following model from our clinical work with children

> spelling / nonsense word reading
> < decoding words in lists
> < decoding words in text
> < reading comprehension
> < listening comprehension / IQ

with dyslexia. It is consistent with findings from the Colorado Twin Study and with Maggie Bruck's (1990) work with adults who had been diagnosed with childhood dyslexia. The pattern seems to hold for most of the older dyslexic children we have seen in our clinical work, particularly those who have had good remediation. Although not every adjacent difference is statistically significant, the pattern of hierarchical differences appears to hold.

PHASE II: EVALUATION OF PHONOLOGICAL PROCESSING

Three specific phonological deficits are considered markers of dyslexia: (a) rapid automatized or serial naming, (b) verbal short-term memory, and (c) phonemic awareness deficits. Rapid naming is also called "retrieval of phonological codes," and verbal short-term memory is also called "phonological coding in working memory" (Wagner et al. 1993; Wagner and Torgesen 1987). There is evidence in the literature that all three are related to dyslexia, and that each can be present in the absence of the other two (e.g., Wood and Felton 1994). The next phase of testing looks at each of the three.

RAPID SERIAL NAMING

Rapid Serial Naming can predict later dysfluency. It is usually tested using a procedure developed by Martha Denckla and Rita Rudel (1976b). On their Rapid Automatized Naming Test (RAN) children are asked to name five colors (and then numbers, pictured objects, and letters) presented over and over in random order on a 50-item matrix. Scores are presented in regard to time rather than accuracy. Each subtest has age norms in seconds so that a clinician can see how quickly a child retrieves names in comparison with age peers. Evidence of slow retrieval by itself does not mean, necessarily, that a child is dyslexic. This information needs to be used as part of a collection of evidence.

In our clinical practice, we find that being at least one, and usually two, standard deviations slower than peers on more than one RAN subtest is common for children with severe and enduring difficulty in acquiring speed in decoding. The RAN is not commercially available, but a well-normed rapid naming test with standardized scores is now available as part of a battery described below (CTOPP; Wagner, Torgesen, and Rashotte 1999).

VERBAL SHORT-TERM MEMORY

There is less agreement about the optimal way to measure verbal short-term memory. The Digit Span test from the Wechsler Intelligence Scales for Children (WISC-IV) is a measure of recall of digits repeated by a child in both foreword and backward order. The advantage here is that this subtest can be viewed as part of an overall picture of language strengths and weaknesses on the Verbal Scale of the WISC-IV. Another approach is to compare memory for rote material (e.g., lists of unrelated words) to memory for meaningful material (e.g., words in sentences). To do this, standard scores from the Word Sequences and Sentence Imitation subtests of the Detroit Tests of Learning Aptitude (DTLA-4; Hammill 1998) can be compared. Again, this information cannot be used alone to make a diagnosis of dyslexia, but should be presented as part of a pattern of evidence.

PHONEMIC AWARENESS

There are a number of different ways to measure phonemic awareness. Richard Wagner points out that several factors increase the difficulty of phonemic awareness tests and should be taken into consideration when choosing a measure to administer (Wagner et al. 2003). One is the linguistic complexity of the words that make up these tests. For example, it is harder to segment the word *hand* than the word *cast* because the nasal sound after *a* in *hand* makes it hard to pull the /a/ away from the /n/. Another factor is the structure of the task. In a developmental sequence by Marilyn Adams (1990), these measures are leveled by structure to include rhyming, sound sorting (*guinea pig, goat, girl*, but not *hamster; pet, sat, mitt*, but not *hop*), segmenting of onsets (*guinea pig* = /g/-/uinea pig), blending (/g/-/oa/-/t/ = *goat*), full segmentation (*goat* = /g/-/oa/-/t/) and phoneme manipulation ("Say 'smack' without the /m/). Wagner also points out that tasks requiring both memory and an operation such as segmenting are far more complex than tasks without a heavy memory load. Most of these tasks are correlated with each other (Stanovich, Cunningham, and Cramer 1984). Several good measures developed in the 1960s and 1970s are still in use. The Roswell-Chall Auditory Blending Test (1997) has held up very well in terms of reliability according to a 1988 study by Hallie Yopp. Results from this test are presented in terms of whether or not children blend well enough to handle word reading tasks at each grade, 1 through 5.

Jerome Rosner's Test of Auditory Analysis Skills (1974, 1975) was published in a revised version as the Phonological Awareness Skills Program (PASP; 1999) test, with age equivalent norms for ages 4 to 10. Children are asked to delete syllables from words, then to delete initial, final, and medial consonants (e.g., "Say *roast*. Now say it again but don't say /s/"). Note that this complex manipulation task involves conceptualizing the location of the phonemes, deleting one, and then blending the others into a new word. The task assumes facility with consonant clusters, which are complex and difficult units for poor readers (Bruck and Treiman 1990). In our clinical practice, we have found that children who cannot manage these items inevitably have difficulty reading words with consonant clusters and usually benefit from training in consonant cluster *word changes* activities (Elkonin 1963, 1973), which are described in Chapter 5. At even more complex levels, children are asked to substitute medial sounds (*dash* to *dish*; *stake* to *snake*), and finally, to think in sound analogies (*faint* is to *fate* as *band* is to . . .).

Charles and Patricia Lindamood's Auditory Conceptualization Test, now in its third edition (LAC; 2004), requires more training to administer. Designed in a sequence ranging from young children to adults, at its most complex it leads the student through a series of sound changes with small colored blocks representing the sounds. For some adults, as Patricia Lindamood points out, their own phonemic awareness (PA) is challenged by tasks such as asking a child, "If that says *ap*, show me *pa* (e.g., change yellow-blue to blue-yellow).

Several PA measures were developed by researchers during the 1990s and early 2000s. Researcher Joseph Torgesen and his Florida colleagues have made major contributions in this area by publishing tests developed as research measures of PA growth for their longitudinal training grant from the National Institute of Child Health and Human development (NICHD). The Test of Phonological Awareness (TOPA; 1994b) is a screening test that measures the ability of children in grades K to 2 to match pictures of words by initial or final sound. More recently, Wagner, Torgesen, and Rashotte's Comprehensive Test of Phonological Processing (CTOPP; 1999) has provided a comprehensive collection of phonological processing tests, supported by extensive research and normed on 1,656 individuals. There are two versions of the test, one for ages 5 to 6 and another for ages 7 to 24. They draw from the same pool of subtests with seven subtests for younger children (i.e., Elision, Rapid Color Naming, Blending Words, Sound Matching,

Rapid Object Naming, Memory for Digits, and Nonword Repetition.) For older children and young adults there are six subtests in the standard battery (i.e., Elision, Blending Words, Memory for Digits, Rapid Digit Naming, Nonword Repetition, and Rapid Letter Naming) as well as norms for older individuals administered the tests designed for young children. Results are presented in standard scores for subtests as well as subtest composites (i.e., Phonological Awareness, Phonological Memory, and Rapid Naming). This battery is complex to administer and score and is best administered by evaluation specialists. Its advantage is that where blending, segmenting, sound manipulation, rapid serial naming, and digit memory have formerly been administered using multiple measures, it is now possible to use a single instrument with subtests normed on the same individuals. Only in these circumstances is it possible to say that a child is strong in one form of phonological processing and significantly weaker in another.

Keep in mind that none of these tasks should be used as the only measure in making instructional decisions and that while children with dyslexia typically demonstrate weak phonemic awareness, not all children with weak phonemic awareness are dyslexic. Be sure to use multiple sources of information about discrepancies and phonological processing in making a diagnosis of dyslexia. Keep in mind, too, that dyslexia is not an either/or syndrome. Using a medical analogy, dyslexia is more like high blood pressure than pregnancy. It can be mild or severe. Like mild high blood pressure, mild dyslexia responds well to a treatment plan and should not be ignored. And of course, severe dyslexia can have devastating consequences if left untreated.

PHASE III: INVENTORY OF STRENGTHS AND WEAKNESSES, AND PLANNING FOR INSTRUCTION

Phase three of an evaluation should be carried out in preparation for instruction and as a baseline for measuring progress. This phase is similar to what good teachers do in the classroom and involves an inventory of strengths and weaknesses in regard to skills and strategies. It involves generating lists of mastered material and lists of what needs to be taught next. Careful observation of oral decoding in connected text is crucial. We often videotape reading episodes for careful analysis of strategies. We always try to listen to a child read a familiar book from home or school. We also use a set of graded reading passages such as the Analytical Reading Inventory (ARI; Woods and Moe 2002) or the Qualitative Reading Inventory (QRI; Leslie and Caldwell 2001) to establish both independent and instructional reading levels, and to note strategies through miscues. Observations can tell us whether the child is using a full range of cue systems (e.g., letters, pictures, contextual meaning, and prior information) and whether these systems are being used in isolation or in an integrated manner. Trial teaching using both phonetically controlled text and trade books can be useful in planning instruction.

Some practitioners use published tests to construct a record of which letter names, letter sounds, and sight words have been mastered by a child. Marie Clay's *Observation Survey* provides a helpful structure for working with younger children. Measures such as the Brigance Diagnostic Inventories (Brigance 1977, 1991) or Florence Roswell and Jeanne Chall's Diagnostic Assessment of Reading (DAR; Roswell and Chall 1992) provide procedures for collecting this data. The DAR has a particularly well-constructed sequence of word types. However, the same information can be garnered by an experienced clinician through observations of miscues in text.

Analysis of spelling errors, both from test lists and from a writing sample, provides insight about phonological awareness and phonics knowledge that is useful in planning remediation. It makes sense to follow a standardized spelling test such as the WIAT with the phonetically organized Spellmaster lists (Greenbaum 1987) in order to inventory basic letter-sound patterns. As outlined in the Screening section above, phoneme segmentation can be measured in the classroom using young children's invented spellings (Mann, Tobin, and Wilson 1987; Morris and Perney 1984). Morris's (1999, Morris et al. 2003) 12-word spelling list with its developmental scoring system is not normed, but provides a source of good descriptive information about linguistic development for kindergarten or first-grade children.

In looking at writing in the absence of a comprehensive model for standardized assessment of written expression, Hooper suggests an informal measure such as a writing sample administered with "think-alouds" involving a dialogue with the child as she works at getting ideas down on paper, and trial teaching structured to focus on the presenting problem (Hooper et al. 1994). This is a sensible and workable suggestion.

An effective evaluation should clarify the nature of a child's reading difficulty, but should also provide specific information for remediation. We like to end an evaluation with trial teaching, and we like to demonstrate possible methods and materials for parents and teacher/tutors as well. For example, we often administer a reading passage from an alternate form of an informal reading inventory at a student's instructional level, and ask the student to write a short essay under several conditions. We begin by asking the student to summarize the passage, and then we contrast this piece with a second one written with much more direct guidance. We ask the student whether any of the guided strategies we used were helpful, and if so, we include them in the educational plan.

During the first two phases of a formal evaluation it should be possible to diagnose dyslexia. If there are discrepancies in test scores with IQ or oral language significantly stronger than reading ability in the absence of other causes, we can say that a student has dyslexia or reading disorder at the word reading level. Use of phonological processing tests should confirm characteristic linguistic deficits. In the third step of the evaluation we have gathered information telling us where and how to begin instruction. To illustrate the above principles, we conclude this chapter with several case studies, the first carried out in a clinic and the others in schools.

CASE STUDY OF A FORMAL EDUCATIONAL EVALUATION: KM

This discrepancy-based evaluation was carried out over ten years ago. At the time we considered it a good example of theory and research put into practice. We still believe that the evaluation met the child's needs in terms of resulting in appropriate instruction and growth in reading (see Chapter 25).

BACKGROUND INFORMATION AND PSYCHOLOGICAL PROFILE

KM first came to the Child Study Center, a university clinic for evaluating and tutoring children with special needs, when her school suggested testing at the end of her first-grade year because of reading difficulty. Counter to our own advice earlier in this chapter, we did not begin with an initial consultation with a psychologist because her school supplied results from the Wechsler Preschool and Primary Scales of Intelligence (WPPSI-R; Wechsler 1989[9]). KM's IQ was reported to be in the superior range. Information provided in an initial family interview indicated that her father had experienced difficulty in reading as a child, and that her mother thought that she herself had had attention deficit disorder as a child. Her parents were divorced, which ordinarily would have presented the possibility of emotional issues interfering with the development of reading, but all sources reported an amicable relationship between the parents with successfully shared custody.

KM had attended kindergarten and first grade in an independent school with small classes and assistant teachers which meant that she had received a great deal of personal attention in an enriched and supportive atmosphere. She was first identified as being at risk for reading difficulty when her school administered a kindergarten screening (Uhry

---

[9] There is now a newer edition of this IQ test. The WPPSI-III was published in 2002.

1993a). Results indicated mild difficulty with phonological awareness (e.g., segmenting, blending, invented spelling), and with recognition of environmental print (e.g., names of classmates and other classroom words). Results from the Rapid Automatized Naming Test (RAN; Denckla and Rudel 1976a) indicated extraordinarily slow response time in naming letters. KM was not immediately referred for assessment, but her school did provide some small-group help during first grade. She had not been provided with systematic direct instruction in letter-sound associations because her school used a whole language approach to reading. A visit to observe KM's classroom convinced us that while lack of direct instruction may have exacerbated her difficulties, it was not the cause; many other children read quite well. KM's restless behavior during reading time suggested the possibility of attentional issues, but she was extremely well focused during math instruction. Her teacher considered her to be talented in math.

DISCREPANCIES

Because her family history, weak PA on a kindergarten screening, and failure to learn to read suggested the possibility that KM was dyslexic, we wished to look at possible discrepancy scores. We began the evaluation by asking her to read a word list from the Wechsler Individual Achievement Test (WIAT). Her standard score on this test was 81, which is a standard deviation below average (i.e., the average range is 85-115) and more than three standard deviations below her IQ score. Because word reading is so idiosyncratic during first grade, we administered a second test to see if she might score higher on a different set of words. A single standardized test should never determine diagnoses or important decisions. KM's standard score was 78 on the Word Identification test of the Woodcock Reading Mastery Test, with, again, a large discrepancy between reading and IQ. We realized that we were basing a judgment on just a few words in both cases. However, we had confirmation of her very poor reading from her school's end-of-year standardized testing where she scored in the 7th percentile (roughly a standard score of 78) on a group administered reading achievement test, and from the less formal reading assessment we administered using her own books (see below).

To confirm our sense that KM was dyslexic, we wanted to see if spelling and nonsense word reading were especially low. KM's Woodcock Word Attack (nonsense word) standard score was 61. The pattern here was consistent with a diagnosis of dyslexia, with nonsense word reading significantly lower than word reading, which, in turn, was significantly lower than IQ. KM's spelling was also low; she earned a standard score of 84 on the WIAT.

Because of possible attentional and emotional issues, it was important to establish reading as a specific rather than general academic discrepancy, so we wanted to see if reading and math were discrepant from each other. We like the Test of Early Mathematics Ability (TEMA-3; Ginsburg and Baroody 2003) for young children because it is interactive, uses manipulative materials, and includes follow-up probes for all items. Had KM's score not been so high we would have also administered the WIAT math tests to establish a discrepancy on tests normed on the same sample. With KM's score in the 99th percentile on the TEMA-2, this was not necessary; the discrepancy was clear. KM was quite talented in math and her disability was specific to reading.

PHONOLOGICAL PROCESSING
Phonemic Awareness

Because phonological processing deficits are associated with dyslexia, we expected this to be a weak area for KM. Weakness here, together with the above discrepancies, would have made a strong case for the hypothesis of dyslexia. We were surprised to find that KM's phonemic awareness skills were only moderately weak. She could blend phonemes into words on the Roswell-Chall Auditory Blending Test, scoring well above the first grade criterion level. On Rosner's Test of Auditory Analysis Skills she scored at the first grade level. She could delete many (but not all) initial and final consonant sounds from words. Keep in mind, though, that her school's kindergarten screening had indicated weakness in this area a year earlier. Her ability here was atypical. This relative strength in phonological awareness, together with our questions about ADD, made us question a diagnosis of dyslexia at this point.

Rapid Serial Naming

Our next finding, however, was consistent with a diagnosis of dyslexia. KM took an extraordinarily long time to complete serial naming tasks on the Rapid Automatized Naming Test (RAN). We knew from KM's school that she had done quite poorly at retrieving color names (the only subtest administered) when she took the RAN in connection with her school's kindergarten screening a year earlier. During our assessment KM scored in the average range on object naming, but was at least two standard deviations slower than age peers on each of the other subtests (colors, numbers, and letters). These results provided strong evidence that KM's reading difficulty was linked with slow retrieval rate. It explained the difficulty she had had in learning to say both letter names and letter sounds in kindergarten.

The discrepancies between reading and IQ, and between reading and math, as well as KM's extraordinarily slow retrieval rate pointed to a diagnosis of dyslexia, but we could not rule out ADD or emotional difficulties at this point.

INVENTORY OF STRENGTHS AND WEAKNESSES

Note that the following inventory is arranged into categories that ultimately became areas for remediation.

Letter knowledge

We began the final phase of the evaluation by taking an inventory of the letter sounds that KM knew. She could provide the appropriate sounds for almost all single consonants in isolation; exceptions were the sound of v and the soft sounds for *c* and *g*. She was less secure on vowel sounds; short *a* was her only consistent vowel. Her letter sound knowledge was about that of a child entering first grade. Even though KM knew most consonant sounds she was quite slow to respond, which was consistent with her slow naming speed on the RAN. This was an area in which we wanted to provide remediation; KM needed to learn short and long vowels and she needed to increase response time on consonant sounds.

Spelling

We asked KM to write a story for us and she wrote the following, accompanied by a drawing of a brightly patterned Easter egg:

> This agg is aestrtagg
> a vere gudagg

This story seemed minimal when we consider that KM was a highly verbal child who had spent her kindergarten and first grade years in classrooms where writing was a daily event and where many children were prolific writers. Story writing was particularly hard for KM; her isolated spellings on the WIAT were easier to decipher. Several phonetically regular words were spelled correctly and the relationship between spoken and written language is clearer in her WIAT errors (below) than in her story.

lok	for	*look*
pay	for	*play*
rit	for	*right*
adt	for	*eight*

Right from the beginning KM had an easier time spelling and reading words in isolation. She seemed overwhelmed when asked to use several strategies at once in connected text. As with reading, we felt that she would need practice on letter-sounds to the automatic level before writing became comfortable. Vowel errors and omissions of consonants from consonant clusters in her spellings told us where to begin instruction.

Oral Reading

KM read passages from the Diagnostic Reading Scales (DRS) in order for us to establish the level of appropriate text that should be used for her instruction in school and in tutoring. We have transcribed the primer or beginning first grade passage on the left with KM's reading on the right. We introduced the passage by saying, "This is a story about a girl named Mary who is on her way to school."

Mary was on her way to school.	Milli was on her way to school.
She came to the corner.	She could to the church.
She saw a red light.	She saw a red all.
Then she saw the green light.	Then her science saw, said . . . God! . . . all.
Then she went on to school.	Then she was on to school.

Her performance here indicated that she was not ready yet to read primer level text, and that she was not self-correcting when text made little sense.

Because we wanted to see how KM handled more predictable text, we used a book that she had brought with her from school. This was a picture book from New Zealand with just a few, often repeated, words on a page. KM had memorized the text and "read" it without looking at the words. At no point, even when we modeled this for her, did she *finger-point read*, or point at a word as she said it from memory. When she read incorrectly and we asked her to figure out another possible word, she looked around the room rather than at the printed word and became quite distracted. In fact, her attention span for any form of reading was short.

Probably the most striking thing about KM's reading was her failure to integrate appropriate reading strategies. Given unfamiliar text with little context, she used only letter cues and did not correct herself to make sense of what she had read. With familiar, predictable text, she used only prior knowledge of the content and failed to use letter cues at all to monitor herself. This dichotomy continued to characterize KM's reading for the first year of her remedial work with us. We hypothesized that retrieving letter sounds was so tedious for her that she had little energy to devote to other cue systems, and that if any other source of information was available, she used it instead.

UNANSWERED QUESTIONS

Diagnosing dyslexia is a complex process. KM's assessment left several questions unanswered. Her squirminess and short attention span during the evaluation (and during later tutoring) made us wonder if she had ADHD. Keep in mind that this was a suspected family pattern on her mother's side. We ended KM's evaluation report by stating that this was an unresolved issue and encouraged her family to follow up with a psychological evaluation.

When this was done during KM's second grade year, the psychologist confirmed KM's superior IQ score, stating that she was not especially low on those WISC-III subtests that are vulnerable to attentional issues. The psychologist concluded that KM's reading difficulty was not caused by ADHD or by issues related to the divorce. Her recommendation was for tutoring.

When we finished our evaluation, we were convinced that KM was dyslexic based on the large discrepancy between IQ and reading and on her difficulty with rapid retrieval. While we needed a psychologist's opinion to ascertain possible need for either therapy or medication for ADHD, we knew that in any event, KM would need intensive, alphabetically oriented, direct instruction in reading.

The final chapter of this book describes the process of planning a tutoring program for KM based on these evaluation findings, and on the principles and techniques for remediation outlined in the chapters that follow.

CASE STUDIES FROM CLASSROOM TEACHERS

The discrepancy model served KM well because the discrepancy between her IQ and reading achievement was so large. KM would have been diagnosed as having dyslexia using either the phonological-core-deficit model or the response-to instruction-model. Kindergarten screening revealed dramatically slow automatic naming and moderate weakness in phonemic awareness. By the end of first grade phonemic awareness was stronger, but she was still very slow at naming. KM struggled to read in a setting in which her classmates thrived. Meaning-based instruction worked for most, but was not explicit enough for her. She appeared to need direct instruction in phonics. These additional findings provided additional evidence to support a diagnosis that could have been made based on the discrepancy model alone. Not all children are as well served by this model.

FAILURE OF THE DISCREPANCY-BASED MODEL: JP

Following is a case study of a struggling reader taken from notes kept by his teacher. This story is an example of a child who was not served well by evaluation using the discrepancy model. Because he was held back a grade, and because his school district provided special services only once a child was two years behind grade expectations, JP struggled for three years before being provided with special services.

Background

JP was a student in Ms. Green's second grade in a public school in the Bronx in New York City. His school district is what New York State calls a "high-needs" district. The school is under-resourced and its families are economically disadvantaged. Although he grew up in New York, JP was born in Puerto Rico. He and many others in his school speak Spanish at home. JP was repeating second grade. Like many poor urban children in high-needs schools, JP struggles with reading.

Failure for children in these schools is not unexpected. To figure out the cause is complex. I do not know JP's early teachers, but I have heard kindergarten teachers say that teaching letter names is a "lost cause" if children speak a language other than English, and, "He needs to learn English first. Then I'll teach him about reading." I have heard first grade teachers of impoverished children say, "How can I teach them to read? Their parents don't even read to them at home." I have heard teachers say that holding a child back in the same grade a second year would provide "time to catch up." The research on repeating a grade by holding back is poor (e.g., Jimerson and Kaufman 2003). The psychological effect can be devastating and time, alone, has never taught a struggling reader to read. To hold a child back without changing the curriculum is to see apparent progress early in the year relative to year-younger children, but with a slower growth curve this advantage is almost always lost by the end of the repeated year. None of the above reactions to struggling readers (i.e., waiting until English is learned, blaming the parents, holding over) is helpful. I do not know what happened to JP before he entered second grade for the second time, but luckily for JP, his second-time-around Grade 2 teacher was Ms. Green and she did help.

Unlike many teachers in high-needs, hard-to-staff, under-resourced, urban schools, Ms. Green was already certified. Unlike many certified teachers, she continued to seek out professional development experiences. She felt a real sense of responsibility for all children in her classroom and wanted to learn more about beginning reading. Luckily for JP, Ms. Green learned how to teach phonemic awareness and phonics when she took several post-master's reading courses. The following story comes from her notes on JP over the course of a yearlong case study she carried out as practicum work during these courses.

JP lived with his mother and several siblings who all read well. There was no family history of dyslexia and his mother did not remember any developmental delays in JP's language acquisition. He had difficulty with reading in both first and second grade, and attended a school-based, remedial after-school program. He attended summer school after second grade but made little progress and was not promoted to Grade 3.

Evaluation

By October of his second year in Grade 2, JP was seen by a school evaluation team to see if he was eligible for special education services. A classroom visit by the team described a compliant child who listened to directions and carried out his work. During an interview with a social worker, JP's mother reported that homework took up to three hours and often produced angry tears and yelling, although he was usually cheerful in less frustrating situations. He was disorganized about keeping track of assignments and books. His mother saw this behavior as reactive to being held back and to the apparently easier progress of classmates.

The team's school psychologist described JP as friendly, cooperative and productive. Projective assessment indicated that he was well adjusted emotionally and related well to others but was (appropriately) anxious about schoolwork. During IQ testing, he was on-task, involved, and monitored his own performance through self-corrections. His IQ on the WISC-III was in the high average range. An educational evaluator carried out academic testing and did an unusually thorough job of observing and reporting decoding and spelling errors pointing to a specific problem in learning and using letter-sound information. Although his math composite score on a standardized academic achievement battery was average, his low average reading composite score was a full 20 standard score points lower than his IQ. This difference is large enough to be considered a discrepancy. However, the discrepancy formula that was used involved comparing his reading grade equivalent of 1:8 to his actual grade placement, which was 2:5. Had he not repeated second grade the grade-level discrepancy still would not have been a full two-year difference. Testing of decoding-related phonological processing skills (i.e., phonemic awareness, rapid naming) was not carried out.

In a summary report written by the team in November, his reading was reported to be at a late Grade 1 level. Although there had been a classroom visit, there was no record of consultations with his teacher or collaboratively developed plans for trial teaching in the classroom or any special services. He was labeled "nonhandicapped," with no follow-up plan to improve reading.

Informal Classroom Assessment

Luckily, his teacher rose to the challenge and took on responsibility for finding solutions. Ms. Green had suspected that JP was dyslexic because he seemed bright but he also seemed to struggle with word-level reading. JP was referred in the early fall and seen by the school evaluation team in January. Without waiting for evaluation results, Ms. Green began informal assessment. Based on observations, she was able to see that he struggled to sound out new words. She learned from the Rosner Test of Auditory Analysis Skills that he could segment and delete initial phonemes in words but did not seem to be aware of phonemes in other positions. This was consistent with his decoding; he sounded out initial letters and made guesses that made little sense in terms of either meaning or other letters. While he was the age of an early third grader, he scored on this phonemic awareness test at a level attained by early first graders.

Ms. Green began working with JP, providing short phonemic awareness and phonics lessons one-to-one whenever she could find five minutes to work with him during the day. She included direct instruction in these areas in JP's small reading group. She felt confident about doing this without a diagnosis because this instruction is useful for all young children. Even with this direct instruction, JP's progress was slower than that of other children in his reading group. Ms. Green stayed in close touch with JP's mother about his progress. At the end of the year, she told his mother that she knew he was bright and that he tried hard. She suggested an outside evaluation and JP was eventually seen by a university reading clinic and diagnosed with dyslexia at age nine.

Diagnosis Based on Failure to Thrive with Appropriate Instruction

Lynn and Douglas Fuchs' failure-to-respond model would have provided JP with special services much earlier; he had struggled more than others in his instructional groupings during first grade, both in class and in his after school program. He had struggled during second grade to the point where he was assigned to summer school. While some children made good progress with this intense, morning-long literacy instruction, JP did not, and in September he was retained in Grade 2. We do not have descriptions of his instruction in these early settings, but we do know that Ms. Green's Grade 2 instruction was appropriate and that other students with low reading achievement thrived. This model would have served JP better, as would have Torgesen and Wagner's (1998) and Fletcher et al.'s (1998) phonological core deficit model. It was clear to Ms. Green that phonological processing was a deficit area for JP.

THE PHONOLOGICAL CORE DEFICIT MODEL OF ASSESSMENT: AT

This last story has a happier outcome. This case study comes from an inclusion classroom where Ms. Goldman and Ms. Field share responsibility for 23 kindergarten children. Both teachers are certified in special as well as regular education. New York City routinely administers criterion-referenced testing[10] to all primary-grade children to track progress in letter knowledge, phonemic awareness, and early reading skills. The Early Childhood Literacy Assessment System (ECLAS) is administered early in the fall, at the end of the school year, and in between where warranted. Screening is discontinued somewhere between kindergarten and grade 3 once criterion is met for each language area.

Early Identification and Intervention: AT

AT is the younger child of Eastern European parents and English is her second language. Her older brother, who struggled with both English and reading in the early grades, is now the lowest achieving reader in his fourth grade class. AT entered kindergarten as a general education student. When Ms. Goldman administered the ECLAS she found that AT knew only a few letter names and no letter sounds, and was unable to perform phonological tasks, even at the rhyming level. She was concerned about AT because of her brother's struggle with reading and because AT's knowledge of letters and phonemic processing was weak.

AT was not Ms. Goldman's only concern. In this school, in which many children receive free or reduced lunch as Title I services, many children come to school with little letter or phonemic knowledge. Ms. Goldman stated that all children in her class receive "daily direct, explicit phonemic awareness and phonics training. It was my hope that this direct instruction would help bring the at-risk children in the class up to grade level by the end and that they would be able to move on to first grade prepared for the literacy challenges." Both of AT's teachers observe their children closely every day. Both make subtle adjustments to curriculum on an ongoing basis to be sure that their children are learning. By spring, in this nurturing and focused environment, AT had responded well to instruction. She knew almost all letter names, could segment spoken words into phonemes, could sound out and blend in simple decodable texts, and could use other cue systems to read a few simple, predictable trade books.

Is AT dyslexic? Probably not. Might she have struggled to read without this direct, explicit instruction? Her early profile fits that of many children with ongoing reading difficulty. The wonderful thing about successful early intervention is that it really does not matter what

---

[10] Criterion-referenced early literacy testing measures performance in terms of tasks believed to be precursors of literacy. Where norm-referenced testing compares a child to a group norm, criterion-referenced testing tells us whether or not a child has mastered a task believed to be a benchmark, such as being successful at 4/6 rhyming items.

might have been. If she has dyslexia, it is very mild. With the right instruction, AT is doing well. We do not know what would have happened had KM or JP been in this kindergarten class, but we can guess that it would have helped them to have had the right instruction from the start.

In New York City and across the United States, there is more and more focus on ongoing, day-to-day and month-by-month assessment by the classroom teacher. In the best of all possible worlds, teachers would observe carefully, keep portfolios of children's work, administer informal, curriculum-based measures on an ongoing basis, and have the knowledge and skills to analyze this data frequently to use in planning instruction. In this world, all children at-risk would learn to read.

II

Instruction for Dyslexia

4

Principles and Techniques of Instruction for Students with Dyslexia

This chapter begins by looking at principles and techniques of instruction for students with dyslexia from an historical perspective. Then it documents the trend toward scientific research in the teaching of reading for all children. It closes with short summaries of principles and techniques that are discussed in more depth in the chapters that follow.

Until the past 20 years, reading disabilities research has been justifiably criticized for focusing disproportionately on the search for causality and all but neglecting inquiry on correction or prevention of the problem. The reading disabilities field has, in fact, been referred to as "deficit driven" (Poplin 1983). Rachel Gittelman, a psychologist at the College of Physicians and Surgeons, Columbia University, reviewing the research on the remediation of reading disorders, stated that, "The literature on the treatment of children with reading retardation is full of opinionated practices devoid of even barely adequately controlled treatment research" (Gittelman 1983).

The Teachers College task force (Peister et al. 1978–1980) drew attention to the fact that even where control or comparison groups exist, the instruction applied in these groups often has not been adequately described, making it difficult to determine which instructional components are actually being compared. The nature of choice of outcome measures frequently is not given adequate consideration in planning program evaluation or in interpreting findings from studies that have been carried out. As Gittelman (1983) pointed out, most standardized tests are not designed to pick up small gains over short periods of time; thus, with short term or "one shot" studies the possibility of failure to detect treatment effects statistically where they exist is greatly increased.

SCIENTIFIC RESEARCH ON INSTRUCTIONAL TECHNIQUES

At the time of the second edition of this book in 1995, Gittleman's assessment of the situation had begun to change. Large-scale longitudinal studies of children with specific reading disabilities had been funded by the National Institutes of Child Health and Human Development (NICHD) and had provided a more comprehensive description of dyslexia. This research is described in Chapter 2. From this research we learned that dyslexia is related to specific deficits in phonological processing, that it runs in families, and that it involves differences in brain functioning.

A second wave of NICHD-funded studies was carried out during the 1990s, this time focused on effective instruction. Early reports from these longitudinal treatment studies were described in the 1995 edition of this book. Barbara Foorman in Texas and Joseph Torgesen in Florida headed two research teams. Both teams worked with large numbers of children who were randomly assigned to a variety of instructional groups. Careful records were kept documenting response to treatment over time, considering factors such as IQ, socioeconomic group, and age. Sophisticated statistical techniques were used to sort out questions such as what kind of instruction worked well for what children and under what conditions (e.g., Foorman et al. 1991, 1997, 1998, 2003; Torgesen et al. 1997, 1999; Torgesen, Wagner, and Rashotte 1997)

Other research teams addressed many of these same issues during the 1990s. Some of these other studies, like the NICHD studies, were what we call *scientific research* (i.e., quantitative designs with random assignment to comparison groups and with thorough descriptions of the participants, treatments, and research procedures). Others were more descriptive in nature, with finely drawn qualitative analyses of case studies or individual classrooms.

By the mid 1990s, the U. S. Department of Education and the U. S. Department of Health and Human Services had asked the National Academy of Sciences to create a committee to review the research on preventing reading difficulties. This committee of the National Research Council, made up of both qualitative and quantitative researchers, looked at both types of research studies, and as a team, synthesized their response to these findings. The report, titled *Preventing*

Reading Difficulties in Young Children, suggested, in brief, combining systematic phonics with many opportunities to practice new words in meaningful text together with opportunities to write in the classroom, and for struggling readers, one-to-one or small group help from a reading specialist employing these same methods (Snow, Burns, and Griffin 1998).

In 1997, the U. S. Congress approached both the NICHD and the Secretary of Education with a request to create a National Reading Panel (NRP) to "assess the status of research-based knowledge, including the effectiveness of various approaches to teaching children to read." Unlike the National Research Council report, which was a review of research, the NRP carried out a meta-analysis of scientifically conducted studies. From literally thousands of studies, they categorized studies by topic, and then selected those deemed to be scientific: those with random assignment to treatment and control groups and with adequate descriptions of procedures employed. For the included studies, the Panel subcommittees converted scores to the same standardized system, and were able to make comparisons of instructional elements and of students varying in characteristics. They looked at what is called *effect size*, a statistical technique used in meta-analyses that provides information about the strength of a significant difference in group scores. For the first time questions about the features of best instruction for children with dyslexia could be answered with some degree of scientific confidence.

INSTRUCTIONAL PRINCIPLES
DIRECT INSTRUCTION

Historically, one of the most often acknowledged principles of instruction for children with dyslexia is direct instruction. N. G. Haring and B. Bateman in their book, *Teaching the Learning Disabled Child* (1977), made the point that these children do not learn "by osmosis," as other children seem to do. Rather, they need direct, intensive, and systematic input from, and interaction with, the teacher.

Under the scrutiny of scientific research, this principle holds up well, particularly in regard to phonemic awareness and phonics instruction (see Chapters 5, 6, and 7). In children with deficits in awareness of the sound structure of words in spoken language, it makes sense that this awareness will not be learned through informal exposure. Rather than assuming that a child will notice rhyme and alliteration when listening to good literature, the teacher needs to teach this directly and to reinforce it as she reads aloud.

FREQUENT FEEDBACK

Academic feedback has been considered to be an essential instructional component of learning to mastery (Berliner 1981). Rosenshine and

Stevens (1984) cite immediate feedback from the teacher as one of the five most important contributive factors to academic achievement. They subdivide the feedback process into four instructional components: demonstration, guided practice, feedback, and independent practice. Although little research has specifically investigated the effects of this variable on students with dyslexia, some provision for teacher feedback is incorporated in all established programs employing direct instruction, as exemplified by the *DISTAR* program (see Chapter 17). In some programs a *guided discovery* or *Socratic* method is used under careful teacher supervision to ensure correct responses (see Chapter 20, *Alphabetic Phonics* and Chapter 24, the *Lindamood Program*). Providing standards against which to measure their performance helps students to become self-monitors and take on more responsibility for their own progress (Bandura 1982). This is not an area that has been explored by the National Reading Panel Report (2000) but many of the features of feedback are implicit in programs that provide direct instruction.

PACING

Careful pacing of instruction has been considered an essential feature of effective teaching for students with dyslexia in order to prevent information overload, which occurs when the amount of information to be processed within a given time span exceeds the individual's capacity (Bryant et al. 1980). The successful teacher or practitioner working with students with dyslexia, regardless of instructional setting, must provide for this contingency in planning each lesson (Cox 1992; Gillingham and Stillman 1960; Slingerland 1976). Most established remedial methods and programs use a structured, hierarchical approach to learning, breaking down tasks into small units taught in order of difficulty (Bryant et al. 1980).

One difficulty for teachers in making on-the-spot decisions about pacing is that the slow response time of many children with reading difficulties can create too much waiting time to maintain interest in the lesson. The training of teachers in *Success for All* (Chapter 16) places emphasis on the pacing of small group instruction to maximize time on task and to minimize time wasted on monitoring behavior. Instruction can be fast-paced but still break down learning into small, manageable pieces so that students are not overloaded. Another technique, oral unison response is incorporated in several programs (e.g., see the chapters in Part III on *DISTAR, Slingerland, Success for All*) to ensure that each student is fully involved in the lesson at hand. Hand signals used to cue group response, as in the *DISTAR* program (see Chapter 17) and Enfield and Greene's *Project Read* (1983; see Chapter 23), serve as attentional devices to trigger learned behaviors and to cut down on management time.

Pacing as a discreet variable in reading instruction was not examined by the National Reading Panel. This is an indication that there are not enough research studies to draw conclusions about this instructional variable.

SYSTEMATIC, STRUCTURED PROGRESSION FROM THE SIMPLE TO THE COMPLEX

Planning instruction around small steps that build on and reinforce the known and that introduce the unknown in tiny increments of learning are an important feature of many of the programs outlined in Part III. One example of this is the use of the six basic syllable types to structure the learning of letter-sound associations in the Wilson Reading System (see Chapter 23). At only six points in the program is there a real conceptual shift from the known to the unknown as each new syllable type is introduced. Most new learning provides just one more example of a mastered syllable type. Moving in manageable steps that connect old learning to new learning is an important component of systematic phonics. It is easier to manage a fast-paced and engaging lesson when students are not overwhelmed with new material. Probably the strongest finding of the Report of the National Reading Panel (2000) is the effectiveness of systematic phonics instruction (see Chapter 7, *Phonics*).

LEARNING TO MASTERY

Historically, mastery has been considered an extremely important factor in remedial or preventive instruction for disabled readers. Barak Rosenshine, a proponent of direct instruction, states that to insure retention, mastery needs to reach levels of 70 to 80 percent when new reading skills are acquired; in independent practice, mastery should be 100 percent, especially for learners with disabilities (Rosenshine 1983). This is a common sense approach that parallels thinking about independent and instructional levels in reading. Mastery of close to 100 percent of the words in a passage or short story is considered optimal when children read to themselves. Books with as few as 5 percent unfamiliar words are reserved for guided instruction by a teacher. Text with only 90 percent mastery is considered *frustration level* or text too difficult for the reader under circumstances other than listening.

Gaining automaticity is a critical component of mastery learning in remedial reading instruction. Automatic processing at the word level frees up working memory to allow for more efficient processing at the sentence and passage levels of text (LaBerge and Samuels 1974; Perfetti

1985b; Stanovich 1984). See Chapter 8 for more information on automaticity. Readers with dyslexia tend to be slower at word recognition than good readers (Perfetti 1984; Stanovich 1980). Most of the established remedial programs, therefore, make ample provision for extended practice to attain automaticity beginning at the letter-sound level. Barbara Bateman, in particular, stresses the need for repetition with all new learning, a concept termed *overlearning* (Bateman 1979). However, as Dale Bryant and his associates at Teachers College pointed out, practice needs to be carefully distributed over time, rather than massed. They suggested that massed practice reinforces short-term memory at the expense of long-term memory (Bryant et al. 1980). The majority of remedial programs for dyslexic students provide for systematic review of previously learned material at the beginning and end of each lesson.

Mastery learning is an important feature of a number of programs described in Part III. For example, in *Alphabetic Phonics* (see Chapter 20) a new sound is not introduced until the current letter-sound has been mastered. *Success for All* (see Chapter 16) is another program in which mastery learning plays an important role. In this program, six-week units of study are sequenced to coincide with the needs of small groups of students. At six-week intervals, all students are assessed and regrouped for instruction. Only students at mastery level for the current unit proceed to the subsequent unit. Those not at mastery level repeat the unit within the new grouping.

MULTISENSORY INSTRUCTION

The use of multisensory techniques in remedial reading interventions is widespread and dates back to the 1920s and to Grace Fernald who instructed students to trace letters or words while saying the names aloud (Fernald and Keller 1921). This procedure came to be known as the *VAKT approach* (i.e., visual, auditory, kinesthetic, tactile). Fernald maintained that this reinforcement would help to produce a memory schema for the stimulus information. Samuel Orton's hypothesis that dyslexia is caused by incomplete cerebral dominance, resulting in reversal and sequencing problems, led to the adoption of multisensory teaching methods by his many disciples (e.g., Cox 1992; Gillingham and Stillman 1960; Slingerland 1971; Traub and Bloom 2000; Wilson 1988b). Another example of multisensory instruction can be found in the field of speech remediation. The Lindamoods (Lindamood and Lindamood 1998) stress the importance of developing oral-motor awareness in children and adults with deficits in auditory conceptualization (see Chapter 24).

Perhaps the most interesting research to date on the effects of multisensory instruction is that conducted by Charles Hulme. Seeking to understand the rationale for multisensory instruction with readers with disabilities, Hulme carried out a series of carefully controlled studies during the early 1980s to answer questions about the underlying processes affected in multisensory reading and writing instruction. In one of these studies, for instance, he found that tracing letters significantly enhanced the ability of disabled readers to remember the names of letters they have seen, and that this brought their recognition performance up to that of typically developing readers. However, tracing had little improvement effect on typically developing readers (Hulme 1981). He proposed that the benefits gained from letter tracing by disabled readers but not by good readers are attributable to disabled readers' failure to employ a speech code to memorize letters. This is a credible explanation in light of what is known about the phonological coding deficits in individuals with dyslexia. That is, multisensory instruction provided a way around the use of the phonological code in children with dyslexia.

In another exploration of multisensory instruction, Hulme and Lynette Bradley (1984) used an Orton-Gillingham technique called "Save Our Spelling" (SOS) in which a student reads a word and then copies it three times, saying each letter aloud as it is written. Both young, typically developing readers and older, poor readers learned to spell more words correctly using the multisensory SOS technique than when using a comparison technique in which lettered tiles were selected for spellings. Ultimately, however, Hulme was not able to determine whether or how information processed in one sensory modality might enhance the processing of information in another.

Three more recent studies provide examples of treatment research using multisensory instruction. Barbara Wise, who works with Richard Olson in Colorado, has incorporated features of the Lindamood Program (see Chapter 24) into instruction that includes a computer-based component for young children with reading problems. Children are taught to recognize pictures of mouth positions in regard to the sounds made when their own mouths are in those positions (e.g., top teeth on lower lip producing the sound /f/). These new skills are then practiced on a computer program that incorporates both mouth movements and synthesized speech. Speech sound training is eventually extended into reading recognition training that also has a computer-practice component. Words that children cannot read can be highlighted for computer-based speech-synthesis production, segment by segment. The computer-based segmentation training is called ROSS, or Reading with Orthographic and Speech Segmentation. Children in the ROSS group outperformed a control group after this multisensory training (Wise 1995).

Joseph Torgesen, Richard Wagner, and Carol Rashotte at Florida State University also used the Lindamood method. In their

NICHD-funded longitudinal study, these multisensory techniques were used in connection with a synthetic phonics program in an intervention with first-grade children at risk because of poor phonological awareness skills. Three additional instructional groups included: (a) implicit phonics instruction using basal-reader text, (b) one-to-one support for regular classroom instruction, and (c) regular classroom instruction alone. The multisensory direct instruction synthetic phonics model was more effective than the other instructional models in terms of phonological processing tasks such as phonemic awareness and non-sense word reading (Torgesen et al. 1999).

Barbara Foorman and her colleagues, with funding from an NICHD grant, also used multisensory instruction as a treatment component in two of the three reading instructional systems she compared in her work with second and third graders with reading disabilities. This study is described in more detail in Chapter 7, *Phonics*. The important point here is that both methods using multisensory instruction were effective, but the study was not controlled in such a way that the role of multisensory instruction could be examined systematically (Foorman et al. 1997).

Despite the widespread inclusion of multisensory techniques in remedial programs for students with dyslexia and the conviction among both practitioners and researchers that the techniques work, there is little scientific research to suggest that it is the multisensory component that makes these systematic reading programs effective. This is because these particular competing variables have not been well controlled. Because of this, the National Reading Panel did not examine the multisensory aspect of instruction.

ONGOING ASSESSMENT

Monitoring and evaluating student progress is an essential component of successful academic treatment, although not all treatment methods for students with dyslexia include evaluation procedures. Naomi Zigmond and Sandra Miller (1986) have reported studies that show significantly greater academic gains for students whose teachers monitored student progress, as compared to students whose teachers collected no ongoing progress data. However, these reviewers emphasized that to be effective, progress evaluation must be frequent and systematic and teachers must use the data constructively to modify instruction when needed. Furthermore, a data-based approach has been found to be more effective in improving pupil achievement than informal observational procedures, though the data analysis need not be elaborate to provide adequate information on student progress. Note the systematic daily record taking in *Reading Recovery* (see Chapter 15), the frequent curriculum-based evaluation (i.e., benchmarks) in *Alphabetic Phonics* (see Chapter 20), and the periodic assessment and regrouping for instruction in *Success for All* (see Chapter 16).

The remaining chapters in Part II of this book describe how these principles and techniques can be applied in instruction in specific areas of reading and writing instruction. The chapters in Part III look at the principles and techniques as used by particular programs.

5

Phonemic Awareness

This chapter provides information about the nature of phonemic awareness, how it impacts reading, and how it differs from phonics instruction. Because it is considered a precursor to reading, the research studies of effective phonemic awareness training that are included in this chapter are organized in sections on emergent, beginning, and remedial reading, as are the suggestions for teachers at the end of the chapter.

Phonics and phonemic awareness are considered to be important aspects of learning to read words, and the two terms are often confused. *Phonics* is defined in *The Literacy Dictionary* as, "a way of teaching reading and spelling that stresses symbol–sound relationships, especially in beginning instruction" (Harris and Hodges 1995, p. 186). Phonics involves connecting printed letters to the sounds that are associated with them.

Phonological awareness, on the other hand, involves just sounds. Being aware of phonology means being able to listen to a spoken word and to analyze what Russian psychologist D. B. Elkonin called its "sound structure" (1973, p. 560). This involves being able to identify sounds in spoken language and to understand the sequence of these sounds. This can involve analysis of speech at several levels, such as:

1. words in sentences (e.g., /I/-/am/-/going/-/to/-/a/-/birth-day/-/party/
2. syllables in words (e.g., /At/-/lan/-/tic/ in Atlantic)

3. onsets and rimes[11] in words (e.g., /b/-/eak/ in *beak* and /str/-/etch/ in *stretch*)
4. individual phonemes in words (e. g., /a/-/t/ in *at*).

The final two, analysis of initial phonemes and analysis of all the phonemes in a word, are the most critical to learning to read.

A *phoneme* is the smallest unit of sound in a word that can affect its meaning. For example, the contrast in the phoneme sounds /t/ and /p/ allows us to differentiate the meanings of the words *mat* and *map*. You need auditory discrimination in order to tell these words apart, but phonemic awareness is more than discrimination of differences in sounds. It involves, for example, being able to produce the final sound in *mat* and the final sound in *map* and being conscious of the sequence of sounds and of the final sound in each of these words as the different sound. Phonemic awareness is a subset of the larger category, phonological awareness, and it is phonemic awareness that is especially important to the acquisition of reading.

What makes phonemic awareness difficult is that phonemes in speech are *coarticulated*, or spoken together, with their surrounding phonemes. Although spoken words break apart fairly naturally into syllables, they do not break apart into phonemes very easily. Individual phonemes are difficult to differentiate in the speech stream. Vowels can exist alone in natural speech, as in the words *oh* and *eye*, and in the syllables *o-pen* and *a-pron*. Vowels are what linguists call sonorants, or continuous speech sounds that can be held for a period of time. Only a few consonant sounds are sonorants (e.g., /m/, /r/, /l/). Most consonants are *obstruents* or sounds that obstruct or close off the stream of air crossing the vocal folds. Notice that you can draw out or continue the sound of /a/ in *at*, but that the sound /t/ lasts a very brief time and closes off the vowel sound.

Some obstruents have such a brief duration that they are difficult for some people to discriminate. The initial consonant *d*, for example, lasts for such a tiny amount of time that it cannot be said without a vowel after it. Teachers tend to pronounce obstruents as /duuuh/ or /tuuuh/. According to Paula Tallal (see Chapter 2) word reading disorder can be the result of difficulty discriminating these rapid sounds. To complicate matters for all children, each coarticulated phoneme can have a subtly (or not so subtly) different sound depending on the surrounding phonemes. The sound /r/ distorts preceding vowels (e.g., note the sounds of the letter *a* in *cat* and in *car*). In her book, *Speech to Print: Language Essentials for Teachers*, Louisa Moats suggests that teachers

---

[11]An "onset" is the opening consonant or consonant cluster or digraph in a syllable, such as *m* in *meat* or *tr* in *treat* or *ch* in *cheat*. The "rime" portion of a syllable consists of the vowel and final consonant unit, in this case, the unit *eat*.

watch their mouths in a mirror as they listen for sound contrasts in the initial consonants in the words *tap* and *trap* in order to better understand the principle of coarticulation (Moats 2000). Learning to read in English and other alphabetic languages involves learning to understand the alphabetic principle, the idea that sequences of sounds in speech are represented by sequences of letters in written words. This is difficult for young children because of the abstract nature of phonemes.

PHONEMIC AWARENESS DEVELOPMENT

Phonemic awareness skills develop over time. Researchers have used a variety of tasks to demonstrate that children grow in ability to understand the sound structure of spoken words. Some of the following tasks can be observed during routine literacy activities at home and school, and others are tests developed by researchers. Two pioneers in the field of phonemic awareness carried out research in the 1960s and 1970s. Their studies were critical to the notion that the development of phonemic awareness in young children was key to the development of reading. The first, D. B. Elkonin, carried out training studies indicating the causal role of phonemic awareness in later reading ability. His task involved using a picture to generate oral language (e.g., a picture of two geese) and a diagram of the sound structure of the word (e.g., four squares to represent the four phonemes in *guzi* the Russian word for *geese*.). The child was asked to say the word aloud, stretch out the sounds, and then to say each phoneme's sound while placing a cardboard counter onto each of the squares below the picture. This provided a concrete model of the individual phonemes and of their order in the word (Elkonin 1963, 1973). This procedure is discussed in more depth in the section on beginning reading later on in this chapter. The second researcher, Isabel Liberman, was a professor of reading education at the University of Connecticut. Working with a group of psychologists and linguists, including her husband, Alvin Liberman who was an expert in speech, she carried out studies at Haskins Laboratories in New Haven. Her work indicated that prereaders could analyze spoken words and that this skill could be used to predict later reading (Liberman 1973). Her tasks involved asking young children to tap out syllables and then phonemes in words. For example, two taps would represent the two syllables in the word *pencil*.

Several researchers have carried out studies of the relative difficulty of phonemic awareness tasks (e.g., Schatschneider et al. 1999; Stahl and Murray 1994; Uhry and Ehri 1999; Yopp 1988). Ordering the tasks is complicated by the complexity of the task (i.e., blending versus segmenting) as well as by the complexity of the words used (i.e., *at* versus *stretch*). Phonological awareness tasks are listed here in approximate order of difficulty. All but the syllable task are considered phonemic awareness tasks, and the order is based on a phonemic awareness hierarchy by Marilyn Adams (1990).

1. *Response to Rhymes.* Three- and four-year-olds can memorize nursery rhymes and rhyming songs. They can provide the final word in rhyming text when listening to a story. In a British study, researchers assessed preschoolers each year until they learned to read. Those who were most skilled in memorizing nursery rhymes were most skilled, later, in learning to read (Maclean, Bryant, and Bradley 1987).

2. *Classifying or Matching by Phonemes.* Many 4- and 5-year-olds can match words by rhyme or alliteration. A classroom task involves, "Line up if your name sounds like Michael's at the beginning (e.g., *Marco, Melissa*). One research task involves picking the "odd-man-out" from a set of words (e.g., *bat, baby, table, boot*) with initial, final, or middle sound the focus. Another task, common to workbooks, is to hunt for a picture that matches the first picture in a row (e.g., Find the picture that begins like *bear* from a choice of *car, bat, dog*).

3. *Segmenting Part of a Word.* Five-year-olds can usually segment or isolate out the first sound in a word. They can tell you that the word *dog* starts with the sound /d/. Kindergarten teachers know this from listening to children say /k/ as they invent spellings such as K or KT for *cat*. Invented spelling is a form of phoneme segmentation because the sound needs to be stretched out and identified before it is matched with a letter. By age five many children can blend sounds into words. The teacher says the phonemes in isolation and the child synthesizes the sounds into a word (e.g., /c/-/a/-/t/). Variations include an easier version, blending an onset with a rime (e.g., /c/-/at/) and a harder version, blending a nonword (e.g., /z/-/a/-/t/).

4. *Full Phoneme Segmentation.* This task involves tapping out the number of phonemes, or saying phonemes aloud in order, or pulling tiles into a linear sequence while saying each phoneme in order. By the end of kindergarten or early in Grade 1, most children can segment all the sounds in short words. Teachers notice that children usually begin to include vowels (not necessarily spelled correctly) in their invented spellings around the time that formal reading instruction begins early in Grade 1. Children who can represent all sounds in their invented spellings usually do well on research tasks such as saying aloud the sounds in a word presented by the researcher. Phoneme segmentation tasks vary in difficulty depending on the linguistic structure of

the word that is being segmented. For example, two-phoneme words are easier to segment than words with three phonemes, and two-phoneme words starting with vowels are easier than those starting with consonants (i.e., *age* is easier to segment than either *same* or *say*; Uhry and Ehri 1999).

5. *Phoneme Deletion or Elision.* Deleting phonemes from words (e.g., "Say *same* without the /s/") is a good example of a task that varies in difficulty depending on the complexity of the chosen word and the position of the phoneme to be removed. Many kindergarten and first grade children are successful with the example above. The task becomes markedly more difficult when, as in an assessment tool developed by Jerome Rosner, the phoneme to be deleted is part of a consonant cluster (e.g., "Say *stale* without the /t/)," an item at the third grade level (Rosner 1975, 1999). Marilyn Adams (1990) lists this task as more difficult than full phoneme segmentation in her discussion of phonemic awareness tasks, while Christopher Schatschneider and his colleagues found it to be easier (Schatschneider et al. 1999).

PHONEMIC AWARENESS AND READING

Research shows the relationship between phonemic awareness and reading to be complex. There is evidence that phonemic awareness is causal in the development of early word reading, but there is also evidence that learning to read words supports the further development of phonemic awareness. To suggest a causal relationship two kinds of research are needed. First, there needs to be a correlation between early phonemic awareness level and later level of word reading skill. That is, researchers need to be able to demonstrate that children rank order on one task in much the same way they rank order on the other. Second, they must be able to demonstrate in a training study with controls that changing the level of phonemic awareness in one group increases its later success in reading in comparison with controls. Lynette Bradley and Peter Bryant were the first to demonstrate both of these findings in a single, large-scale longitudinal study described later in this chapter (Bradley and Bryant 1983, 1985).

Phonemic awareness training contributes to ability in phonological processing tasks including word reading and spelling, but it also contributes to reading comprehension. Linnea Ehri, a member of the National Reading Panel, reports that its meta-analysis identified ten studies in which this training had a positive effect on reading comprehension (Ehri, Nunes, Willows et al. 2001). Most likely this is because increasing word reading ability through phonemic awareness training facilitated comprehension.

Phonemic awareness is developmental, but it also responds to instruction. This instruction is most effective when it takes advantage of Lev Vygotsky's *zone of proximal development*, that is, when it is a match for the developmental level of the child and when a teacher scaffolds performance just beyond the level at which the child can perform independently. In children who are slow to develop phonemic awareness, this carefully planned instruction is critical. It needs to be planned from on-going assessment, both formal and informal. Assessment of phonemic awareness is a complicated issue because different kinds of items are appropriate at different levels of development.

Training in phonics has been part of classroom instruction for centuries. Teachers trained in the Orton-Gillingham approach have used phonics for many years in the remediation of dyslexia (Gillingham and Stillman 1960). This has not been the case for phonemic awareness. The Russian psychologist D. B. Elkonin and the University of Connecticut professor Isabel Liberman published evidence of the link between early phonemic awareness and later reading as early as the 1960s and 1970s. However, it was only during the late 1980s and 1990s that phonemic awareness began to be a regular part of early literacy programs and remedial programs for children with dyslexia.

The Executive Summary of Snow's *Preventing Reading Difficulties in Young Children* recommends that teachers in the early grades include "explicit instruction and practice that lead to an appreciation that spoken words are made up of smaller units of sound . . ." (Snow et al. 1998, p. 7). The National Reading Panel also recommends that phonemic awareness training begin early, as its effects are greatest in preschool and kindergarten. There is good evidence from a number of studies that early phonemic training increases a child's level of phonemic awareness prior to reading instruction. The following phonemic awareness training studies have been arranged into a sequence with three levels (i.e., emergent literacy, beginning reading, and remedial reading). Following this, there is a short section with ideas for teaching phonemic awareness.

TRAINING STUDIES WITH PREREADERS

Before exposure to formal reading instruction, kindergarten children who are not at risk typically can match spoken words by rhyme and alliteration, can provide a rhyme at the end of a sentence in predictable text read aloud by the teacher, can match words based on alliteration (common initial sound), can say the first sound or the last sound they hear in a word, and can segment and represent beginning and ending consonants in invented spellings (e.g., LK for the word *like*). Many prereaders can blend phonemes into words. A variety of training tasks have been used successfully to increase ability in these areas.

Two important, large-scale, longitudinal studies of phonemic awareness training were carried out with prereaders in the 1980s. Ingvar Lundberg and his Danish colleagues studied 235 kindergarten children whose classroom teachers provided phonemic awareness training throughout the school year. Training involved rhyming stories and games, rhythmic movement to syllabic patterns, and phoneme segmentation practice. By the end of the year, these children were superior to controls on phonemic awareness measures, with particularly strong effects for phoneme segmentation. The study is important because it followed these children to the end of the second-grade school year. Although training was limited to sound analysis and did not involve reading, the children who were trained were superior to controls on reading and spelling measures two years after training ended (Lundberg, Frost, and Petersen 1988). Lundberg's tasks have been published in the United States as a guide for teachers, *Phonemic Awareness for Young Children: A Classroom Curriculum* (Adams et al. 1998). Ideas for classroom PA instruction from this book are included at the end of this chapter.

In another seminal study, Lynette Bradley and Peter Bryant undertook phonemic awareness training in England with 4- and 5-year-old children considered to be at risk for reading failure because of low levels of phonemic awareness (Bradley and Bryant 1983, 1985). The training involved practice in what they called *sound categorization*, which requires selection of the "odd man out" from a set of four pictures, three of whose names match in regard to alliteration (*bun, bus, rug, bug*), rhyme (*bun, hut, gun, sun*) or medial vowel (*hug, pig, dig, wig*). Training took place in 40 ten-minute sessions over a two-year period. Note that while instructional sessions were quite short, instruction was effective. Toward the end of training some of the children used plastic letters to segment and spell words. The sixty subjects were in four groups: (a) sound categorization, (b) sound categorization with letters, (c) categorization by concepts rather than sounds, and (d) controls. The group with a significant advantage in reading and spelling at the end of the study was the sound categorization group whose training included plastic letters, and this advantage held two years after the study ended (Bradley and Bryant 1985).

This finding leads to the question of whether or not to include letters in phonemic awareness training. Linnea Ehri's work suggests that this should be done. She trained kindergarten children to segment with both blank tokens and with letters. Her results indicated that using letters for segmenting produced superior ability in both segmenting and blending (Hohn and Ehri 1983). In a later study (Ehri and Wilce 1987b), kindergarten children were taught to read using segmentation in combination with letters. These children had a significant advantage over controls trained in letter-sounds but not trained in segmenting words. Ehri makes the point that spelling (segmenting using letters) leads into reading. This is a finding that is consistent with the National Reading Panel's meta-analysis.

Benita Blachman, who studied with Isabel Liberman, later worked with her own students Eileen Ball and Darlene Tangel on phonemic awareness training studies. In one study, they used both phoneme segmentation and letter-sound training with children whose kindergarten teachers taught them to segment phonemes, and, as a consequence, to read and spell better by the end of the kindergarten year in comparison with a sound-only group and a control group. The training involved groups of five children, for 20 minutes, four times a week for seven weeks. They used a "say-it-and-move-it" activity similar to Elkonin's pictures and boxes (e.g., saying a word in response to a picture, saying each sound in that word, and sliding a token down for each sound). This was done first with blank tiles and later with a mix of blank and lettered tiles. Other activities included a sound-sorting task based on the Bradley and Bryant task described above, as well as training in letter-sound associations (Blachman et al. 1994). Eileen Ball used the say-it-and-move-it task to teach phonemic awareness to kindergarten children (Ball and Blachman 1991), as did Darlene Tangel who reported improvement in invented spelling as a result of this training (Tangel and Blachman 1995). Blachman has published a book of teaching suggestions, called *Road to the Code*, based on the instruction in these studies (Blachman et al. 2000). Several of these ideas are presented at the end of this chapter.

Susan Brady, another of Isabel Liberman's students, combined a number of research-based phonemic training methods in her work with urban kindergarten children. Training for 21 children from two intact classes included the Lindamoods' (1975) training in awareness of articulatory gestures, Ball and Blachman's (1991) "say-it-and-move-it" technique, and other letter-free activities. By the end of the school year, the trained group was significantly stronger at segmenting and rhyming tasks in comparison with controls, and at follow-up a year later, they surpassed controls on measures of word reading (Brady et al. 1994).

Brian Byrne and Ruth Fielding-Barnsley used a program called *Sound Foundations*. Preschool children in Australia received intense instruction in small groups, as did controls. The experimental group was taught what Byrne called "sound sharing" through the use of posters with pictures of objects whose names shared either beginning or ending sounds (e.g., *sun, seal, sailor; bus, house, dress*). They were taught to search for all the same-sound words. Instruction also involved phonemic awareness games with cards, and letter-sound association training. Controls were taught classification by non-phonemic categories as in the Bradley and Bryant (1983) study. At posttest the children were taught to read word pairs (e.g., *sat*, *mat*) and then tested for transfer of knowledge (e.g., "Does the written word *sow* say 'sow' or 'mow?'"). The experimentally trained children had a significant advantage over controls in the development of phonemic awareness as well as in the ability to learn written words (Byrne and Fielding-Barnsley 1991). In a follow-up study of these children at the end of the first-grade year, Byrne found that those who had entered first grade with the highest levels of phonemic awareness were the most successful readers (Byrne and Fielding-Barnsley 1993). In a later follow-up study they found that the experimentally trained children were superior in non-word reading in Grades 1 and 2, and by the end of Grade 2, were significantly better at comprehension (Byrne and Fielding-Barnsley 1995).

In a short-term supplementary study, the above researchers repeated their 1991 experiment with a new set of preschoolers (Byrne and Fielding-Barnsley 1995). This time, however, classroom teachers provided instruction using the *Sound Foundations* posters with around 20 children twice a week. Classroom training was planned by the teachers using the *Sound Foundations* manual and did not cover the full curriculum covered in the 1991 study. At post-test, there was an advantage for experimental classrooms over controls, but these children did not do as well as the 1991 preschoolers who were trained more intensively in small groups. Note that this is one of the studies used in the National Reading Panel's meta-analysis and is consistent with the Panel's finding that small group phonemic awareness instruction is most effective.

Joseph Torgesen has carried out a series of training studies funded by the National Institute of Child Health and Human Development (NICHD). In one of these studies, Torgesen and his colleagues identified 42 children with low phonemic awareness scores (i.e., 15th-50th percentile) and provided them with roughly seven weeks of PA training in groups of three to five children late in the kindergarten year. Three training conditions involved: (a) segmenting and then blending words, (b) blending words alone, and (c) listening and discussing stories. Both phonemic awareness groups did better at posttest in regard to the specific skill or skills that were taught. That is, the segmenting and blending group scored higher in these areas than controls and the blending group scored higher in blending than controls. Of particular interest was the large advantage the segmenting and blending group had over the blending-only group in terms of ability to learn to read new words. The authors interpreted this finding to indicate that phonemic awareness does not generalize well across tasks and needs to be taught at both the synthesis (blending) and analysis (segmenting) levels (Torgesen, Morgan, and Davis 1992).

In another study, Torgesen and his colleagues provided four 20-minute sessions a week of one-to-one instruction to kindergarten children who were weak at letter naming and in the lowest 12 percent in phonemic awareness. This study is complicated to interpret in terms of the effects of PA training because both PA and phonics instruction were used. The Lindamood Program (Chapter 24) was used for PA training. This is an intensive program with direct instruction involving listening to phonemes and associating them with what the Lindamoods call *articulatory gestures* or the positions of tongue, teeth, and lips as phonemes are formed. The significant advantage in PA post-test scores for children with this direct instruction, in comparison with several control groups, is consistent with the findings of the Report of the NRP that PA training is effective when PA is taught directly (Torgesen et al. 1999).

Rollanda O'Connor and her colleagues also explored the specificity of effects of phonemic awareness training. They trained urban kindergarten children with low phonemic scores (i.e., 0–30th percentile) in two phonemic awareness treatments, both of which included letter-sound training (O'Connor, Jenkins, and Slocum 1995). One treatment was specific to segmenting and blending. She refers to the second instructional treatment as *global* phonemic awareness skills. It involved a wide variety of tasks, including segmenting and blending, and was predicted to result in a higher degree of generalization than the training focused on segmenting and blending alone. A third group received training in letter-sounds alone. A fourth group of high achieving children receiving no extra treatment but served as another control group. Training was carried out over a 10-week period, twice a week for 15 minutes, in groups of three to five children. At post-test, both experimental groups were superior to controls on measures of phonemic awareness and word reading, but the two groups did not differ from each other on measures of segmenting and blending, nor did they differ from the initially high-achieving controls, with whom they had caught up. Children in the two phonemic awareness conditions tended to make more substantial progress in comparison with low achieving children in other studies. O'Connor attributes this to two treatment factors. The first is integration of the same sounds and words into segmenting and blending instruction. That is, when a phoneme was used for segmenting instruction during a session, it was also used for blending instruction. This means that the same words were both deconstructed and constructed. The second instructional factor noted is the use of letters as a component of sound training. Note that the successful use of letters in phonemic awareness training here is consistent with the National Reading Panel's findings.

study O'Connor and her colleagues worked with en with and without disabilities (O'Connor, Notari-sy 1996). Intervention activities were taught by the 1 teachers and lasted six months. Training involved d activities from their program, *Ladders to Literacy* (O Connor, Notari-Syverson, and Vadasy 1998a). The sequence included clapping syllables, shared reading with finger-point reading, and ended with the full segmentation of three-phoneme words using letters to represent sounds. Again, children who were trained were superior to controls in segmentation, blending, and word reading. In an end-of-first-grade follow-up study, with no special treatment during the intervening year, children without disabilities were no longer significantly higher achieving than their controls. This was not the case, however, for children with disabilities in regular education classrooms. These children continued to have a significant advantage over untreated controls, this time in regard to word and nonword reading and spelling. The effect size of 2.11 for spelling was large (O'Connor, Notari-Syverson, and Vadasy 1998b). Keep in mind that a moderate effect size is roughly .50. This finding is consistent with the report of the National Reading Panel regarding particularly strong effect sizes for phonemic awareness training for young prereaders at risk.

TRAINING STUDIES WITH BEGINNING READERS

Phonemic awareness is rarely taught to reading-age children without being linked to phonics instruction. The use of letters and of linkages with phonics training are among the recommendations of the National Reading Panel (2000). The studies in this and the following section on remedial readers are really about the effects of phonemic awareness training in combination with phonics.

Around the time that children are exposed to formal reading instruction in first grade, there is an increase in ability to segment phonemes in spoken words. Where invented spellings in kindergarten usually involve more consonants than vowels, early in first grade there is often a dramatic increase in ability to represent the presence of vowels. Ability to separate vowels from consonants and, then, consonants from each other within consonant clusters, are the important phonemic segmentation milestones during the early primary grades. Catherine Snow and her colleagues on the Committee on the Prevention of Reading Difficulties in Young Children for the National Research Council suggest continuing phonemic awareness training into Grade 2 and linking it to explicit instruction in phonics for children who have not yet learned to read independently. They also suggest continuing phonemic awareness training for Grade 2 independent readers through linking it to spelling instruction (Snow, Burns, and Griffin 1998).

D. B. Elkonin and his colleagues used one of the first procedures designed to promote phonemic awareness in beginning readers in the 1960s and 1970s in what was then the Soviet Union. Their training tasks used pictures to help children remember the target word and boxes to help children conceptualize the sound structure of a spoken word. Small blank tiles were moved from the picture to the boxes as the word was said aloud, one phoneme at a time. Elkonin's task has provided a model for a number of researchers (e.g., Ball and Blachman 1991; Uhry and Shepherd 1993a). See the illustrated example provided here.

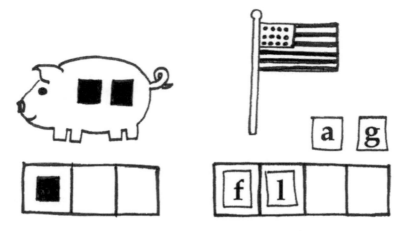

Elkonin-type boxes with unlettered and lettered tiles to move into boxes to represent the phonemes in spoken words.

As Elkonin's training progressed, colors were used to differentiate vowels from consonants. Eventually, letters were provided on the tiles, beginning with vowels. With the introduction of vowels, an activity known as *word changes* was added to the basic segmentation exercises. An English equivalent would involve changing the word *cat* to *cut* by exchanging the *a* tile for one with *u*. Patricia and James Cunningham's *Making Words* technique uses this method (1992). Consonants were added later and the word-changing exercises continued. Word changing is an especially effective way to teach children awareness of consonant clusters (e.g., clap-lap-cap-clap; sit-slit-split-spit-pit). Several training studies by various Russian researchers are described briefly by Elkonin and reported as successful in the translated reviews of this literature, but none of the research methods is described in detail (Elkonin 1963, 1973).

Benita Blachman includes phoneme segmentation in a five-part lesson she has used in several studies of beginning reading in inner-city schools. The lesson includes these five components: (1) letter-sound practice, (2) segmenting and blending activities similar to Elkonin's *word changes* using letters in a pocket chart, (3) reading phonetically regular words and sight words, (4) reading from phonetically controlled as well as trade story books, and (5) writing from dictation. There is evidence from several of Blachman's studies of a significant advantage in reading for children who were trained, in comparison with controls (Blachman 1987; Blachman et al. 1994, 1999).

In a study carried out with Margaret Jo Shepherd, we used segmenting and spelling training in a school setting with 22 first graders (a mix of at-risk and normally developing readers). Using a sequence of cvc (e.g., *map, hit*) and ccvcc words (e.g., *flap, milk, blast*), the children were taught in small groups to segment with blank blocks and later with lettered blocks, to type these words into a computer from dictation, and to play computer spelling games such as Reader Rabbit (The Learning Company) with these words. All activities stressed analyzing phonemes in spoken words. Elkonin-type *word-change* activities were used to teach consonant clusters. After seven months, these first graders had a significant advantage over controls taught in small groups using traditional phonics strategies on a variety of reading skills. The most dramatic difference being in phonetic reading of nonsense words (Uhry and Shepherd 1993a).

We found this training to be effective in a clinical setting as well. Twelve first and second graders were trained in an after-school-tutoring center. Note that KM was one of these children (see Chapters 3 and 25). The children were considered to be at risk because of poor phonemic awareness skills, family history of dyslexia, and, in the case of the second graders, failure to acquire reading. After-school tutoring twice a week included letter-sound training, segmentation and spelling training, and guided reading in both phonics–controlled (decodable) and narratively controlled (meaning based) children's literature. Over a five-month period, they made significant gains in phonemic awareness as well as in sight word reading, nonsense word reading, and spelling tests. Although remediation was not complete at the end of this initial training period in terms of catching up with age peers, the anticipated discrepancy between word reading, viewed in the literature as remediable, and nonsense word reading, viewed as a chronic deficit, did not develop. In fact, after training, nonsense word reading was stronger than word reading for the group as a whole and for 8 of the 12 children when considered individually. The increase in sight word reading was also substantial. This finding supports Ehri's model, mentioned in Chapter 1, in which phonemic awareness plays an important role as a foundation for the acquisition of even irregularly spelled words (Uhry and Shepherd 1997).

Patricia and Charles Lindamood were early advocates of phonemic awareness training. Their program begins with an emphasis on oral-motor awareness of sound production. Descriptive labels are used to refer to the mouth action used in producing different sound categories. For example, the term *lip poppers* is used for sounds such as /p/ and /b/. Once students are proficient at associating these pictures with sounds, training moves to exercises involving the manipulation of markers representing phonemes in spoken words (see Elkonin 1963, 1973). These exercises also incorporate the descriptive labels mentioned above. One research study of this method reports that second- through fifth-grade scores rose over a five-year period for children who began this training in first grade (Howard 1982). The program can be used with prereaders as well as much older students for whom oral word analysis is integrated with phonics instruction. This program is described more fully in Chapter 24.

The Lindamood Program was an important component of Joseph Torgesen's tutoring treatment in the longitudinal kindergarten prevention study reported in the previous section. Phonemic awareness training via the Lindamood Program continued into Grades 1 and 2. After an initial period of focus on sound analysis and articulatory gesture, the program involves the use of letters to represent phonemes. Word building is linked to text reading in several phonics-based readers. The group with phonemic awareness and systematic phonics instruction did significantly better on Grade 2 measures of phonemic awareness as well as on measures of word and nonword reading in comparison with the three other groups (i.e., embedded phonics, classroom reading support, and nontutored controls). That is, kindergarten phonemic awareness training, in combination with later phonics instruction continued through Grade 2, had a positive effect on word reading (Torgesen et al. 1999)

Barbara Foorman and her colleagues carried out several large-scale longitudinal training studies in Texas supported by the National Institute of Child Health and Human Development. In one, they explored the question of what type of phonics instruction was effective (Foorman et al. 1998). Close to three hundred children in Grades 1 and 2 qualified for this study as Title I students scoring in the lowest 18th percentile on a kindergarten literacy screening. The ethnicity of the participants was 60% African American, 20% Hispanic, and 20% White. One of the three classroom-based treatment groups involved Direct Code (DC) instruction using direct instruction in phonological awareness and phonics through use of the Open Court Reading Program (Open Court Reading Program 1995; Adams, Bereiter et al.

1995). Open Court emphasizes phonological awareness in the primary grades and teaches it in Kindergarten and early Grade 1 without use of letters (e.g., clapping syllables, singing songs using alliteration, blending phonemes said aloud by puppets). Even once phonics instruction begins, phonemic awareness instruction is kept separate and does not involves the use of letters, with letter-based phonics training following in later lessons. The second treatment, involved phonemic awareness training together with embedded code (EC) instruction using an onset-rime (i.e., word family) program developed by Elfrieda Heibert and her colleagues (Heibert et al. 1992). The third program involved whole language activities without emphasis on phonemic awareness. The children in the direct code (DC) group using the Open Court phonemic awareness program had an advantage on PA measures at the end of the year-long training in comparison to the children receiving embedded instruction or no instruction in PA. Note that while these children held an advantage in PA, their word-reading scores did not exceed those of children in the embedded code (EC) onset-rime phonics treatment, which is discussed in the chapter on phonics that follows.

PA TRAINING STUDIES WITH REMEDIAL READERS

As with beginning reading programs, remedial reading programs are rarely based on phoneme segmentation training alone. It is more usual to find phonemic awareness training included as one component of a phonics program. This makes it hard to isolate the specific effect for phonemic training.

The Lindamood program is widely used in remedial programs with older children. A team working with Joseph Torgesen in Florida used the 1984 version of this program, Auditory Discrimination in Depth (ADD), in an after-school-tutoring program to train ten dyslexic children (Alexander et al. 1991). This successful project is reported in more detail in Chapter 24. Of particular note was the dramatic growth in both phonemic awareness and nonsense word reading, contrary to the widely held opinion that poor nonsense word reading is an enduring and hard-to-remediate characteristic of the reader with dyslexia. The program is distinctive in that it initially teaches sounds without letters, even with older children and adults.

Maureen Lovett has also carried out studies with older remedial readers (Lovett and Steinbach 1997). In a study reported in Chapter 7 in greater detail, both phonemic awareness and phonics training were used with a range of ages, including children in Grades 5 and 6. One instructional group received training in direct instruction in phonemic analysis and oral blending taught in combination with phonics (PHAB/DI). As in the Lindamood-based study above, this group surpassed controls in both phonemic awareness and nonword reading by the end of training.

The connections between segmenting and spelling, suggested by Snow, Burns, and Griffin (1998) for Grade 2 children, appear to work, as well, for older children with dyslexia. There is evidence from a year-long classroom-based case study of three bright fourth-grade children with dyslexia, segmenting was linked with spelling techniques. This method was used to see whether increasing letter-based phoneme awareness could help these children become more skilled with vowel digraphs and trigraphs (e.g., *au*, *igh*) in reading. Using a single-subject design with multiple measures taken over baseline and treatments, several different traditional phonics-based training conditions failed to produce improvement in ability to generalize vowel patterns to the reading of nonwords. The improvement in generalization to these unfamiliar nonwords was dramatic only when spelling-based phoneme analysis training of new vowel patterns was used (Uhry 1993b).

Joanna Williams was an early advocate of phonemic awareness training. Her ABD's of Reading (analysis, blending, and decoding) was used with older learning disabled students in New York City public school special education classes (Williams 1980). The program began with auditory syllable analysis, followed by phoneme analysis using only nine phonemes, in an adaptation of the Elkonin technique. At the next step the phonemes, which were represented by wooden squares, were blended into bigrams and trigrams. Later, letters were introduced on the squares and the children manipulated the squares to form words. Eventually, six more letters were added to the original nine, and practice on ccvc and cvcc words was introduced. Williams reported significantly greater improvement in phonemic analysis and blending skills for these children in comparison with controls. Skill transfer was noted in superior ability to read nonsense words.

Although the overall meta-analysis of the National Reading Panel indicated relatively small effect sizes for older children with disabilities, these particular treatments are encouraging. Although not all used letters for phonemic awareness training at the beginning, all used letters eventually, and all integrated this training into work with phonics for reading or spelling or both.

IDEAS FOR INSTRUCTION IN PHONEMIC AWARENESS

In planning instruction in phonemic awareness, keep in mind the following principles developed from the findings of the National Reading Panel:

1. Start early. Phonemic awareness training is most effective in kindergarten.

2. Phonemic awareness training is most effective for young children at risk for reading failure, but is also effective with young emergent and beginning readers, and with older remedial readers.

3. Phoneme awareness does not take much time to teach. Research shows the effectiveness of around 20 hours over the course of a year (e.g., 2-3 times a week for 10-20 minutes a session). Time should vary depending on children's needs.

4. In studies reported by the National Reading Panel, there was no evidence that instruction needed to be on a tutorial basis to be effective. In fact, in the studies reported, those with small group instruction were more effective than one-to-one or large group work.

5. Include letters as representations of phonemes as soon as children know some letter names. That is, teach letter-sounds together with phonemic awareness.

6. Teach only one or two tasks at a time rather than using many different formats. For example, at mid-kindergarten, blending and initial phoneme segmentation might be the focus, while early in grade one the task might involve full phoneme segmentation and spelling of short-vowel words.

7. Choose tasks that are a good match for a child's phonemic development as well as a good match for current level of literacy. Stretching and segmenting initial sounds helps kindergarten children learn to invent spellings. Word change tasks help Grade 2 children learn to use word family knowledge in conventional spellings.

Following are classroom ideas for increasing phonemic awareness. They are not arranged systematically but are included to provide an idea of the sorts of activities used in studies of effective instruction. Many of the activities are based on the training research outlined above and are available in publications for teachers. Be cautious about jumping from idea to idea. Keep in mind that being systematic and sticking with a few formats works best. It is important to follow a systematic progression of sounds, with activities to support this progression.

EMERGENT READERS

- Use reading aloud as an opportunity to sensitize children to the sounds in words. Use books with rhyme and alliteration. Emphasize these sound elements with your voice. Slow down and let the children predict an end-of-line rhyme. Slow down and stretch out the first sounds in pairs of alliterative words. Hallie Yopp has many good suggestions for the use of literature in developing phonemic awareness (Yopp 1995).

- Use puppets to sort by initial sound. "This is Ralph Raven and he really, really likes rrrraisins. And rrrrulers. And rrrrocks. Do

you think he likes iiiice cream? Or rrrrice? Or mmmmustard?"
Set up centers for sound sorting once a phoneme has been
introduced. Use a small bin or shoebox to collect small objects.
While this activity begins with the focus on sound alone, it can
be used as a way of introducing a letter. The bin or box can be
labeled with the letter. Some children will need additional direct
instruction from a teacher in these centers and others will be
able to practice sounds independently.

- Coordinate consonant name learning with phonemes used in
  sound matching and initial segmentation training. Use key word
  pictures and short jingles to teach the names and sounds of letters.
  Benita Blachman's book includes large reproducible alphabet picture cards for coloring. For example, in one, the letter *r* is embedded in a picture for coloring while reciting, "red rooster in red
  running shoes" (from *Road to the Code* by Blachman et al. 2000).
- Pretend to be an imaginary troll who talks a "funny way" (e.g.,
  "I'm going to give you a /b/-/ike/" (from *Phonemic Awareness in
  Young Children* by Adams et al. 1998).
- Play the "fix it" game. Use a puppet to read aloud a story with
  some words stretched out (e.g., /f-aaaa-t/). Have the children
  blend the sounds or "fix" them so they sound like real words
  (from *Road to the Code* by Blachman et al. 2000).
- Play *Mrs. Magic Mouth*. Start with simply moving one chip from
  the pictured mouth down to the line below while repeating a
  phoneme said aloud by the teacher. Once the task is clear, practice listening for multiple sounds with multiple chips (e.g., /t/-
  /t/ or /a/-/t/. Eventually, model breaking apart the phonemes
  in a word said aloud and pulling down a chip for each segmented phoneme. The sequence should proceed from two and
  then three phoneme words with short /a/ and then to words
  with short /a/ and consonant clusters (Uhry and Ehri 1999).

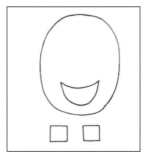 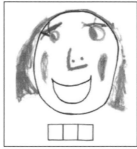 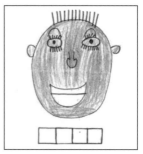

Each child will need a template for designing his or her Mr. or Mrs. Magic Mouth. Begin with
two boxes for two-phoneme words and add boxes as the child develops greater sophistication
with phonemic segmentation. Linnea Ehri is credited with the idea of tokens moving from a
mouth to a sequence of boxes as phonemes are said aloud by the child (Uhry and Ehri 1999).

- Once children know letter names, model inventing spellings for short, simple words. Stretch out the sounds. "Mmmmmike." Ask, "What letter sounds like /mmmm/"? Write the letter *M*. Ask, "Mike, does that look like part of your name?
- Read *The Hungry Thing* (Slepian and Seidler 1967) aloud. In this picture book the Hungry Thing is fed foods such as *schmancakes* (i.e., pancakes). Use a center to encourage children to fix pretend lunches of plastic foods that they can re-name by rhyming. This is a form of phoneme deletion and substitution (Yopp and Yopp 2000).
- Songs for teaching phonemic awareness are suggested in an article by Hallie Yopp (1992).

BEGINNING READERS

- *Use Sound Bingo to Introduce Vowel Sounds.* Use bingo cards with pictures of objects beginning with a few designated phonemes, including a few familiar consonants and vowels and a new vowel sound. Roll a lettered die, which can be made from a small square wooden block. Children take turns rolling the die and pronouncing the letter sound. Have all of the children use a blank disk to cover pictured objects beginning with the rolled sound. This game combines phonics (i.e., making letter-sound response more automatic) with phonemic awareness (i.e., saying the names of pictured items and then analyzing them for designated phonemes). Blachman's book has reproducible bingo cards for a range of developmental levels (from *Road to the Code* by Blachman et al. 2000).
- *Use Spelling to Teach Segmenting.* Encourage stretching of sounds to invent spellings during process writing. Remind children to use patterns that have been taught. That is, help them link the short /a/ sound in an invented spelling to short /a/ spelled *a* in a known word.
- *Integrate Phonemic Awareness, Phonics, and Spelling Instruction.* Develop a sequence of weekly spelling words to use for learning in all three areas. Start with review of just a few consonants and a single short vowel. The usual first short vowel is a and there are a number of phonics controlled readers and trade books that focus on words such as *cat, sat, Sam,* and *Dad. Recipe for Reading* has wonderful word lists for this.
- *Teach Blending Using a Puppet Who Talks in Sound Segments.* Coordinate this blending game with other phonemic awareness training by using the same sounds across activities (from Open Court 1995; Adams et al. 1995).

- *Teach Blending as you Move Children through Routines.* Short periods of instruction can be fit into routines such as lunch lines. "Line up for lunch /J/-/o/-/s/-/e/."

REMEDIAL READERS

- Many of the game-like formats for teaching phonemic awareness to pre-readers and beginning readers can seem babyish to older students. Many older students can be better motivated by keeping charts as records of their own progress.
- Use assessment to identify exactly what needs teaching. Be particularly sensitive to the reteaching of previously taught material because of issues of demoralization. Be certain that older children understanding the difference between initial understanding and mastery at the automatic level, and of the importance of both.
- Integrate phonemic awareness with phonics instruction for both reading and spelling.
- Older readers with severe difficulties in phonemic awareness may need an intense and extensive program such as the Lindamood program (Chapter 24) in order to make the dramatic progress needed in order to catch.

COMPUTER ASSISTED INSTRUCTION IN PHONEMIC AWARENESS

One advantage of computer assisted instruction (CAI) is that systematic, carefully sequenced instruction can be individualized and matched to a child's needs and pace. Another is the strong motivation provided by computer game formats. Computers provide the practice afforded by workbooks but, unlike workbooks, are interactive and provide sound, a critical component of phonemic awareness. A number of researchers have provided effective instruction in phonemic awareness using CAI. Two examples follow:

- *Daisy Quest* provides opportunities to match words by rhyme and by beginning, ending, and middle sounds. Its companion program, *Daisy's Castle,* provides practice in recognizing words blended by onset-rimes and from a sequence of phonemes. Children trained in phonemic awareness using Daisy Quest were superior in word reading compared to controls trained on the computer in phonics (Torgesen and Barker 1995).
- *Reader Rabbit* includes a spelling format with segmentation training (The Learning Company). Children listen as the computer "speaks" a word matching a pictured object. Then they segment its sounds and type a letter that appears in an Elkonin-type box

for each of the phonemes. This Reader Rabbit game was part of a collection of activities used by first graders who were superior to controls in word reading after eight months of training in a study carried out with first graders (Uhry and Shepherd 1993a).

Several phonemic awareness intervention programs for young children are reviewed in Chapter 14, *Early Interventions*. Most of the programs for older readers reviewed in Part III incorporate phonemic awareness instruction.

6

Spelling to Read

This chapter on the spellings of emergent readers and the role of developmental spelling in early reading acquisition is placed here because many researchers have provided evidence that early spelling is the link between phonemic awareness and reading. Regularities in these spellings are an indication of the developing awareness of the phonemic structure of spoken language, an important prerequisite to early reading.

Frith's stage theory (see Chapter 1) is supported by research indicating that spelling precedes reading at what she calls the *alphabetic phase* of reading acquisition. To spell, one needs to use a left-to-right, letter-by-letter strategy, the very strategy that is so important to the acquisition of the *alphabetic* or *cipher* decoding strategy (Ehri and Wilce 1987b; Morris 1993; Morris et al. 2003; Uhry and Shepherd 1993a). According to Frith, it is the transition to the alphabetic stage through the strategies practiced in spelling by ear that is such a struggle for children with dyslexia.

INVENTED SPELLING

The terms *invented spelling* and *creative spelling* are used for spellings that children construct themselves, in contrast with spellings memorized from conventional models. There is evidence that children do this by listening for the sounds in spoken words and representing them with letter names (Treiman 1994). The letter name *m*, for example, sounds like the /m/ sound at the beginning of *monkey*.

Maria Montessori (1964) was an early advocate of the theory that writing precedes reading developmentally and that it is thus more natural for children to begin reading instruction by composing their own words, rather than by attempting to read the words of others. Use of children's compositions (and dictated stories from prereaders) as text for reading instruction was the foundation of the Language Experience Approach so popular as part of the American Open Classroom movement of the early 1970s. Sylvia Ashton-Warner was widely read during that period. She encouraged her young New Zealand Maori students to express themselves in what she called *organic writing*—writing chosen by the children themselves and based on topics of great personal interest. She wrote that both content and spelling belonged to the realm of the child and "the vent of creativity" (Ashton-Warner 1963, p. 52). Her work provided many of the principles of process writing developed and popularized by Donald Graves (1983) and Lucy Calkins (1983).

The term *invented spelling* has its foundation in constructivist theory, which proposes that we are active participants in building our own learning. Although five-year-olds are still limited in terms of being able to memorize conventional spellings, many are quite adept at creating spelling systems based on what they know about speech sounds and letter names.

Carol Chomsky (1971, 1979) believes, as did Montessori, that building an awareness of the communicative purposes of written language is an important advantage of having children write before teaching them to read. Both Chomsky and Charles Read (1971) realized a second advantage. Through extensive samples of preschool children's writing, they realized that children's very early spellings are created, not from knowledge of orthography, but from their emerging understandings of the sound structure of spoken language. They realized, too, that these spellings were related to phonemic awareness and that they are developmental. That is, they unfold in predictable patterns.

INVENTED SPELLING IS DEVELOPMENTAL

Edmund Henderson and his students at the University of Virginia developed a model of five developmental spelling stages. Richard Gentry describes these stages in regard to writing samples collected by Glenda Bissex as her young son, Paul, taught himself to write (Bissex 1980; Gentry 1982). See Templeton and Morris (2000) for more information about the Virginia studies. The following discussion uses Henderson's and Gentry's work and is illustrated with spellings that I have collected from children over time.

Pre-Phonetic Stage: Random Strings of Letters

The earliest stage involves random strings of letters. Children at this stage understand that speech is represented with print, and they know how to write some letters, but they do not use letters to represent specific speech sounds. The following example of Maddie's preschool writing shows an understanding of writing as a form involving a letter string with a period at the end.

ZSRJXPHOGCANMDDLFEIt.

Another of her writing samples demonstrates situational understanding of writing. When asked what she had written, she said it was her homework. Note the mix of letters and numbers.

HOVLEUFI411

Maddie's grocery list below shows understanding of one function of writing. Although most of the items were nonspecific ("It's stuff to buy"), she asked her mother to spell two of the words aloud before she wrote them down, indicating that she knew that the other items were not spelled in enough detail to be understood.

ADESS
OHIiL
SSSSS
MILK
ICECREAM
Xtp
tOtO
tOtO

The following was written by another preschooler and then dictated ("Dear Nanny, I am coming to see you. Love, Emily"). The letter E at the end may stand for her name; she knew how to write E for Emily.

TWAE

These mostly random strings of letters are typical of the pre-phonetic stage of spelling. Some children begin writing letters and playing at writing text as early as 2 or 3 while others come to school without letter knowledge. This stage of spelling and writing is not based in phonemic processing. Coming to school without the ability or inclination to write random strings of letters as a playful and pleasurable activity is not necessarily an early indicator of dyslexia. Rather, it could be an indication of lack of exposure and opportunity. A lack of the ability to remember letter names is, however, an early indicator.

The Semi-Phonetic Stage: Letters Represent Phonemes

At this stage children begin to understand the alphabetic principle, the idea that a temporal sequence of speech sounds maps onto a spatial sequence of letters. Typically they begin by representing whole words with sound-alike letter names as in Maddie's valentine below. She begins with a random string of letters but uses the letter I for the word *I* and the letter U for the word *you*. She also uses the letter L to stand for the word *love*. In doing this, she has demonstrated beginning ability to segment phonemes.

PGCAD ILU   Happy Valentine's Day. I love you.

There are two indicators of the alphabetic principle here. First, phonemes are represented by letters. Second, the sounds are represented sequentially from left to right. The letters, while not always conventional representations, are perceptually logical.

Spellings in kindergarten typically progress from random strings of letters (pre-phonetic) to use of letters to represent initial consonant sounds, and later, both initial and final sounds (semi-phonetic). For example, typical spellings for *cat* are either K or KT. Some spellings seem confusing to teachers, but are quite logical from a child's point of view. For example, the spellings J and JS for the word *dress* are logical given that the initial sound in *dress* is closer to the sound made by the letter name J than the letter name D. Teachers need this linguistic knowledge in order to keep track of their children's progress.

During kindergarten, children typically begin story writing with drawings and the addition of a few words. Teachers expect the stories to lengthen and to become more logical in terms of letter representations of sounds. Analysis of these spellings draws on linguistic knowledge and illustrates the importance of Louisa Moats' stance that this knowledge base is important to teachers. The following kindergarten drawing of a car, complete with muffler, includes the story," I want to drive."

Following is teacher detective work:

1. *I* is used to represent the sound of long /i/. This is not only logical but conventional.

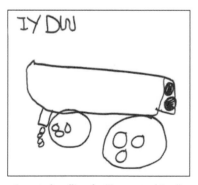

Invented spelling for "I want to drive."

2. *Y* is used to represent the word *want*. The name of the letter Y is close to the sound that adults usually represent with the letter W. Y is a common kindergarten spelling for the /w/ sound. He has segmented off the sound /w/ and represented it with the letter name Y, which is his best available perceptual match for this sound.

3. *D* is used to represent the word *to*. Using a D rather than a T for the /t/ sound is also common in young children. The sounds /d/ and /t/ are formed in the same manner, with the tip of the tongue against the roof of the mouth. The difference between them is that one is voiced and the other is not.

4. *W* is used to represent the word *drive*. This is harder to explain than the above spellings. The name of the letter W could be written as "doubleyou," and words beginning with this name's initial sound could be spelled D. However, this isn't a good explanation in this case because the /dr/ sound in *drive* is closer to /j/ than /d/. This could be a random representation. Many children include spellings typical of more than one stage in a single word.

Teachers of young children need to teach themselves to do these sorts of analyses of invented spellings. It is important to be able to keep track of linguistic development. Lack of progress in invented spelling is an important and reliable indicator of early struggle in learning to read. While random letter representation is typical early in the process, we expect change toward more logical representations. Difficulty making progress in invented spelling is a strong predictor of dyslexia. See the section below on using invented spelling as a predictor.

Instruction at this stage involves both explicit phonemic awareness and letter name instruction. For some children short periods of large group instruction may be enough. For children at risk for dyslexia, additional small group work and individual support in segmenting phonemes during writing is crucial. It doesn't take a teacher long to help a child with, "Stretch it out. What letter makes that sound?"

The Phonetic Stage: All Phonemes Are Represented

At the phonetic stage, all phonemes are represented in spellings. The word dress might be written as JRAS. Although this is not conventional, all four of the phonemes are mapped onto letters whose names are perceptually reasonable matches for the word's phonemes. Progress from the Semi-Phonetic to the Phonetic spelling stage is gradual. Typically developing children can usually represent a few vowels in their spellings by late kindergarten or early first grade and can sequence sounds in words and words in sentences. Use of vowels in spellings is a good indicator of developmental readiness for learning a few short vowel sounds to use in reading.

In the following spelling, note that the missing letters are all consonants that occur in clusters (i.e., *n* in *want*, both *l* and *t* in *oldest*.) It is harder to segment a consonant within a cluster than a consonant surrounded by vowels (Treiman 1993; Uhry and Ehri 1999).

I WAT to BE The aDis   I want to be the oldest.

Nasal consonants, such as the missing *n* in WAT (i.e., *want*) are particularly hard to segment in this situation. The sound of the letter *n* is actually perceived as a change in the sound of the preceding vowel, in this case the /a/. In his book on teaching spelling, Richard Gentry provides other examples of this phenomenon (e.g., *jump* as JUP, *stamp* as STAP) (Gentry and Gillet 1993).

The two first graders who wrote the following were responding after listening to their teacher read aloud from *Charlotte's Web*. These two children are in the same grade, but at very different levels of phonemic awareness.

BLIbud   I liked when he said she was blood thirsty.
I lace Shrlit's Wib   I like *Charlotte's Web*.

The first sample is difficult to read. Not all sounds are represented. The I is in the middle rather than at the beginning. There are six letters and nine words. The writer of the second sample represents all speech sounds. The vowels are not conventionally spelled, but all vowel sounds are represented. Keep in mind that the vowel before an *r* is hard to perceive. Notice the *e* at the end of *lace*. This child is already showing awareness of orthographic conventions.

The Transitional Stage: Beginning Use of Orthographic Units

Orthographic spelling makes use of spelling conventions with units of sound represented by units of letters. This is a visual rather than phonetic strategy but it builds on phonemic awareness as a frame for sequencing and for identifying the sound units that need to be spelled. Children at this stage are responsive to memorizing words and remember spellings rather than sounding them out. They are learning to visualize print as well as to listen for sounds.

The following sample accompanied a detailed picture of two people watching a crocodile, a dinosaur, and two fish swimming in a pond.

The PePL r WOCHeN The POD.

It is transitional in its correct spelling of *The* and its use of *ch*. The sound /ch/is more typically spelled with just an H in young spellers. The child does not include the *n* in *pond*. Nasal sounds before other consonants are hard to hear and develop during this period of transition to orthography.

The transition to orthographic spelling can be conceptualized as learning to use memory for visual patterns rather than phonology, but it involves morphology, or units of meaning, as well. One spelling that is almost universal in phonetic spellers is use of the letter t to indicate some past tenses (e.g., stopt, kisst, walkt) (Bryant, Nunes, and Bindman 1997). Learning that the unit -*ed* indicates the past tense is characteristic of the shift to orthographic spelling. This involves use of morphology as well as orthography.

Conventional or Correct Spellings

This fifth stage involves orthographically correct spelling. This stage is accomplished little by little over long periods of time as orthographic conventions (e.g., the igh in sigh and light) and rules for endings (e.g., hoping, not hopeing) are taught. All of these conventions and rules are supported by the early ear-spelling strategy of sequencing sounds and listening to be sure a spelling includes all the sounds.

In older children with dyslexia, conventional spelling takes a long time to develop. Spellings often do not reflect a strong foundation in either the sounds or orthographic units necessary to success. Earlier stages of spelling have not been mastered. The following is a short story written by a fourth grader in a class for gifted children with dyslexia.

> Time 500,00,00 bc The gobs sent
> amastr to er da
> cristulbolso went
> hey gum and They in Flamostr

What is worrisome about his spellings is that he is still not representing all of the sounds in words, or even all words in sentences. Leaving out sounds is a red flag in children beyond first grade.

INVENTED SPELLING IS RULE BASED

One thing that is apparent from the above sequence of spellings is that pre-conventional, invented, rule-based substitutions and omissions are constructed by children much as grammar is constructed (Chomsky 1971, 1979; Read 1971, 1975, 1986). The use of Y for the /w/ sound by many children is evidence that children construct a rule system in which letter names are paired with phonemes (Treiman 1994). No one tells children to do this. There is remarkable consistency in the patterns of spelling approximations among children (e.g., the letter *H* is frequently used to represent the sound of the letters *ch*; the letter *J* is used to represent the sound of the letters *dr* as in *drum*). Again, these children appear to be constructing a set of rules for spelling by linking the names of letters and the sounds of phonemes.

RESEARCH ON INVENTED SPELLING AND READING

Carol Chomsky maintained that the invented spelling approach enhances phonemic awareness. From her observations of children composing self-generated stories as part of their first grade schooling. Chomsky concluded:

> The invented spellers, during the months that they engage in their writing activities, are providing themselves with excellent and valuable practice in phonetics, word analysis and synthesis, and letter-sound correspondences (Chomsky 1979).

In order to invent a spelling, one must be able to identify and sequence phonemes in spoken language. Sounding out spellings is a form of self-instruction in phonemic awareness and supports beginning reading. A number of researchers have found that instruction in spelling by ear provides an advantage in learning to read. A number of researchers have explored the relationship between invented spelling and reading.

INVENTED SPELLING PREDICTS READING

Several researchers have used invented spelling as a predictor of later reading. Virginia Mann and her colleagues explored the relationship between invented spelling and later reading. They administered a test of invented spellings to 29 mid-kindergarten children. The spellings were scored using a developmental scale with credit given for non-conventional spellings on the basis of phonological accuracy using a scale of 1 to 3 and with 4 given for conventional spellings. These developmental spelling scores were significantly correlated with mid-first-grade scores in both word identification and word attack. One interesting finding was that the degree to which children reversed letters in kindergarten was not correlated with first grade reading. Mann also looked at the relationship between invented spelling and underlying linguistic processes and skills. She found that phoneme segmentation and letter writing accounted for almost all of the variance in invented spelling. That is, no other factors were significantly correlated once these factors were accounted for (Mann, Tobin, and Wilson 1987).

Darrell Morris and his colleague Jan Perney carried out a similar study. Morris was interested in seeing if invented spelling was correlated with later reading because he felt that classroom spellings provided an opportunity for teachers to assess linguistic development on an ongoing basis. They administered both an invented spelling test and the Metropolitan Readiness Test to 75 children in September of the first grade year. Morris used a developmental scoring system for the spellings that was based on Henderson's stages as outlined earlier in this chapter. Again, the developmental spelling scores were significantly correlated with later word reading and with the Metropolitan Achievement Test administered at the end of the school year. Interestingly, the invented spellings were a stronger predictor of later reading than was the Metropolitan Readiness Test (Morris and Perney 1984).

INVENTED SPELLING AND FINGER-POINT READING

The above studies indicate that early invented spelling is strongly correlated with first grade reading. It is also strongly correlated with finger-point reading. Finger-point reading is a kindergarten and first grade phenomenon in which children who cannot yet read listen to a story read aloud from a big book. They listen so many times that they are able to memorize it, and then, saying each word from memory, match each spoken word, by pointing, with word in print. Finger-point reading and invented spelling have much in common in terms of the strategies they each employ. Segmenting phonemes and naming letters are utilized in both.

Darrell Morris calls finger-point reading *concept of print in text*. He argues that being able to segment an initial phoneme and to associate it with a printed letter enables children to make this voice-print match. In several studies in which measures were collected on an ongoing basis during first grade, Morris found that segmenting initial phonemes was a pre-condition to finger-point reading. He also found that successful finger-point reading appeared to teach children how to segment beyond the initial phoneme, a pre-condition for true reading (Morris 1993; Morris et al. 2003).

Linnea Ehri carried out a study in which she explored the skills and knowledge necessary for success with different aspects of finger-point reading. She worked with 36 five-year-olds, some of whom could read a few preprimer words, but were not really readers yet. Using regression analysis, she found that knowing how to read a few words contributed to children's ability to learn new words from the finger-point reading activity. She also found that phonemic segmentation ability and letter knowledge contributed to ability to finger-point correctly as text was said aloud, and for finding words in the text designated by the examiner. She made the important point that although this is an effective reading method for children who know letter names and a few words, and who are skilled at segmenting, it is unrealistic to think that this method will be effective with children without these skills (Ehri and Sweet 1991).

There is evidence from a study using regression analysis with urban kindergarten children that skill in invented spelling makes a greater contribution to finger-point reading than either phonemic awareness or letter naming or a combination of the two (Uhry 1999, 2002a). Finger-point reading and invented spelling have these two skills in common, but they also have the alphabetic principle in common. They both use the mapping of sounds onto letters in a sequence. This third characteristic may explain the power of invented spelling to facilitate reading, as demonstrated through the training studies that follow.

INVENTED SPELLING SUPPORTS EARLY READING

Bradley and Bryant's longitudinal study of the effect of PA training using letters is described in detail in Chapter 5, *Phonemic Awareness.* Analyzing sounds in words and representing them with letters is a form of spelling. These children, who were at risk for reading failure because of weakness in PA at the onset of the study, read and spelled better than controls after two years of training in matching oral words by rhyme and alliteration and in segmenting and spelling these words with plastic letters (Bradley and Bryant 1983, 1985).

In a study mentioned in Chapter 5, Ehri and Wilce found that kindergarten children trained for a few weeks in spelling exercises in which orally presented words were segmented and then spelled with lettered tiles had an advantage over controls in reading new words with these letters. These researchers state:

> Spelling might be expected to contribute to reading skill because, in learning to spell, children are taught some of the elements of decoding skill. They learn to divide pronunciations of words into their constituent sounds. They learn to represent sounds and words visually by converting sounds into letters. Both of these elements, phonemic awareness and letter-sound knowledge, are thought to be important components in reading words (Ehri and Wilce 1987b, p. 48).

Clarke (1988) reports a study of four Canadian classrooms using two different spelling approaches for weekly writing activities. In one, children were encouraged to spell correctly with the teacher supplying model spellings. In the other, children were encouraged to invent their own spellings. By March of the first-grade year, the invented spellers had become stronger decoders. Results were particularly striking when the initially lowest achievers from each classroom were compared across groups. Thus, there is support in these three studies for using spelling involving analysis of phoneme segments as a method of teaching beginning reading. This seems to support Frith's model of alphabetic spelling preceding and leading the way into alphabetic reading.

Uhry and Shepherd (1993a) worked with small groups of children twice a week in 20 minute sessions over the course of the childrens' first-grade school year, and taught them phoneme segmentation (e.g., "What sound do you hear at the beginning of *pig*?") in combination with spelling (e.g., "What letter spells the /p/ sound?"). Children trained in segmentation/spelling showed an advantage in word reading, story reading, and nonsense word reading (e.g., *ift, bim*) in comparison with children trained in letter-sound associations and whole word reading. The advantage in nonsense word reading suggests an advantage in alphabetic decoding. Instruction here was carefully sequenced in terms of introducing words composed of relatively transparent letter sounds (e.g., *map,*) early in the training and limiting instruction to words that are phonetically regular. Keep in mind that the training in this study was very explicit. Children were encouraged to listen carefully, to say each phoneme in order, and then to spell the phonemes. In addition, they were provided with feedback and opportunities to practice to mastery.

Rebecca Treiman's book *Beginning to Spell* (1993) documents the developmental spellings of children in a whole language classroom over the course of their first grade year, much in the tradition of Charles Read's work (1971, 1986) and Glenda Bissex's *GNYS AT WRK* (1980). Treiman entered the invented spellings she collected into a specially designed computer program to analyze frequencies of phoneme spellings under different orthographic conditions. Treiman draws several conclusions from analysis of her data: (a) invented spellings do not become permanent misspellings in first graders, and, in fact, they encourage children to think about the relationships between sounds and letters, and (b) the process of inventing spellings helps children acquire the alphabetic principle. This book is especially useful for teachers seeking insight into the linguistic complexities of invented spelling.

READING INSTRUCTION FEATURING SPELLING TO READ
THE WRITING ROAD TO READING

The Spalding Method is a beginning reading program for classroom use that starts with spelling and writing. The teacher's manual, developed by Romalda Spalding, is called *The Writing Road to Reading* (Spalding and Spalding 1986). Spalding was trained in the Orton-Gillingham approach by Dr. Orton and then went on to develop a language arts program that could be used with a whole class. Thus, the Spalding Method incorporates many of the Orton-Gillingham principles, including an emphasis on integrating the various sensory modalities involved in learning to read. However, it differs from the earlier method in many respects, most particularly by teaching writing before reading and by introducing first the most commonly used English words, many of which are not phonetically regular.

Students write all words in notebooks that they add to as they proceed through the program. These spelling books serve as their major reference source. Twenty-nine spelling rules are taught in the program; students write these in their books along with examples of application. In addition, students are taught a marking system to help them identify and remember phonogram spellings and pronunciations: phonograms are underlined and, for those having more than one sound, numbers are used to identify which sound a phonogram represents in a given word. Sylvia Farnham-Diggory maintains in her introduction to the program manual that knowing the seventy phonograms and these twenty-nine rules enables anyone to spell eighty percent of all English words. According to Farnham-Diggory, reading in this method is never taught; children "simply pick up a book and start reading" (Farnham-Diggory 1986).

OTHER PROGRAMS USING SPELLING TO READ

IBM's old *Writing to Read* program (Martin 1985; Martin and Friedberg 1986; see Chapter 21 in the 1995 edition) is no longer available, but was designed to build on the principle of spelling leading to reading. It contained a computer word processing component aimed at promoting reading acquisition among kindergartners and first graders. This worked much like the computer game *Reader Rabbit* in which children say a picture aloud, segment and spell the word and then type the letters into the computer in order to see and read the word.

Benita Blachman includes both segmenting and spelling in a program for at-risk beginning readers. Spelling is taught through the use of a pocket chart with letters for sounding out and spelling orally presented words (Blachman 1987; Blachman et al. 1994). This activity is part of a sequence that moves from segmenting and spelling to word and story reading.

Patricia and James Cunningham use a technique that they call "making words" in regular primary level classrooms to enhance the relationship between invented spelling and decoding (Cunningham and Cunningham 1992). A restricted set of letters on cards is used to build words from oral directions in an activity that is something like the Elkonin *word changes*. Children are asked, "Now, change just one letter, and change *sing* to *ring*. Now we will make a five-letter word. Add a letter to change *ring* to *rings*." Each child works with a set of her own letters and then each word is spelled with large letters for the whole class to see. Note that this gives children a chance to correct their invented spellings. A range of words, from two to five letters, provides instructional opportunities for children with a range of abilities.

The after school tutoring program used by Fordham's Ennis William Cosby Graduate Certificate Program provides support for first graders who are in the bottom quartile of their class in a high-needs urban school. This instruction includes a sequence of six activities linking spelling with reading: (a) introduction of a new letter-sound, (b) segmenting and spelling words with this sound, (c) reading these words on cards, (d) reading these words in decodable text, (e) reading these words in predictable trade books, and (e) writing about the stories. Thus, before a word with a new letter sound is read, it is deconstructed through segmenting and spelling. Children tutored in this method were significantly better at reading than a comparison group of children who received homework help in reading and writing in their after school program (Uhry 2003).

CONCERNS ABOUT INVENTED SPELLING

One of the major concerns raised about using invented spelling as an instructional approach is that it may perpetuate incorrect spellings. This is the position held by some Orton-Gillingham trained teachers who work with dyslexic children. As mentioned in Chapter 11, *Spelling*, these remedial educators do not introduce free writing activities until their pupils have mastered basic phonics skills, although copying and practice in writing from dictation forms a substantial portion of their curriculum. However, researchers who observe young children without dyslexia (e.g., Bissex 1980; Henderson and Beers 1980; Read 1971, 1975, 1986) have found that invented spellings are gradually replaced with orthographically conventional ones as the children gain reading experience. Note that this is consistent with Frith's notion that orthographic reading precedes and leads into orthographic spelling. That is, seeing words in print eventually influences spellings.

Note that in Linnea Ehri's reading model there is an additional stage between Frith's *logographic* and *alphabetic* stages (see Chapter 1). At this stage children read only some salient features of a word, reading *look* as "like," for example. In the early stages of invented spelling both of these words might be spelled as "LK." An argument could be made that as children become aware of medial vowels and begin to segment and spell the word *like* as "LIK" they will be more apt to look for a vowel when they read the word *look*, and to recognize that it is not a match for the lexically stored word *like*.

Children with dyslexia do not tend to develop sensitivity to the match between phonology and orthography on their own. They need more direct, systematic instruction in this area than do other children. This does not negate the usefulness of invented spelling for children with dyslexia, but it does suggest that they need systematic support in identifying phonemes in words and in associating these sounds with letters as they write.

A second concern about the writing-before-reading approach is that children may be confused by the differences between their own spellings and the printed words they encounter when they begin to read. This is not a problem, according to Chomsky (1979). Reporting on Read's observations (Read 1970), she claims that children appear to have no difficulty making the distinction between their spellings and conventional spellings and that they tend, in fact, to view writing and reading as completely separate tasks, a conclusion that Lynette Bradley and Peter Bryant also reach in their research (Bradley 1985; Bradley and Bryant 1979).

Keep in mind that the practice of encouraging children to invent spellings is not a substitute for a systematic spelling program (see Chapter 11). Invented spellings are appropriate during the time in kindergarten and first grade when children are learning letter formations, names and sounds, and becoming aware of phonemes within spoken words, and applying this learning to mastery of the alphabetic principle. Using the ear to invent spellings works well with words in which there is a simple relationship between letters and sounds. Once all five short vowels are learned, children can invent or create thousands of accurate spellings of consonant-vowel-consonant words that they have never seen or spelled before. My sense is that not only children with dyslexia, but all children, should be taught letter-sounds directly, and then held accountable for spellings using any sounds that have been taught.

Learning spelling conventions for orthographic units becomes more important as the other five syllable types[12] are introduced. Spelling by ear is not efficient with words such as *soap* and *hope*. Once children are developmentally ready to use the more complex orthographic strategy they should be taught to move beyond invented spellings to patterns involving units of orthographically conventional letters.

---

[12]The six syllable types are: (a) closed or cvc as in *sat*; (b) vowel teams as in *coat*; (c) long vowel with silent *e* as in *hope*; (d) r-controlled as in *bird*; (e) open as in *hi* and *o-pen*; and (f) consonant-l-e as in *a-ble* and *ap-ple*).

7

Phonics Instruction

This chapter provides information about phonics and phonics instruction. It begins with a discussion of the relationship between phonics and learning to read in a written language that is built on letter-sound associations, or what is called an *alphabetic language*. It raises issues from both historical and current debates regarding phonics instruction and provides summaries of research in these areas from the Report of the National Reading Panel (2000; Ehri, Nunes, Stahl, and Willows 2001). The chapter closes with a short outline of the Orton-Gillingham approach, the traditional method for teaching students with dyslexia to read and write.

The term *phonics* means the connection between phonemes and letters. Where the term *phonemic awareness* refers to sounds alone—the analysis of phonemes in spoken language—the term *phonics* has to do with connecting phonemes to letters and using these connections for reading and spelling. Both phonemic awareness and letter name knowledge are precursors of phonics and of alphabetic reading.

English is an alphabetic language. Unlike languages such as Chinese, which has thousands of meaning-based characters, alphabetic languages have a relatively small number of letter-sounds that can be combined into an almost infinite number of words. Languages with a direct one-to-one relationship between graphemes and phonemes, such as German, are said to be *transparent* languages. Because English is derived from so many languages, it is complex and far from transparent. Many of its 26 letters have more than one sound (e.g., the letter a sounded as in *Kate, cat, watch, ball,* and *Elizabeth*), and many of its 44 phonemes have more than one spelling (e.g., the long /a/ sound spelled as in *Kate, tail, straight, eight, hey, hay,* and *acorn*).

THE DEBATE ABOUT PHONICS
THE HISTORICAL DEBATE

Up until the 1930s, most children learned to read through phonics instruction. It was John Dewey who influenced the introduction of a more meaning-based approach and the onset of basal readers in which sight words were gradually introduced and memorized through systematic repetition in series such as *Dick and Jane.* Historically, there has been disagreement about whether or not to teach phonics to children learning to read in English. Jeanne Chall (1983a) used the term *The Great Debate* to describe this controversy. One argument runs that English spelling is irregular, making rule-based learning undependable. Given these irregularities, the argument runs, focusing on whole words and their meanings is a more productive route (Goodman, 1967, 1993; Smith 2004). Goodman, who advocates a top-down or meaning-based approach, argues that individual letters are not very important to reading and that new words are best learned as a *psycho-linguistic guessing game,* through using knowledge of syntactical and semantic context. Goodman and Smith's philosophy is exemplified in the whole language approach in which new words are approached contextually rather than through letter sounds.

The opposing argument is that because of the complexities of the English spelling system, it is difficult to figure out the system without instruction, and thus, difficult to read new words independently. While all children benefit from phonics instruction, failure to provide this instruction is particularly detrimental to children with phonological deficits. This argument that phonics should be taught systematically and directly, and not left to children to figure out on their own, is supported by an overwhelming volume of research (Adams 1990; Chall 1983a; Gough and Tunmer 1986; Liberman et al. 1983; National Reading Panel 2000; Olson et al. 1985; Perfetti 1985a; Snow et al 1998; Vellutino 1983).

When the second edition of this book was published in 1995, there was agreement in the scientific research community that phonics instruction should be part of the reading curriculum for all school children (e.g., Adams 1990; Chall 1983a). At that time, however, this conclusion had not generalized broadly to classroom practice where basal reader and whole language philosophy programs predominated. Since 1995, there has been a shift toward more focus on phonics instruction.

#209 02-03-2011 4:22PM
Item(s) checked out to Kim, Deanna M..

TITLE: Dyslexia : theory & practice of i
BC: 31147012354901544tv
DUE DATE: 03-01-11

TITLE: Trainstop
BC: 31157039091773
DUE DATE: 03-01-11

Castro Valley Library
Renewals call 510-790-8096

In some cases this involves *balanced* or *comprehensive* reading instruction with integration of phonics and a whole language focus on oral language, reading/writing links, and authentic, meaningful learning situations. Michael Pressley's *Reading Instruction that Works: The Case for Balanced Teaching* (2003) is a wonderful resource to use in planning classroom instruction based on this integration.

Several events since the mid 1990s are responsible for the movement toward the inclusion of phonics in the early grades. First, two large states moved away from whole language instruction because of low reading scores that were attributed to whole language instruction. In 1995 California, then a whole language state, tied with Louisiana for the lowest Grade 4 reading scores in the country on the National Assessment of Educational Progress. Pete Wilson, governor at the time, set up financial incentives for teacher training in phonics and for phonics-based basal readers, and a bill was passed by the California legislature in 1996 requiring the teaching of systematic phonics (Snow et al. 1998). In Texas, the early results of Barbara Foorman's NICHD-funded research suggested an advantage for phonics instruction for children at risk because of weak phonological awareness and her findings were influential in determining policy at the state level. These two states have wide influence on the design of basal readers, which, in turn, influence reading methodology in other states.

Another source of influence came from two reports on reading instruction, one from the National Research Council and the second from the National Reading Panel. Much of the research in the National Reading Panel's meta-analysis involved large-scale, scientifically designed research funded by the NICHD with clear findings on the effectiveness of phonics instruction, especially for young children and children with disabilities. A third source of influence was the reauthorization by Congress of the Elementary and Secondary Education Act in 2001 as No Child Left Behind, together with incentives through federal funding to states to support schools using scientifically researched programs.

CURRENT DEBATES

Although there is now some consensus in the direction of a balanced or comprehensive approach that includes phonics instruction, exactly how phonics should be taught continues to be a controversial topic. The following should provide a knowledge base for better understanding of this controversy.

Systematic versus Incidental Phonics Instruction

Systematic phonics involves a method of teaching using the following three principles. First, in systematic phonics, instruction is explicit, meaning that letter-sound associations and their application in reading and spelling are taught directly. Rather than simply assuming that children will figure out that the letter *b* represents the sound /b/ after reading text that includes a lot of words starting with *b*, the teacher provides a lesson in which he says, something like, "This is the letter *b* and when you see it in a word, you should say the /b/ sound." Orton Gillingham programs such as Alphabetic Phonics (Chapter 20) and the Wilson Reading System (Chapter 22) use flash cards with key word pictures and letters (e.g., a picture of an umbrella with the letter *u*) to teach and review the association between a letter and a sound.

The second principle of systematic instruction is the use of a preplanned sequence of letter-sounds. This serves two purposes. It assures that all letter-sounds will be taught over time, and it assures that developmentally simple patterns will be taught before more complex patterns. We know from children's invented (developmental) spellings that consonant letter-sound associations, with a few exceptions, are easier to learn than vowels. Rebecca Treiman (1993) points out that many consonant's names are similar to their sounds (e.g., *m, s, t,* but not *w* or *y*). The association between the letter m and the sound /m/ is much easier to learn than associations for short vowels. Alphabetic Phonics bases its sequence on the frequency with which patterns occur in English. For example, hard *c* (as in the word *cup*) is more frequent than soft *c* (as in *ceiling*), and occurs earlier in the sequence. The Wilson Reading System teaches vowels organized by the six English syllable types. Syllables with short vowels are both the most frequent syllable type and the simplest. One syllable words with short vowels (e.g., *at, top, flop, milk*) are relatively easy to sound out once short vowel sounds are learned. The left-to-right, letter-by-letter alphabetic strategy is best exemplified in one syllable short vowel words, and are commonly taught early in phonics sequences.

The third principle of systematic phonics is that letter-sound associations are practiced in text as well as in isolation. Systematic phonics programs tend to include practice in decodable text, a term used for text that can be decoded using letter-sounds that have been taught. Many Orton-Gillingham programs such as the Wilson Reading System program include decodable text, as do commercially available basal programs that are systematic, such as *Open Court* (Adams et al. 1995) and *Success for All* (Slavin et al. 1996).

Incidental phonics instruction, on the other hand, tends to occur in programs that are not so systematic. Incidental phonics assumes a top-down approach in which the content of the story carries the lesson. Harris and Hodges, in *The Literacy Dictionary* (1995) define incidental learning as "change in behavior that is not directly taught or sought." When meaning-based teaching does include phonics instruction, it tends to occur in response to a child stumbling with decoding, demonstrating a need for instruction, using what is often called a *teachable moment*. Reading Recovery (see Chapter 15) uses this approach. The teacher takes a running record as the child reads aloud and then uses miscue analysis to determine which letter-sounds might need a short lesson during an upcoming instructional session. That is, phonics instruction is incidental to particular text. A pattern is taught as it is needed rather than according to an overall plan.

The Report of the National Reading Panel (2000) indicated that systematic phonics provides children with a significant advantage in comparison with both incidental phonics and with approaches that do not include phonics instruction. In one of the studies included in the meta-analysis of the NRP, described in Chapter 5, Joseph Torgesen provided instruction for kindergarten children at risk because they were weak in letter naming and PA (i.e., lowest 12%). In this two-year study, bridging grades K through 2, each of four instructional groups had roughly 44 children. One question was the effectiveness of systematic, explicitly taught phonological awareness and phonics in contrast with what they call *embedded* phonics instruction that results from incidental instruction while learning to read and write words. The first of the four groups received phonological awareness and systematic phonics (PASP) in which the 1984 version of the Lindamood program was used (see Chapter 24). The second group received embedded phonics (EP) activities in which writing activities were used to listen for sounds in words and sight-word learning was used as a vehicle for learning letter sounds. A third group received one-to-one instruction involving support in the child's regular classroom (RCS) literacy activities, and a fourth group of controls did not receive any extra help. The PASP group, which spent 80% of tutoring time on word level instruction, did significantly better at the end of training on measures of phonological awareness, and on reading of both real and nonwords, in comparison with the EP group, which spent 43% of its time on word reading and 57% on text reading activities. Both groups were stronger on these measures than the RCS and control groups. Although the tutored groups were stronger on comprehension than controls, there were no instructional group differences (Torgesen, Wagner, Rashotte, Rose et al. 1999). This and other studies support the use of systematic phonics instruction.

Synthetic versus Analytic Phonics Instruction

Synthetic Phonics is a part-to-whole or bottom-up approach that starts with small units (i.e., letters), and uses them to construct larger units (i.e., words). Once letter-sounds have been learned, they are blended, or synthesized, into words for reading. For example, in Alphabetic Phonics (see Chapter 20) the consonant digraph *ph* is presented on a card with a picture of a phone to help children remember the sound. A child practices by responding with the phoneme /ph/ when shown the card by a teacher or tutor. Once the letter-sound correspondence has been practiced in isolation, the grapheme, in this case the digraph *ph*, is blended with other letters into a word. Synthetic phonics almost always goes together with the teaching of a systematic sequence of letter sounds and is typical of Orton-Gillingham programs.

Analytic Phonics is a whole-to-part approach in which children are taught to read words by sight and then encouraged to recognize phonics elements in the memorized words. For example, after reading the words *bear, baby,* and *book,* a child might realize that the letter *b* is associated with the sound /b/. Analytic phonics can involve discovery learning in which the text provides words with common patterns and children are left to deduce the patterns on their own, or it can involve guided discovery or direct instruction, usually through lessons in which children are encouraged to deconstruct words and find common patterns. Thus analytic phonics can be either incidental or systematic.

Single Phonemes versus Units of Phonemes

Another controversial area involves the size of the unit to be taught. Synthetic phonics programs such as Alphabetic Phonics and the Wilson Reading System teach students to blend single phonemes into words (i.e., /c/-/a/-/t/). The text from *Mac and Tab,* pictured here, is an example of decodable text used in a synthetic phonics approach. Before children are asked to read this page, they are taught the short /a/ sound of the letter *a,* as well as the sounds of the consonants *c, t, m, n, h, b,* and *p.*

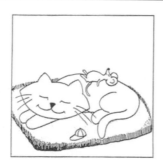

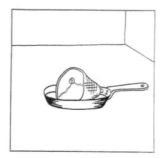

Tab has a nap on the mat.
Mac has a nap on Tab.

The ham is in the pan.
The ham is for Tab.

Excerpt from Primary Phonics: Mac and Tab by Barbara W. Makar. (Reproduced with permission from Educators Publishing Service, 625 Mt. Auburn Street, Cambridge, MA, Telephone: (800) 225-5750, www.epsbooks.com Copyright 1995).

In contrast, several other programs use a *word family* or *onset-rime* approach in which a unit of letters is learned (e.g., -at, -all), each with a series of onsets (e.g., bat, cat, hat; ball, call, hall). A word family approach is used by Reading Recovery (see Chapter 15) for word study instruction but not for text reading. The Merrill Linguistic Readers present an example of text that is organized around a sequence of word families. Notice in the text sample provided here that in the Merrill readers only the initial consonant sound changes from word to word (i.e., *cat, sat, mat*) in contrast with *Mac and Tab*, in which both initial and final consonants vary. The Merrill series is one of a number of linguistic readers on the market.

A Cat on a Mat

Is a cat on a mat?
A cat is on a mat.

Is the cat fat?
The cat is fat.

Is the cat Nat?
The cat on the mat is Nat.

Excerpt from the Merrill Linguistic Reading Program: I Can by Rosemary G. Wilson and Mildred K. Rudolph. (Reproduced with permission from Charles E. Merrill Publishing Co., Columbus, OH. Copyright 1980).

The basic rationale for using any one of these programs with disabled readers has been that a linguistic approach, with its onset-rime break, makes blending easier and enables reading by analogy. Usha Goswami's research indicates that even very young children can read through analogy (Goswami 1986). Having read *cat*, they can read *sat*. However Linnea Ehri's research suggests that the analogy strategy is enhanced by prior phonics knowledge (Ehri and Robbins 1992). In other words, children who can sound out *s-a-t* can read the *at* family by analogy more easily than those who cannot.

We used a two-step model based on this implication in our clinical practice with children with dyslexia at the Child Study Center at Teachers College, Columbia University (see Chapter 26; Shepherd and Uhry 1993; Uhry 2002b) and in school-based tutorials through Fordham's Young Readers at Risk program (Uhry 2003). We use decodable text with a synthetic phonics focus to teach consonant sounds at both beginnings and ends of words, starting with short /a/ words, and then, when each pattern is mastered for accuracy, we switch to short periods of practice in the Merrill readers and other text with word-families to work on fluency. We found that reading whole pages of words in the Merrill readers with the same rime unit helps children *chunk* these units (i.e., read and blend /c/-/at/ rather than /c/-/a/-/t/) for greater automaticity.

Decodable Text versus Natural Language Text

Decodable text is text containing words made up of a systematic sequence of letter sounds, so that almost every word can be sounded out by children who have learned these letter-sounds. *Mac and Tab* and *A Cat on a Mat* are examples of decodable text, also called *phonetically controlled* or *phonics-controlled* text. In using decodable text, the match between text and reader is critical. For example, text with silent *e* words would be decodable for children who have practiced associations for vowels with silent *e*, but not for children who have practiced only short vowels.

There are two other types of text that have been developed, historically, for beginning readers. One type of text, often called *sight-word* text, was developed in the 1930s, and involves the gradual and systematic introduction of whole words. Once a new word is taught, the word is used over and over so that it becomes automatic. The idea is to introduce new words slowly so that a child is never faced with too many unknown words at once. Both decodable text and sight-word text tend to be stilted because word choices are so constrained. A third text type uses more natural language. This *natural language text* uses language that supports the meaning of a story. All three text types could be described as predictable. Decodable text is predictable in terms of the range of phonemes and syllable structures. Sight-word text is predictable in terms of its use of familiar words. Natural language text provides predictability through the use of illustrations related to the text, repetitive language, and rhyme. Both Brian Wildsmith's (2001) *Cat on the Mat* from Oxford and the Wright Group story *Dan, the Flying Man* (Cowley 1990) are examples of well-illustrated, natural language texts often used in whole language classrooms. They use rhyme and repetition, and provide opportunities to practice the letter-sound strategy with short *a* words together with meaning-based strategies. Another example is Scholastic's *Buzz Said the Bee* (Lewison 1992), also rich in rhyme and repetition, and also full of short vowel words. Harper's I-Can-Read-Book, *Grandmas at Bat*, is written and illustrated by Caldecott Medal winner Emily McCully (1993). With the words "coach" and "team" repeated over and over, it is perfect for learning vowel digraphs. Another Harper book, *Hill of Fire* by Thomas P. Lewis, can be used for contrasting short vowel words with silent *e* words.

Use of decodable text has not been as extensively researched as many other aspects of phonics. The National Reading Panel Report lists decodable text as an area in need of research. Many reading experts argue against the use of decodable text because it discourages the use of multiple cue systems. The language in decodable text can be awkward because the choice of vocabulary is so limited, and this hampers the use of meaning to help with decoding. Other experts are enthusiastic about decodable text. They argue that children already know how to use pictures and context to figure out unfamiliar words. Decodable text encourages them to use letter sounds—a cue system that is new to them. There is evidence from research that beginning readers and readers with dyslexia over-use illustrations and context as cue systems and under-use letters. Note that the Merrill Linguistic Readers do not include any illustrations for precisely this reason.

Up to now, there has not been conclusive evidence for or against decodable text. What research there was did not control for instruction carefully enough. That is, the studies really contrasted phonics instruction that included decodable text with other instruction that included other text. The best controlled of these early studies is an often cited experiment by Connie Juel who concluded that children learned what they were taught. Children in phonics instruction reading decodable text learned word attack skills and children with phonics instruction who read sight-approach basal readers learned more sight words. There was no advantage for either group on a standardized reading test (Juel and Roper-Schneider 1985).

A recent study carried out by Joseph Jenkins and his colleagues found no advantage for either phonetically decodable text or for storybook text that was less phonetically decodable when they compared at-risk first-grade children after 25 weeks of school-based tutoring four days a week. Both groups had the same phonics instruction and both practiced reading words before they appeared in whichever text was read during tutoring sessions. While both groups surpassed an untutored control group at posttest, neither tutored group (i.e., decodable versus less decodable text) surpassed the other in word reading or passage comprehension (Jenkins et al. 2004).

Because there is not an abundance of evidence that either decodable text or natural language text is better for teaching reading, until more research is carried out, the common sense approach is to provide children with practice in both text types. With this approach, the alphabetic strategy (i.e., sounding out letters and blending the sounds into words) is practiced in decodable text, and then multiple strategies (i.e., sounding out, using illustrations, using context, using repetition and rhyme for unfamiliar words) can be practiced in natural language text. The important thing, as pointed out by Jenkins, is to provide opportunities to read words with newly taught phonics patterns. Note that *Mac and Tab*, *A Cat on a Mat*, and *Dan, the Flying Man*

all have words with the short /a/ sound and that each supports a particular strategy—alphabetic sounding out, reading units of letters fluently,
and monitoring multiple strategies while reading for meaning. In our
clinical practice, we encourage teachers to coordinate the use all three
text types, each for its own purpose.

Tutorials versus Group Instruction

Historically, it has been considered best practice to provide tutorial instruction for students with dyslexia. It was believed that every
child's phonics program should be individually tailored, with instruction matched with ongoing, assessment-based analysis of individual
needs. This belief has been questioned recently as a result of the
Report of the National Reading Panel (2000). It was found that in the
studies included in the report, there were not significant differences in
effects among large group, small group, and one-to-one instruction.
Phonics instruction that was systematic was effective for all three
groupings.

In thinking about instructional practices in schools, we are
strong advocates of the tutorial, not because this is necessarily more
effective in terms of a child's progress, but because it allows the teacher
to learn so much about instruction. Our practice with both preservice
and inservice teachers at Fordham is built around on-going case studies.
This provides time and focus for teachers to think about making small
modifications to instruction in response to a student's progress.
Teachers say that they develop techniques that they are able to carry
over into instruction with groups. That is, we strongly recommend that
teachers refine their own instructional skills through working with an
individual or two on a regular basis.

PHONICS INSTRUCTION AND DYSLEXIA
The Orton-Gillingham Approach

What is the most effective instruction for students with dyslexia?
Programs with an Orton-Gillingham approach are the traditional remedial approach for these students. The Orton-Gillingham approach,
mentioned in Chapter 4, was designed for one-to-one instruction. In
1960, Anna Gillingham and Bessie Stillman published an instruction
manual for remedial teachers, along with instruction materials. Since
then, the method has become the basic model upon which multisensory remedial intervention programs for dyslexic children have been
built. A number of programs based on the Orton-Gillingham approach
are described in detail in Part III of this book (i.e., *Alphabetic Phonics*,

the *Slingerland Program*, *Recipe for Reading*, Enfield and Green's *Project Read*, and the *Wilson Reading System*.

June Orton, the wife of Samuel Orton, summarized the three most important distinguishing features of the Orton-Gillingham approach as follows:

1. It is a direct approach to the study of *synthetic phonics*, presenting the sounds of the phonograms orally as separate units and then *teaching* the process of blending them into syllables and words.

2. It is an *integrated, multisensory* approach. Each unit and sequence is established through hearing, speaking, seeing, and writing. Auditory, visual, and kinesthetic patterns reinforce each other, a feature that also provides for individual needs among the students.

3. It is a *systematic*, step-by-step approach, proceeding from the simpler to the more complex in orderly progression in an upward spiral of language development. (Orton 1964, p. 11).

As Gillingham and Stillman (1960) described it, the method is built on the close association of visual, auditory, and kinesthetic aspects of language to form what they called the *language triangle*. In strong contrast to an analytic phonics method, the Orton-Gillingham approach teaches letter sounds and the blending of these sounds into words. It should never be used, according to its authors, as a supplement to sight or basal reader approaches. Furthermore, any reading outside of Orton-Gillingham material is forbidden. Complying with this restriction obviously presents a problem, and tutors using this method have had to deviate to some extent from the method with any child who remains in a regular classroom. Gillingham and Stillman placed considerable emphasis on the need for older children to break old habits. In order to *establish the alphabetic principle* among these children, words must no longer be viewed "as ideograms to-be-remembered as wholes" (Gillingham and Stillman 1960), and all guessing must be eliminated.

In the Orton-Gillingham approach, letters or phonograms are introduced as visual symbols printed on cards. First, the letter name (or names, in the case of digraphs) is taught. The teacher says the name, the child repeats it. Then the teacher asks what letter it is, and the child gives the name. When this is secure, the letter sound is taught in the same manner. The association between visual and auditory characteristics of letters is made in this way. Then *auditory-to-auditory* association is established—the teacher says the letter sound and asks the pupil for the letter name. This is followed by *visual-kinesthetic* and *auditory-kinesthetic* associations. The teacher writes the letter, carefully explaining its formation and orientation, and the student traces the letter, then copies it, then writes it from memory, and finally writes it from memory with eyes averted. This last step will internalize the visual and kinesthetic image of the letter. For auditory-kinesthetic reinforcement, the teacher gives the letter sound and asks the student to write the letter that makes that particular sound. When writing, however, the student always says the letter name, not the sound, a procedure that has been called *Simultaneous Oral Spelling (SOS)*.

The introduction of letters and letter combinations is carefully sequenced. Initially, ten letters are taught: two vowels (*a, i*) and eight consonants (*f, h, b, j, k, m, p, t*). Each letter is introduced with a *key word*, for example, *i-igloo*. The difference between vowels and consonants is taught, drawing the student's attention to the open and closed positions of the mouth in pronunciation, and reinforced using different colored cards for vowels and consonants. These cards are used to bring learning to mastery in drill exercises. Once letter names and letter sound knowledge are secure, reading begins. Three letter cards are laid out (for example, *b-i-t*), and the student is asked to produce each sound in succession, repeating them with increasing speed and smoothness, until able to pronounce the word. The same associations are established with words as with letters; the child traces, copies, and writes each word. Printed cards for each word, provided in a file box referred to as the *Jewel Case*, are used in word recognition drill exercises. *Recognition speed* is encouraged through use of a stopwatch or egg timer, and the teacher keeps a progress graph for words learned. In this way, the student builds his reading lexicon.

Orton-Gillingham lessons are intended to be conducted within forty- to sixty-minute periods. A guide for developing a daily routine is provided in the teacher's manual. New phonograms are introduced gradually, usually not more than two in one lesson, and must be taught in invariant order to match the word cards and other materials provided.

In the Orton-Gillingham approach, reading of text begins only when the student is able to read c-v-c (consonant-vowel-consonant) words perfectly (presumably to a highly automatic level), as well as phonetic four letter words with digraphs such as *th* and *ph*. Stories containing words the student has learned are printed in the teacher's manual. Phonetically irregular sight words, which the student has not previously encountered, are underlined and told to the student by the teacher. The student reads each sentence silently first, asking for help if needed. In oral reading, he is encouraged to read with inflection, although no attention is paid to word meaning or comprehension. Gillingham and Stillman contended that the pleasure children derive from finally being able to read justifies the bland contents of these phonics-controlled texts. The same stories are used for dictation exercises.

Syllabication is taught to all students and particularly encouraged for those who previously used a whole-word approach. Practice begins with students reading words with syllables separated, followed by their rearranging jumbled syllables to form real words. Students are taught to place stress marks on accented syllables.

Additionally, the Orton-Gillingham approach describes the evolution of written language. As an introduction to remedial instruction, the dyslexic student is given a brief history of the development of written language, from pictographs to ideographs to alphabets, which helps him to understand the concept of an alphabetic system. For teachers, a brief history of the English language is provided to increase their understanding of word derivations. The information is intended to help teachers develop knowledge of spelling patterns, and thereby transfer this knowledge to their students.

A number of sites for training in the Orton-Gillingham approach are listed in the Resource and Teacher Training Guide at the end of this book. Many of them can supply information about tutoring and evaluation resources for children and adults with dyslexia. The Reading Disabilities Unit at Massachusetts General Hospital in Boston has provided this training for many years. Training includes both lectures and practical work. Dr. Edwin Cole, a neurologist who was also instrumental in starting the Carroll School in Lincoln, Massachusetts, started the program. This school for children with dyslexia uses the Orton-Gillingham method and also serves as a training site. Barbara Wilson, author of the Wilson Method, trained at Massachusetts General (see Chapter 22).

RESEARCH ON PHONICS INSTRUCTION FOR STUDENTS WITH DYSLEXIA

Although it has been used extensively with children and adolescents who are dyslexic, until recently little research has been conducted to validate the effectiveness of the Orton-Gillingham approach, as described above. Probably the primary reason for the lack of systematic data collection is that the method has been used almost exclusively in tutorial situations or in small schools for children with dyslexia. In neither case are controls available for comparison.

However, during the 1990s, large-scale treatment studies funded by the National Institute for Health and Human Development compared versions of Orton-Gillingham phonics with other instructional approaches. In one of these studies, for example, Barbara Foorman and her colleagues contrasted three instructional methods carried out in small resource-room groups with second and third grade children of average intelligence and with word-reading scores in the lowest 25th percentile. An Orton-Gillingham based synthetic phonics program,

Alphabetic Phonics (Cox 1992), was contrasted with analytic phonics instruction using an onset-rime approach and with a sight word approach. The three treatment groups were taught by existing resource room teachers who were provided with special training. For example, the Neuhaus Center in Houston provided training for teachers working with the Alphabetic Phonics group. Children trained in this Orton-Gillingham method held a small advantage at posttest in phonological processing, orthographic processing (i.e., spelling recognition), and in word reading. Only the advantage in phonological processing was significant once IQ and socioeconomic status were taken into account. That is, Orton-Gillingham instruction was effective in teaching phonemic processing, but failed to transfer to word reading in this study (Foorman et al. 1997).

Foorman's 1997 study was one of 11 using Orton-Gillingham instruction and carried out with students either at-risk or with reading disability and included in the National Reading Panel's Report (2000). The effect sizes for these studies were small relative to those with other instructional approaches, but the NRP authors remind us that the students in some of these studies may be older, "low achieving" students (i.e., slow learners rather than children with specific reading disability and average IQ). The largest effect sizes for all of these studies was for younger (i.e., K-1), at-risk students and students with specific reading disability and average IQ.

One difficulty with Orton-Gillingham programs is that there is relatively little research that focuses on the specific components of this complex and well integrated instruction. For example, while systematicity is well researched, we know little about the effects of multisensory instruction. Much time is spent in Orton-Gillingham establishing the various multisensory linkages (i.e., between the visual, auditory, and kinesthetic modalities) and almost no time on learning to generalize techniques into reading regular text (i.e., text that is not decodable). More research is needed in this area.

Additional information about research findings for specific phonics programs is included in Part III of this book.

SUMMARY

To summarize, research has demonstrated that instruction built on the following principles of phonics instruction is effective:

- Teach letter-sounds and other aspects of the alphabetic principle (e.g., blending for reading, segmenting for spelling) using direct instruction rather than incidental learning.

- Use a preplanned sequence to insure that you progress from the simple to the complex and that all 98 letter-sound combinations are taught in roughly their order of usefulness.
- Provide lots of time for practice of new letter-sounds in words in text. Until research demonstrates that one or the other approach is more effective, provide both decodable text and real stories containing the new pattern, and teach students how to generalize word-reading strategies.
- Both letter-by-letter and onset-rime phonics approaches are effective so long as they are taught systematically. Again, both approaches can be useful at various stages in the development of beginning reading.

8

Rate and Fluency

The term *fluency*, when applied to reading, indicates several attributes. Fluent reading is accurate. Fluent reading is quick; words are recognized automatically, without the need for sounding out or figuring out from context. And fluent reading is expressive, as if the reader comprehends and is helping the listener comprehend through phrasing and inflection. Reading rate is considered to be a critical factor in fluency. Just as phonemic processing issues can cause problems with word reading accuracy, lack of speed and automaticity can cause difficulties in fluency. This chapter reviews research-based theories regarding rate and fluency and makes suggestions for instruction.

THEORY AND RESEARCH ON FLUENCY
READING SPEED AFFECTS COMPREHENSION

There is research indicating that children who read slowly put so much effort into decoding that, even if they pronounce words accurately, there is little processing space left for comprehension. The theory that fast, as well as accurate, word recognition is related to proficient reading was first proposed in 1974 by David LaBerge and S. Jay Samuels (see Chapter 1). Charles Perfetti elaborated upon this hypothesis by suggesting a *limited capacity mechanism* within children's information processing systems. Perfetti contends that poor decoding hampers comprehension by creating a *bottleneck*; the more time and effort required for decoding, the less processing capacity available for comprehension. Perfetti (1985a) refers to this hypothesis as the *verbal efficiency theory*. Using multiple regression analysis, Keith Stanovich and his associates have provided substantial support for the verbal efficiency hypothesis by determining that decoding speed is the highest contributing variable to reading comprehension (Stanovich, Cunningham, and Feeman 1984).

RAPID SERIAL NAMING

Rapid Serial Naming and Dyslexia

Martha Denckla carried out seminal early studies on the speed at which a series of colors, numbers, pictures, and letters could be named using her Rapid Automatized Naming Test (RAN; Denckla and Cutting, 1999; Denckla and Rudel 1974, 1976a, 1976b). As mentioned in Chapter 2, children become faster at these tasks as they grow older, and children who are slow at naming letters in the early grades turn out to be slow at reading words later on. Other researchers have confirmed this (Mannis, Seidenberg, and Doi 1999; Uhry 2002b; Wolf 2001; Wolff, Michel, and Ovrut 1990a). There is even evidence that the development of kindergarten finger-point reading of memorized text is hampered by letter-naming rate. However, there is not clear evidence on the underlying cause of reading rate deficits. That is, researchers have several explanations.

Rapid Serial Naming as a Form of Phonological Processing

One explanation is that weakness in phonological processing causes weakness in word-reading accuracy. Wagner and Torgesen (1987) refer to rapid naming as *phonological recoding in lexical access*. They conceptualize this as a form of phonological processing in which visually presented stimuli are stored and retrieved phonologically. Inefficient retrieval, in their view, can be affected by weak phonological awareness. Note, in a section below, that they include rapid naming subtests in their Comprehensive Test of Phonological Processing (CTOPP) (Wagner, Torgesen, and Rashotte 1999).

Rapid Serial Naming as Orthographic Processing: A Second Deficit

Other researchers have argued against this point of view and consider rapid serial naming to be a measure of orthographic processing speed, and distinct from phonological processing. Bowers and Wolf have presented a model in which the rapid naming task taps separate, non-phonological functions related to speed of processing (1993;

Bowers, 1995, 2001; Bowers, Sunseth, and Golden, 1999; Bowers, and Swanson 1991; Wolf, 1991; 1999, 2001). Bowers (2001) reports that phonological awareness is strongly associated with word reading accuracy and that rapid serial naming is associated with word reading speed. Both are critically important for reading fluently and understanding text.

This differentiation between reading accuracy and reading speed is consistent with Chall's (1983b) reading stage theory. At Stage 1, the Decoding Stage, phonemic awareness supports learning to map tiny units of sound onto letters. Words are sounded out and spellings are invented. At this stage, children learn to decode accurately. At Stage 2, Confirmation, words begin to be recognized automatically. Bowers proposes a detailed account of what may happen when children make this transition. They begin to recognize strings or units of letters that occur over and over. Some teachers call the process chunking and encourage the recognition of *word families* or commonly occurring letter patterns. Evidence from Uhry (2001) supports the notion that strings of letters commonly occurring together in English words (e.g., *m-a-s-t-a-t-i-m*) are recognized more quickly than letters in strings that occur infrequently or not at all (e.g., *m-g-s-r-m-g-m-r*).

Wolf and Bowers (1999) view slow naming as a second core deficit. When children are weak in both phonological processing and rapid naming they are said to have a *double deficit*. Weak readers with the double deficit have been found to be more difficult to remediate than readers weak in only one or the other of these deficits. Historically, not as much is known about remediating word reading rate as about phonological awareness remediation.

RESEARCH ON INSTRUCTION FOR INCREASING RATE AND FLUENCY

In a meta analysis carried out by the National Reading Panel (2000) there was an overwhelming advantage for reading methods carried out in a guided oral reading format. That is, direct instruction is effective. A number of instructional techniques appear to be effective.

Repeated Reading

Repeated reading is a technique with a long history. S. Jay Samuels, an early advocate of repeated reading, suggests that it should be used as a supplement to developmental reading instruction. He compared repeated reading to developing musical or athletic abilities that require practicing basic skills until they can be performed with adequate speed and smoothness (Samuels 1979).

Samuels (1986) suggests several techniques for implementing repeated reading. One technique is the *use of audio support*, in which a student reads silently while listening to a tape-recorded narration of the passage. Another technique is to have the student read for one minute and count the number of words read in that time and then record that number on a graph; after criterion level is reached, the student moves on to another passage. *Paired reading*, having two students read alternately and record for each other the number of words read, is yet another approach.

William Henk, John Helfeldt, and Jennifer Platt suggest several additional variations of the repeated reading model, one being *imitative reading*—the teacher reads a segment of text aloud while the student follows along silently before reading the segment himself, imitating the teacher's intonation and phrasing (Henk, Helfeldt, and Platt 1986). This technique is appropriate for the most disabled readers, according to Henk and his associates. *Radio reading*, in which the student, acting as announcer, reads a script aloud to the rest of the class, can avoid embarrassment, since only the student and the teacher share the script. *Chunking*, or reading in phrases, is another method suggested by these educators to promote fluency. A multisensory technique, referred to as *neurological impress* (NIM), involves the teacher and student simultaneously reading a passage aloud. The teacher forces the pace with her voice and by moving her finger along under the text, refusing to allow any pauses. Group use of this technique resembles the audio support method suggested by Samuels, but has not been found to be as effective as the one-to-one system, according to Henk and his colleagues.

Repeated Exposure to Words

Another element is rapid word identification. If rereading is effective in helping readers become more fluent, it may be because it gives them opportunities to reread the same words until they are automatic. Carol Rashotte investigated the question of whether repeated or non-repeated reading of passages by learning disabled students produces greater fluency and comprehension and whether degree of word overlap between passages is an influential factor (Rashotte 1983). Results of her study indicate that repeated reading is more effective than the equivalent amount of non-repeated reading only when large numbers of words are shared across passages.

Annette Tan and Tom Nicholson carried out research using a flashcard technique to increase automatic word identification and actually increased children's comprehension ability. The children in their study were below-average readers whose ages ranged from 7 to 10. One instructional group used flashcards with single words, with training sustained until a word could be recognized in one second. A second group read the same words embedded in phrases or sentences on flashcards. A third (control) group discussed the meanings of the words but did not read them. After each of five training sessions, each with its own set of words, the three groups were timed on reading these words in lists and in passages where the list words occurred, then asked comprehension questions and asked to do a retelling. The two-flashcard groups read the word lists and the same words in text more accurately and more quickly than controls. In addition, they were both superior to controls on comprehension questions (Tan and Nicholson 1997).

Tan and Nicholson include three points in their discussion of this study. First, *overlearning* is critical to automaticity. Items are repeated over and over until they are mastered. Second, with each successive training session in this study, words were learned to the automatic level more quickly. An effect of overlearning is that on successive training sessions, learning became more efficient. The third and most important point is that flashcard training is not a substitute for good, early training in phonemic awareness and phonics. Flashcard training is appropriate as a supplement to this in terms of rapid recognition. Tan and Nicholson's (1997) study provides strong support for the idea that accurate and rapid word identification is an important component of reading comprehension.

In a discussion of Tan and Nicholson's study, Torgesen, Rashotte, and Alexander (2001) point out that reading words on flashcards is a form of repeated reading, and that repeated readings at the single word, sentence, and text level all appear to be effective in increasing rate. In this same literature review Torgesen and his colleagues point out that their own intervention studies have been more effective than their remediation studies. In other words, it appears to be easier to correct a tendency toward rate and fluency difficulties when addressed very early. They comment on Wolf and Bowers' premise that children with a naming rate deficit have difficulty constructing orthographic images by suggesting that an advantage of repeated readings is that the same word occurs over and over during a short period of time.

Integration of Word Meaning and Rapid Word Recognition

Maryanne Wolf and her colleagues at Tufts University have carried out research on their fluency-based intervention program. Titled *Retrieval, Automaticity, Vocabulary Elaboration, and Orthography*, or RAVE-O, it was developed as pullout instruction for children with reading disabilities. Training involves word meanings as well as multiple exposures to recognizing words in print. Wolf states that the program is unique in terms of teaching word meanings; most fluency training programs focus on rereading. The program also differs from others in that it provides instruction in automaticity of underlying skills such as left-to-right scanning and recognizing letters and patterns of letters, which Wolf calls "sight letter chunks," (p. 378). Connections between root words and their orthography are systematically built. Early reports indicate that the program is more effective than phonetic accuracy training in terms of producing gains in fluency (Wolf, Miller, and Donnelly 2000).

Computer Assisted Instruction (CAI)

A number of researchers have used computer-assisted instruction to increase reading rate. Carol Rashotte and Joseph Torgesen have studied the effects of computer administered repeated reading of passages on learning disabled fourth-grade students (Rashotte and Torgesen 1985). They found that students enjoy this activity because they receive immediate feedback on their improved reading speed and take pleasure in their ability to read the passages with increasing fluency. The major effect of this practice, however, has been to enable students to identify individual words in the passage with greater speed. Particularly encouraging is the finding that learning to read words in context seems to generalize to reading these words out of context.

Guided Reading versus Independent Reading

The National Reading Panel Report uses the term *Guided Reading* in describing repeated readings and other fluency instruction methods that are guided by a teacher working directly with a student or small group. They found this to be more effective than structured independent reading time such as Drop Everything and Read (DEAR) or Uninterrupted Sustained Silent Reading (USSR). Although time-on-task spent reading may have a positive effect on both motivation to read for pleasure and on learning to respond to words rapidly through multiple exposures, it is not as effective a method as guided reading and should never constitute the only experiences a young or weak reader has reading a text in school.

How Fast is Fast Enough?

Armbruster, Lehr, and Osborn (2001) provide suggestions for reading rate in the early grades. They suggest 60 words read correctly per minute at the end of Grade 1, 90 to 100 by the end of Grade 2, and about 114 by the end of Grade 3. Their formula involves following the same procedure in three reading passages and then finding an average for words read correctly. The formula involves computing the total number of words read in one minute, and then subtracting the number of errors.

Torgesen, Rashotte, and Alexander (2001) used standard scores from the Gray Oral Reading Tests (Weiderholt and Bryant 2001) to establish typical reading rates for 10-year-old children in a remediation study. They found that to earn a standard score of 100 these children would need to read roughly 135 to 150 words per minute on the seven stories up through their reading level. What they found, though, was that not only were these remedial readers much slower (i.e., 78 wpm) than the average rate for 10-year-olds, their reading was not accurate. When provided with easier text, which was closer to their independent reading level, their rate rose to 122 wpm. The point here is that text that is too hard greatly reduces reading rate.

In all of the three sources cited here, word accuracy is a factor in word reading rate. Words that are accurately and automatically read can be read much faster than words that must be laboriously decoded. Relatively easy text supports fluency.

ASSESSMENT INSTRUMENTS FOR RATE

Martha Denckla's Rapid Automatized Naming Test, with its four subtests (colors, numbers, objects, and letters) has been available since the 1970s. The RAN has been used widely in research and in the past few years, several commercially available tests of rate have become available (Denckla and Rudel 1974, 1976a, 1976b). The Comprehensive Test of Phonological Processing (CTOPPS; Wagner, Torgesen, and Rashotte 1999) includes rapid naming subtests that are similar to the RAN (i.e., colors, digits, objects).

The Test of Word Reading Efficiency (TOWRE; Torgesen, Wagner, and Rashotte 1999) is a standardized measure with two subtests, one for sight word reading and one for sounding out unfamiliar words. On the Sight Word Efficiency subtest students are asked to read as many words in a list as they can read in 45 seconds. On the Phonetic Decoding Efficiency subtest they are asked to sound out as many nonwords in a list as they can in 45 seconds. Subtest comparison can be carried out for a profile of a student's strong and weak areas.

A newer series of tests called DIBELS have been developed to assess fluency. The Dynamic Indicators of Basic Early Literacy Skills (DIBELS) (Kame'enui et al. 2001; Kaminski and Good 1996) is a series of one-minute fluency measures for use in kindergarten and first grade. Letter Naming Fluency (LNF) measures how many letters can be named in one minute.

The Gray Oral Reading Test–Fourth Edition (GORT-4; Wiederholt and Bryant 2001) is a standardized test that provides a sequence of leveled passages, each with comprehension questions, for ages 6:0 to 18:11. Oral reading is timed and standard scores are provided for accuracy and rate as well as for comprehension. This allows for comparisons of a student's relative strengths and weaknesses.

SUGGESTIONS FOR FLUENCY INSTRUCTION

Some of these suggestions are specific to reading rate and some are aimed at more expressive oral reading.

- *Model Reading Fluently and Expressively.* Read aloud and model the thinking process you use in making choices about phrasing and prosody. Encourage children to repeat what you've read. This provides support for expressive reading, but not necessarily for repeated exposures to orthographic patterns.
- *Choral Reading.* Reading together with a group of peers provides support for weak readers in both word accuracy and pacing. Direct instruction in this method, with the teacher leading the reading, is sometimes called the *neurological imprint model.* Again, it provides a model for expressive reading.
- *Partner Reading.* Taking turns rereading the same passage provides opportunities for repeating words, for modeling and for socializing as motivation.
- *Audio Support.* Provide a book on tape, earphones, and a print copy of the book, so that a child can "rehearse" reading a few paragraphs or a short chapter over and over using the tape as a model for expression.
- *Provide Easy Text.* Although accuracy in reading new words is built into instructional situations where guidance for decoding is provided, fluency is built through reading text that is either familiar or easy and predictable. This can involve text at the *independent reading level* (i.e., 95-100% accuracy), or in an instructional situation, text at the *instructional reading level* (i.e., 90-95% accuracy) so long as unknown words are taught before rereading occurs.
- *Provide Text in which Target Words Make Multiple Appearances.* Keep in mind that many children need to see a word over and over before it will be recognized automatically. Over learning requires multiple readings of the same words.
- *Short Passages.* Repeat short passages often rather than longer passages fewer times. This increases the number of times that a word will be reread and increases the likelihood of retention of the word's orthographic pattern.
- *Flashcards.* Work with words that can be read accurately to make word recognition more rapid. This can be done with decodable words as well as words that are irregular. In the tutoring work I have supervised at Fordham University through the Ennis William Cosby Graduate Certificate Program, children learn to sound out decodable words (e.g., sat, thin, strap) and then they learn to read them quickly using flashcards. Flashcards alone will not produce fluency. Words must be practiced in text and read with expression.
- *Practice Short Plays.* Rereading plays without memorizing them provides practice in fluency. This commonly involves the use of

dialogue from children's literature and is called *Readers Theatre* (Martinez, Roser, and Strecker 1999). Preparing a play for an audience can be highly motivating and provides an authentic context for multiple rereadings.

- *Practice Poems for Expression.* Rereading a poem can be more motivating than rereading a paragraph. Poetry with end rhymes provides a supportive structure. Timothy Rasinski describes a "poetry party" where children practice reading poems dramatically and then perform for each other (Rasinski 2000). Again, for maximum exposure to the same words, keep poems short and reread often.

- *DEAR and USSR.* Drop Everything and Read and Uninterrupted Sustained Silent Reading can provide an opportunity to develop the habit of reading for enjoyment as a regular part of each school day. While the National Reading Panel reports that this practice is not validated by research showing a positive effect, neither does research show a negative effect. In a booklet developed by the Center for the Improvement of Early Reading Achievement (CIERA; Armbruster, Lehr, and Osborn 2001), it is suggested that direct instruction is the best environment for learning to read fluently. Independent reading should never take the place of direct instruction.

9

Vocabulary Instruction

Jeanne Chall (1987) talked about the difference between vocabulary that involves being able to recognize words in reading, commonly called *sight vocabulary*, and vocabulary that involves word meaning, or understanding words when listening and reading. Chall compares these two aspects to Marshall McLuhan's distinction between the *medium* and the *message*. Learning to read words by sight, quickly and automatically, is the medium by which we are brought to the message, or the content of the word. This chapter is about the latter—word meaning

This chapter on vocabulary and the following one on comprehension are based on the premise that spoken language is the foundation of written language. Oral vocabulary and listening comprehension need to be in place before reading can be understood. The early portion of this chapter describes, briefly, models of language and language learning that support both vocabulary and comprehension. The chapter also describes how meaning vocabulary has been taught historically, methods supported by current research, and special considerations for helping individuals with dyslexia build meaning vocabulary.

LANGUAGE DEVELOPMENT

This section provides a short explanation of models of language and of the developmental stages babies and toddlers go through in developing language before they come to school. It begins with a look at how oral vocabulary fits into an integrated view of the components of oral language. Bloom and Lahey (1978) conceptualize oral language as having three components: form, content, and use.

LANGUAGE FORM

Form, the first component of language, is about the way in which a message is delivered, rather than the message itself. There are three aspects of language form to consider: (a) phonology, (b) morphology, and (c) syntax.

Phonology

Phonology refers to rules for units of sound and their sequences. Phonemes, the smallest units of sound in words, are an aspect of phonology. Phonology develops early; babies are noisy. Through responding to involuntary crying, cooing, and babbling sounds, parents help their babies refine the sounds of their particular language, and in Skinnerian terms, they also extinguish sounds not specific to English by not responding to these sounds. For example, although English speaking babies can produce a Spanish /r/ sound, not all older children and adults can do this. During their first year, children learn to recognize patterns of sound and to attach meaning to these patterns, which we call receptive or listening vocabulary. They also learn to exert some control over expressing patterns of sounds, also necessary for their first spoken words.

Morphology

Morphology, the second component of language form, refers to rules for units of meaning within words. Where phonemes are units of sound within words, words are also made up of units of meaning. These small units of meaning are called *morphemes*. The word cats, for example, is composed of two morphemes, the base word *cat* and the *affix* or added morpheme -*s*. What we called root words, prefixes, and suffixes in high school are all morphemic units. Root or base words are called *free morphemes*, or morphemes that can stand alone, such as the verb *fry*. *Bound morphemes* are prefixes and suffixes, or morphemes that are added at the beginning or end, such as *re-* and -*ed* in the word *refried*. Bound morphemes cannot stand alone as words.

Syntax

Syntax, the third component of language form, simply put, involves the order of words in sentences. It has been argued that language learning, especially at the sentence level, is much more complex than simply repeating adult utterances and having them reinforced. The fact that children say sentences they have never heard before indicates they are creating rather than copying word combinations. For example, children learning to speak typically combine morphemes to forms verb tenses rather than just copying the adult words they hear. A sentence such as "I walkted" indicates that they are using a rule system of their own invention, rather than mimicking (deVilliers and deVilliers 1979). Word order affects the meaning of sentences. The meaning of each of the two sentences, "Mommy tickle me" and "I tickle Mommy," is controlled by word order. Lois Bloom (1999) refers to these early sentences as having an agent-action-object form. Once the representation of actions or verbs is used, young children's sentences can be said to have grammar.

Noam Chomsky talks about the deep structure of language that is common across all languages and the surface structure or form, which is language specific (e.g., English or Spanish). Deep and surface structure are related through *grammatical transformations* (Chomsky 1972). Toddlers' language often reflects meaning at the deep structure level (e.g., "Baby eyes") long before the surface structure of the language is complete (e.g., "My baby doll has soap in her eyes."). Young speakers often need an interpreter who must depend on both immediate context and past shared experiences.

Single words are typically uttered around the time of the first birthday and are almost always tangible objects (e.g., *Dada*, *duce* [juice], *bop* [bottle], *manana* [banana], *milk*). Early combinations typically begin to develop around 18 months, and to involve two objects (e. g., "baby eyes") or *object states* such as possession or negation (e.g., "my duce" or "no duce"). True sentences develop through the use of verbs during the third year. Representing an action with a word is more cognitively complex than representing a noun (Bloom 1999). Verb forms are also complex (e.g., the invented past tense *walkted*) and mastery goes on far beyond the early school years.

All three aspects of form are important to vocabulary development. The sounds of language support learning to distinguish and to say words. Morphemes or units of meaning within words help build nuances of meaning. Word order rules provide understanding for assembling units of vocabulary.

SEMANTICS

The second of the three interactive components of language is *semantics*, or the language rules that determine meaning. Semantics can refer to the meanings of words or the meanings of combinations of words in phrases or sentences and the relationships among words. Semantics involves concepts, or categories of objects and experiences. In other words, semantics is the content or meaning communicated through language forms.

Concepts are complex ideas with multiple attributes. School-age children are often taught to look for common attributes across examples of a concept in order to expand their word knowledge. Owens (2001) provides an example in which the word *dog* represents a concept with multiple exemplars. However, young children are very concrete in using words as labels. In building a vocabulary they tend to use words as labels for specific objects, such as a specific dog. At 15 months, Maddie called all dogs "Dodo," her word for her family's dog, "Hobart." Eleanor at 22 months still used the word "ducks" to talk about both ducks and chickens, apparently categorizing winged, egg-laying creatures as having features in common. Vocabulary acquisition is not a matter of simply memorizing labels, but of deepening understandings of the concepts they represent.

PRAGMATICS

Language use or *pragmatics* is the third interactive component of language. In a videotape I use in my classes with teachers, two brothers are playing in a wading pool. When 2-year-old Willy learns to say, "No!" to his older brother Sam who is propelling plastic toys out of his mouth at him, he is learning to use language to negotiate his needs. The common kindergarten directive, "Use your words," is a reminder that language can take the place of physical action and can be causal in social relationships. According to Vygotsky, language develops in a social environment and is scaffolded by language "experts"—parents, teachers and older children who model both form and usage.

Most definitions of language include the key terms that I have italicized in the following definition from Bloom and Lahey: "Language is a *code* whereby *ideas* about the world are *represented* through a *conventional system* of *arbitrary signals* for *communication*" (1978). Form, meaning, and use are all critical to this definition, and must work together for language to be effective.

According to Bloom and Lahey (1978), language disorders occur when any one of these three important components is poorly developed. Brilliant understanding of ideas cannot be communicated well by a person with a speech disorder or communicated in writing by a person with severe phonological processing problems (dyslexia). Perfectly mimicked sentences, common in some autistic children, are not really well integrated language because they have not been generated and because they are not used for effective communication.

LANGUAGE AND SCHOOL LEARNING

The developmental course of language in an individual can be an early indicator of need for special help. As outlined in Chapter 5, difficulty with phonological processing can be observed in the 3-year-old who has difficulty memorizing nursery rhymes and can be an early symptom of dyslexia. Three-year-olds typically have 900 to 1000 word expressive vocabularies and use 3 or 4 word sentences (Owens 2001).

By the time children begin Grade 1, most of their pronunciations can be understood. Children who will become typically developing readers can segment the phonemes in short words and represent them with letters in readable (if not conventional) invented spellings. By age 6, most children are generating complex complete sentences that use all parts of speech. First graders typically use around 2,600 words expressively and have a receptive vocabulary of over 20,000 words. William Nagy estimates that students know 45,000 words by the time they graduate from high school (Nagy 1988).

Just as children at risk for dyslexia need intensive early intervention with direct instruction in phonemic awareness and phonics, children with noticeably smaller-than-typical oral vocabularies need intensive instruction. The question is, what are best methods of instruction for both typically and atypically developing children?

Historically, vocabulary has been associated with intelligence. Early research on vocabulary was carried out by Terman (1916) who found that vocabulary was the best single predictor of verbal intelligence while developing the Stanford Binet Intelligence Scale. Reading vocabulary has also been found to be the strongest predictor of reading comprehension in individuals who can read (Chall and Stahl 1985). Keep in mind that reading comprehension is best predicted by word reading in combination with listening ability, which is sometimes measured in research by verbal IQ. Thus ties between meaning vocabulary and high-level verbal tasks including reading comprehension are well established.

Consider, too, that when we say that vocabulary is a strong predictor of comprehension, the opposite is also true. As a number of researchers have pointed out, we do not know the direction of the relationship between oral vocabulary and reading comprehension. It may be that a large vocabulary helps students comprehend what they read, and it may be that being able to understand during reading helps students to acquire new vocabulary words from context while reading (e.g., Baumann et al. 2003). Most likely, both are the case.

In a chapter on *Vocabulary Processes* in the third *Handbook of Reading Research* William Nagy and Judith Scott report that vocabulary is not currently a "hot topic" with the International Reading Association (Nagy and Scott 2000). Indeed, while the National Reading Panel targeted vocabulary for a subgroup, this committee had difficulty finding enough studies that met the panel's criteria for measurement of vocabulary to carry out a meta-analysis (National Reading

Panel 2000). The subgroup report does, however, summarize studies by method of instruction and it offers implications for instruction that are integrated into the following discussions.

VOCABULARY INSTRUCTION

A question that was researched over half a century ago and is being researched still is whether vocabulary is best taught through definitions, most likely involving direct instruction (e.g., looking up words in the dictionary or being presented with definitions to memorize), or through exposure to words in the context of conversations, listening to stories, or reading.

DEFINITIONS

The easiest way to teach vocabulary is to give children words and their definitions to memorize. This is a long-time tradition and a common educational practice. While this method is an easy one for the teacher, it is not necessarily a method by which words are easily or deeply learned and remembered by students. Memorization sometimes lasts through a Friday test but not often beyond.

William Nagy, in a monograph titled *Teaching Vocabulary to Improve Reading Comprehension*, argues against limiting instruction to definitions, particularly dictionary definitions, because they can be misleading. They often use words that are less familiar than the word they are defining. They do not usually provide examples and they can encourage a rigidly narrow understanding of the word. Keep in mind that children with language disorders can be as concrete as much younger children in their use of words. Nagy suggests, instead, that the teacher should provide opportunities to discuss the word, its definition and examples of its usage.

Another argument against definitional approaches is that there are simply too many words to teach directly. Researchers have provided estimates that through direct instruction, children can be taught about 10 to 12 words a week or 300 to 400 words a year (Stahl 1998, 2004), but there are also estimates that children learn 2000 to 3000 words a years through context while reading (Beck, McKeown, and Kucan 1991; Nagy and Herman 1987; Stahl 1998). Learning through context is necessary if children are to learn the volume of words we know that they will need to do well with language related tasks.

CONTEXT

The counter argument says that context is not always dependable. For vocabulary to be learned in context, children must read widely and they must read material with challenging vocabulary words. Not every third-grade level text has unfamiliar vocabulary words in it. Furthermore, not all text provides meanings from context. For example, in the first chapter of E. B. White's *Charlotte's Web* (1952) the meaning of the word *sopping* can be derived from its context (i.e., "The grass was wet and the earth smelled of springtime. Fern's sneakers were *sopping* by the time she caught up with her father"). However, in the same chapter, when Fern tries to rescue a baby pig, the context for the word *injustice* might lead the reader to *meanness* as easily as to *unfairness* (i.e., "'I see no difference,' replied Fern, still hanging on the ax. This is the most terrible case of *injustice* I ever heard of.'"). Beck refers to context cues that help provide meaning for a new vocabulary word as *directive contexts* (Beck, McKeown, and Kucan 2002). In this same chapter, E. B. White uses a directive context for the word *runt* (i.e., "'Well,' said her mother, 'one of the pigs is a *runt*. It's very small and weak, and it will never amount to anything. So your father has decided to do away with it'"). Text written especially for the acquisition of vocabulary could use directive context in a conscious way, but not all brilliant children's literature is written with such clear contextual clues.

In a review of research on vocabulary instruction with poor readers, Joanne Carlisle distinguishes between definitional approaches to vocabulary, in which new words are learned in isolation, and several other approaches in which new words are learned in the context of meaningful reading (Carlisle 1993). She suggests embedding vocabulary instruction in lessons in which the teacher reads stories aloud. Carlisle also suggests learning vocabulary through instruction in which decoding and word origins are taught together. In this approach, Anglo-Saxon words are taught before ones derived from the romance languages, with initial emphasis on letter-sound associations for decoding words with short and long vowels, followed by syllable division, and then morphemic knowledge of roots and affixes. Thus connections between letter patterns and word meanings are built into instruction (Henry 1988).

MIXED MODELS

Nagy's Model

William Nagy argues for a three-part program of vocabulary instruction, one that combines context with definitions and examples (Nagy 1988). He cites a research review indicating that what he calls a *mixed method* of vocabulary instruction can improve comprehension (Stahl and Fairbanks 1986). Nagy calls for *intensive vocabulary instruction* with the following four characteristics.

1. *Integration.* Vocabulary instruction should be integrated into the study of content and the study of other words. This is in keeping with constructivist views of building new information into existing schemas.

2. *Semantic Mapping.* Vocabulary can be enriched through word discussions in which new words are related to known words, and in which children brainstorm attributes of the concepts that are represented by vocabulary words. Several new related words can be learned at the same time. This method takes advantage of sociolinguistic theories of learning in which language is internalized through social experiences.

3. *Semantic Feature Analysis.* The teacher, acting as the Vygotskian *expert*, scaffolds learning through organizing contributions from many children into a graphic organizer that helps emphasize patterns. Nagy includes a number of ideas for this. Graphic organizers could involve a matrix of related concept words and their attributes. Analysis could involve a Venn Diagram of shared and unshared attributes, or a number of other organizational displays.

4. *Concept Formation.* Nagy warns teachers not to teach vocabulary as "new labels" for existing concepts. Explaining new words with synonyms does not always convey the full meaning. He suggests focusing on the concept and its attributes first, and then providing the new vocabulary word to the students once the concept is understood. Deepening conceptual knowledge prior to labeling it with a vocabulary word is a Piagetian approach, with cognition preceding language. Asking for examples and playing sorting games with words (e.g., "Is this or that an example of injustice?") can continue to deepen understanding once the label has been introduced (Nagy 1988).

Once new words have been learned through definitions, context, and examples, it is important for students to have multiple exposures according to Nagy. As with sight vocabulary, meaning vocabulary needs to become automatic. The more quickly words are recognized and understood the more processing space will be available for comprehension. It is also important that the words are used in meaningful contexts for ongoing refinement and deepening of understandings (Nagy 1988).

Beck and McKeown's Model

Researchers Isabel Beck and Margaret McKeown have worked for many years in the area of vocabulary and comprehension instruction at the University of Pittsburgh's Learning Research and Development Center (LRDC). Their book, *Bringing Words to Life: Robust Vocabulary Instruction* (Beck, McKeown, and Kucan 2002) provides theoretical background as well as rich examples of direct and contextualized instruction through literature.

Beck and her colleagues suggest that there are several levels to word knowledge on a continuum from having no knowledge of the word to understanding its multiple meanings in varying contexts and being able to understand it receptively as well as to use the word precisely. Their discussion of the deep levels of word knowledge make clear the limitations of the old-fashioned practice of having children simply memorize dictionary definitions.

The book also uses a system of *tiers* for choosing words to teach. Tier 1 words are easy words that most children know when coming to school. Tier 2 words are, "high frequency words for mature language users" that can "add productively to an individual's language ability." These words differ by age. The teacher must use judgment in choosing text and in choosing appropriate words for vocabulary study. Tier 2 words can be conceptualized as being in Vygotsky's *zone of proximal development* in which students can be successful with the support or scaffolding provided by a teacher, but cannot on their own. Tier 3 words are low frequency words (i.e., rarely used in general reading text) that might be studied in a specialized context, but are not an efficient use of students' time outside of the specialized content area (i.e., geography or biology lexicons). Criteria for choosing Beck's Tier 2 words, words for instruction, include usefulness in reading and other situations as well as conceptual understanding. The above-mentioned word *injustice* from *Charlotte's Web* would be a good Tier 2 word for discussion. Third graders understand the general concept of fair and unfair but they will need to continue deepening their understanding of the implications of justice and injustice in a democratic society through high school. In addition, the word is pivotal to the unfolding of story and theme, unlike the word *sopping* which does not occur again in the book after this chapter.

Teaching words directly, in Beck's model, involves several steps. First, a very simple definition needs to be provided. This is best provided by the teacher, who uses his or her judgment about what will help students make sense of the word. Examples using familiar situations should be included, and the teacher should be sure the word makes sense in the context of the story as well. Children can generate examples outside of the story context. The teacher can ask whether a situation could be described by the new word, and then ask why.

Follow up includes multiple exposures to the new word and frequent extensions beyond the story. The important point here is that the teacher should use these new words in multiple conversations and situations throughout the day and week, and should encourage the children to use their new words. This is not unlike what parents do with toddlers as they learn new words in a picture book or on an outing.

This kind of instruction is what whole language teachers call "authentic." It is richly contextualized and could not possibly be scripted because it is built on such a high level of knowledge of each child's abilities and interests and on experiences that the teacher and students hold in common. Beck and her colleagues use the term *richness of instruction*, which they define as "instruction that goes beyond definitional information to get students actively involved in using and thinking about word meanings and creating lots of associations among words" (Beck, McKeown, and Kucan 2002).

The book includes multiple examples of teacher-student conversations in chapters focused on both younger and older students. For younger students, the books tend to be read-alouds. Books easy enough for young children to read themselves do not have challenging words. Older students are encouraged to read short passages and then to deconstruct text in terms of what can and cannot be derived from context in terms of word meanings. As with Beck and McKeown's comprehension book *Questioning the Author* (see Chapter 10) students are taught to read text closely to try to figure out what the author is trying to say.

An Appendix of what Beck et al. (2002) call *Text Talk Books* is included. Each book has three vocabulary words listed as appropriate suggestions for instruction. Read-aloud books are listed by grade from Kindergarten through Grade 3. The lists include books of high literary quality such as the classic picture books *Caps for Sale* by Esphyr Slobodkina (*ordinary, refreshed, imitate*) and *Amos and Boris* by William Steig (*timid, morsel, protect*).

Nagy's and Beck's programs are consistent with the findings of the National Reading Panel Report (2000). The NRP subgroup report on vocabulary suggests combining methods rather than limiting instruction to what they call direct and indirect instruction. Findings from the studies they reviewed also indicate, as suggested by Nagy, that repeated exposures to new words are beneficial, and that active learning and use of new words in context are important.

VOCABULARY INSTRUCTION FOR STUDENTS WITH DYSLEXIA

Do children with dyslexia need special vocabulary instruction? The answer to this is yes and no. By definition, children with dyslexia have average or above average intelligence, and intelligence is closely tied to vocabulary, which suggests that they should not have special needs at the time that they enter school. We know that bright young children learn words easily from the context of conversations and listening to stories.

On the other hand, by the time that most children are reading fluently and reading to learn, they are picking up new word meanings from reading. This is one example of Keith Stanovich's *Matthew Effect* (1986b). Stanovich argues that although word-level reading disability begins with a specific problem—the phonological core deficit—it can cause global problems. Because they cannot decode, children with dyslexia are cut off from developing both new vocabulary and strategies for reading comprehension. The vocabulary scores of children with decoding difficulties can actually become lower over time if alternate methods of new word acquisition are not provided for them.

Listening to Books

The following suggestions are for use in addition to the vocabulary instruction suggested for all children in the sections above. An opportunity to listen to books is crucial for children with dyslexia. One of the findings of the Report of the National Reading Panel (2000) is that vocabulary can be learned in the context of books, and that listening to stories is an effective method for this. Another finding is that multiple exposures to new words help children increase vocabulary. In a study by Claudia Robbins and Linnea Ehri, kindergarten children who listened to several readings of a storybook with unfamiliar vocabulary knew more of the new story words at posttest in comparison with words that did not appear in the story (Robbins and Ehri 1994).

Multiple exposures to words help children learn their meanings. This can be in a number of contexts such as in classroom conversations following the introduction of new vocabulary in books. The use of new vocabulary in classroom conversations and authentic learning situations will benefit all children in a class, but it will be of particular benefit to children whose reading skills are limited.

In addition to listening to whole-class read-alouds, listening to taped books provides another solution to being sure that children with dyslexia are exposed to vocabulary. Tapes of necessary educational materials are provided free of cost by the Library of Congress to children and adults with vision impairment. Children with dyslexia are entitled to the same free services. These tapes need to be ordered and they take time to be delivered. They are a good solution for older students faced with five or six large textbooks in a given semester. For younger students, who read many short books, most bookstores and libraries carry children's books on tape. Another solution is to ask other students to record books for a classroom collection. Many schools have a *book buddy* program in which older students routinely visit to read aloud to younger students, and some of this reading can be taped.

Vocabulary Through Computer Assisted Instruction

The Report of the National Reading Panel (2000) indicated that vocabulary instruction delivered through the use of computers "shows positive learning gains over traditional methods." Several studies cited used computer technology to provide aids that the report lists as, "talking software, Hypertext dictionary support, speech prompts, adaptive software, visual representations, and multisensory input." While the studies examined were limited to students without disabilities, features such as talking text provide an ideal learning environment for children with severe decoding difficulties. Bookwise, a CAI literature program described in more detail in the next chapter, includes a feature through which vocabulary words can be defined by a computerized voice.

All children benefit from listening as well as reading in order to enrich their vocabularies (Stahl 2004). This is critically important for children whose instructional reading materials are below their oral vocabulary level. For these children, teachers need to go out of their way to provide listening experiences, and they need to do it in a way that does not take time away from direct instruction in school.

SUMMARY

In a themed issue of the International Dyslexia Association's journal, *Perspectives*, that was devoted to vocabulary and the child with disabilities, Steven Stahl (2004) suggested that definitions without context and examples are soon forgotten. He suggested teaching clusters of related words. Not only should new words be embedded in the context of reading or listening activities, new words will be learned in greater depth if they are compared to similar words. He provides the following example:

> Consider the word "debris." This is a form of "trash," but not all trash is "debris." "Garbage" actually means organic materials, such as leavings from apples peels or leftover and unwanted food. "Debris" means trash left over from some sort of accident or catastrophic event, such as an automobile accident ..." (Stahl 2004).

He suggested that the meaning of a word goes way beyond rote memory of its definition, and that active engagement is required. He also suggested that students need multiple exposures to the word in multiple contexts. These are good suggestions for all students, and especially so for students with limited access to higher-level print.

10

Reading Comprehension

This chapter provides a rationale for comprehension instruction for students with dyslexia and a brief historical perspective of comprehension instruction. Then it compares the specific skills approach historically used with students with reading disabilities with newer, constructivist models in which strategies are taught rather than skills. Finally, it provides information on effective comprehension instruction from the National Reading Panel Report (2000) and provides examples of a number of effective instructional strategies.

COMPREHENSION INSTRUCTION
FOR STUDENTS WITH DYSLEXIA

Comprehension is the goal of word-level reading instruction, but it is often neglected in curriculum for children with word-level reading difficulties. Historically, children with dyslexia have received little training in reading comprehension (Maria 1987). For many years, reading instruction for these children focused almost exclusively on decoding, with minimal attention directed toward reading for meaning. Most children with dyslexia were not taught how to think critically while reading (Baker and Brown 1984; Harste 1985).

The reasoning behind this has been that if dyslexia is a disorder at the word reading level, then instruction should focus on decoding.

The unspoken assumption is that if comprehension rests on decoding and decoding is remediated, then comprehension skills will follow. This reasoning seems faulty. Again, considering the Matthew Effect (Stanovich 1986b), while comprehension may not be the original difficulty, without opportunities to develop comprehension strategies, this, too, can become a real and enduring issue for children with dyslexia. One advantage of whole language instruction is its emphasis on comprehension strategies, despite its lack of direct instruction in decoding.

Weak decoding can have a strong impact on comprehension for students with dyslexia. Probably the single most important factor in increasing their comprehension ability is successful remediation of word-level reading. Chapter 8 (*Rate and Fluency*) discusses the strain that is put on processing space when reading is slow and laborious. Keep in mind Philip Gough's *simple view of reading* (Gough and Tunmer 1986). In this view, decoding and listening comprehension both need to be strong in order for reading comprehension to be strong.

Another impediment to instruction in comprehension is the phonetically decodable text that is often used in teaching phonics to children with dyslexia. This simple text does not lend itself to reading comprehension instruction. The language in these texts is not natural, making it hard to understand. Furthermore, it is difficult to represent complex concepts such as conflict or cause and effect if text is limited to short, phonetically regular words. For bright children who are struggling to read, there is a huge gap between the challenging text they can understand when it is read aloud to them and the simple ideas portrayed in decodable readers.

While all beginning readers have a gap between their listening level and the relatively lower level of text they are able to read aloud and understand, this gap continues to be large for children with decoding problems. It is important that there are ample opportunities for listening to intellectually stimulating books read aloud or on tape during the extended period of time it takes for these students to learn to read words. As mentioned in the previous chapter, listening activities are needed to provide the acquisition of vocabulary. In addition, it is in this format that higher level thinking and comprehension strategies can be taught.

A BRIEF HISTORY OF COMPREHENSION INSTRUCTION

Before the 1980s, there was little focus on comprehension in either regular education classrooms or in reading research. When the first edition of this book was published, Diana Clark wrote, "Reading comprehension instruction has an abysmal record, not just for reading disabled students, but for all learners" (Clark 1988, p. 79). She cited Dolores Durkin's study in which fewer than 50 minutes were spent on comprehension instruction out of 17,997 minutes of the researcher's classroom observation time (Durkin 1978-1979).

David Pearson and Linda Fielding (1991) have made the point that until 1981, there simply were no reviews of research on comprehension. By 1984, in the first edition of the *Handbook of Reading Research*, Robert Tierney and James Cunningham were able to report a dramatic increase. By 1991, when the second volume of the *Handbook* was published, Pearson and Fielding refer to the recent "explosion" in comprehension research and begin with a review of recent reviews. By the time of the third edition (2000), the *Handbook* contained multiple articles describing aspects of meaning-based instruction.

SPECIFIC SKILLS INSTRUCTION

Historically, a bottom-up or specific skills approach has been used for instructing students with reading disabilities. In this approach, comprehension is broken down into skills that typically are pretaught in short exercises before they are practiced in text. Skills include *getting the main idea, finding facts, detecting the sequence,* and *making inferences*. Often, these skills are taught through drills in reading short passages followed by questions. The Barnell Loft Specific Skills Series (Boning 1990) is typical of what is commercially available for this type of instruction. Each skill-type is available in a series of graded texts with a monitoring system that can be carried out by the student as well as by the teacher. A package of these materials allows a classroom of children to work independently on a variety of specific skills at many different reading levels.

Probably one of the most systematic deliveries of this specific skills approach involves computer-assisted instruction (CAI). One example of such application is the program described by Judith Boettcher (1983) that was developed by Control Data Corporation and known as the Reading Comprehension System. It is structured around a five-by-six matrix that enables the teacher to select appropriate lessons for a student depending on instructional needs; there are five levels of difficulty applied to short reading passages written at six vocabulary levels. Each passage includes 10 comprehension questions, two for each of the following five comprehension areas: word meanings, syntax, word relationships, making inferences, and interpreting. Students receive immediate feedback on their answers, and continue working until the computer judges them to be at mastery level on each skill.

One criticism of a specific skills approach is that many of the available materials for this instruction represent something closer to a test than to real instruction (Durkin 1978-79). In other words, instead of breaking a skill down into component parts and providing guided learning experiences with each part, instruction is apt to involve exercises in which students are expected to perform a task over and over without any special guidance. A notable exception can be found in the research of Joanna Williams who uses task analysis and step-by-step teaching to break comprehension down for children with reading difficulty. Her work on main idea identification with children with learning disabilities represents an innovative approach to comprehension skills instruction (Williams 1986). Williams contends that the ability to select main ideas from text requires basic classification skills. Thus, she provides students with initial instruction in categorizing objects and pictures, which is later related to text organization.

When first working at the paragraph level, students are asked, "What is this paragraph about?" (i.e., "What is the general topic?") and then are required to circle the word referring to the general topic. The next question is, "Does this paragraph tell us everything about __?" followed by, "What is the specific topic?" In this way, students learn to identify topic sentences within paragraphs. Later, they learn to determine the main ideas in paragraphs that do not contain topic sentences, the more common type of paragraph according to Williams (1986). All work is carefully sequenced from simple to complex, from choosing titles, for instance, to writing summaries. Investigating the effectiveness of this approach with 11-year-old students with learning disabilities, Williams found that they produced better paragraph summaries than did controls who had not received this training.

STRATEGY INSTRUCTION

Janice Dole and her colleagues described the difference between what they call traditional instruction in comprehension *skills* and a newer approach that involves *strategy* instruction (Dole et al. 1991). They viewed skills as being a rather passively learned set of routines whereas strategies are viewed as cognitive processes requiring decision-making and critical thinking. Indeed, cognitive theory has played a major role in the development of recent comprehension instruction. Pearson and Fielding summarize some of the newer findings as follows:

> (T)he principle seems clear: Students understand and remember ideas better when they have to transform these ideas from one form to another. Apparently it is in the transformation process that *authors'* ideas become *readers'* ideas, rendering them more memorable (Pearson and Fielding 1991, p. 847).

Scott Paris and his colleagues, writing in the second edition of *The Handbook of Reading Research*, call strategies, "personal cognitive tools that can be used selectively and flexibly (Paris, Wasik, and Turner 1991). This is in contrast with skills, which they view as learned to the automatic level and used unconsciously during reading.

Several concepts from the field of cognitive psychology have contributed to this new view of both reading and the reader (Maria 1987). One concept is *schemata*, or psychological frameworks that develop out of an individual's cultural experiences (Rumelhart 1980). According to this view, the reader must fit new facts into an existing mental schema for a particular idea, or if necessary, adjust the schema. Schema theory led to an awareness of the importance of the reader's background knowledge to understanding and interpreting text. The notion of schema building implies that comprehension is an active process with interaction between the text and the reader. Louise Rosenblatt's *Reader Response* theory has influenced the development of schema-based comprehension instruction. In short, Reader Response theory suggests that literary interpretation is constructed by the reader (Rosenblatt 1978; 1989). This reader-text transaction replaces the notion of teacher as expert interpreter guiding the student toward "right" answers.

Another concept that has had tremendous influence on reading comprehension instruction and research is *metacognition*, defined by Linda Baker and Ann Brown as "the knowledge and control the child has over his or her own thinking and learning activities." By knowledge, they refer to the awareness of the processing demands of a particular task, and by control, the ability to check, plan, monitor, or evaluate one's own activities while reading (Baker and Brown 1984).

A third concept that has gained prominence in the reading comprehension literature is the notion of *interaction between student and teacher* in the learning situation. This concept developed out of L. S. Vygotsky's theory of guided learning, in a social context within a student's "zone of proximal development" which he defined as:

> . . . the distance between the actual developmental level as determined by individual problem-solving and the level of potential development as determined through problem-solving under adult guidance or in collaboration with more capable peers (Vygotsky 1978).

Reuven Feuerstein's theory of "mediated learning" has also contributed to our understanding of the teacher-student interaction. Feuerstein maintains that early learning is shaped by interactions in which a parent models problem-solving that eventually allows a child to problem-solve on his own (Feuerstein 1979).

These three ideas—*schema theory, metacognition,* and *socially mediated learning*—have led researchers to a new conceptualization of effective reading comprehension. Support for active learning, self-monitoring, cooperative or social learning, rich contexts, and flexible strategy use can be found in the National Reading Panel subgroup report on comprehension (2000). The executive summary of the Comprehension Subgroup Report lists eight instructional strategies that are supported by scientific research:

1. Comprehension Monitoring
2. Cooperative Learning
3. Graphic and Semantic Organizers
4. Story Structure
5. Question Answering
6. Question Generation
7. Summarizing
8. Multiple-strategy use

The reading comprehension instructional approaches that follow take advantage of these methods. Keep in mind that the National Reading Panel subgroup on comprehension did not include studies of students with disabilities in its meta-analysis. While the strategy instruction methods presented below are appropriate for students with dyslexia (i.e., with decoding problems but with average or above oral language and verbal intelligence), they may not be appropriate for students with more global oral language disorders.

Reciprocal Teaching

Reciprocal teaching is an instructional model designed by Annemarie Palincsar and Ann Brown. This interactive approach to teaching metacognitive strategies has been used successfully with students who are poor readers. This model contains two levels. The first is a sequence of four strategies: 1) generating questions about the text prior to reading, 2) summarizing portions of the text, 3) predicting what will happen next, and 4) clarifying and evaluating after reading the text. The second level of reciprocal teaching involves the instructional delivery, an interactive dialogue between teacher and students, and eventually, among the students themselves (Palincsar 1986; Palincsar and Brown 1983, 1984, 1985).

Reciprocal teaching instruction begins with a teacher-led discussion about the kinds of problems readers may experience in comprehending what they read. It introduces the four strategies, each on a separate day, and explains why they are helpful. Instruction usually begins at the paragraph level, but can involve single sentences for readers who are more disabled. The discussion aims at stimulating metacognitive awareness so that students learn to guide and monitor their own

Aquanauts	
Student 1:	My qustion is, what does the aquanaut need when he goes under water?
Student 2:	A watch
Student 3:	Flippers
Student 4:	A belt
Student 1:	Those are all good answers.
Teacher:	Nice job! I have a question, too. Why does the aquanaut wear a belt, what is so special about it?
Student 3:	It's a heavy belt and keeps him from floating up to the top again.
Teacher:	Good for you.
Student 1:	For my summary now . . . This paragraph was about what the aquanaut needs to take when they go under the water.
Student 5:	And also about why they need those things.
Student 3:	I think we need to clarify "gear."
Student 6:	That's the special things they need.
Teacher:	Another word for gear in this story might be equipment, the equipment that makes is easier for the aquanauts to do their job.
Student 1:	I don't think I have a prediction to make.
Teacher:	Well, in the story they tell us that there are "many strange and wonderful creatures" that the aquanauts see as they do their work. My prediction is that they will describe some of these creatures. What are some of the strange creature that you already know about that live in the ocean?
Student 6:	Octopuses.
Student 3:	Whales?
Student 5:	Sharks!
Teacher:	Let's listen and find out. Who will be our teacher?

"A Reciprocal Teaching Script." Reproduced with permission from the author, Annemarie Palincsar.

comprehension. Once students have caught on to the four strategies, the teacher turns over her role to one of the students who leads the activities and calls on other students. This peer teaching provides the reciprocal teaching component. The teacher subtly guides and provides feedback to the student–as–teacher. After the activities are mastered, they are applied to classroom texts.

Reciprocal teaching involves a number of instructional features studied by the National Reading Panel and found to be effective: cooperative learning, question generation and answering, summarization, and comprehension monitoring. Reciprocal teaching also involves multiple strategies, which the National Reading Panel calls, "a revolution in the field from the study of individual strategies to their flexible and multiple use" (2000). That is, unlike the specific skills strategies described above, students are provided with instruction in integrating a number of strategies for comprehension. They are encouraged to think flexibly and to self-monitor in terms of shifting from one strategy to another.

Palincsar and Brown conducted several evaluations of their techniques and report significant improvement in students' comprehension as measured daily on reading passages. This improvement was maintained over eight weeks following treatment (Palincsar and Brown

1983, 1984, 1985). Moreover, effects carried over into other subject areas such as science and social studies (Brown, Palincsar, and Armbruster 1984).

Transactional Strategies Instruction

Michael Pressley has worked with research colleagues and with teachers to develop teaching methods that he calls *transactional strategies instruction*. Pressley views this instruction as Vygotskian in that comprehension develops as the result of social interactions between students and teacher. Students are provided with direct instruction in a number of comprehension strategies, and are encouraged to talk about and choose a strategy for understanding as they read. Teachers model their own thinking aloud and encourage students to do this for each other. Students are provided with positive reinforcement when a strategy is successful, and are encouraged to attribute success to use of the strategy. Thought processes are valued more than product. Pressley compares transactional strategies instruction to whole language instruction in some regards (e.g., process over product) but comments that whole language is more based in philosophy than in cognitive psychology. Teachers using transactional strategy instruction tend to step in as coaches whereas whole language teachers tend to be in favor of noninterventionist learning. Pressley differentiates it from other strategy instruction models that use direct explanation by the degree to which this model becomes part of the texture of every aspect of school life over a very long period of time (Pressley et al. 1992).

Irene Gaskins of the Benchmark School is a collaborator of Pressley's. Benchmark is an independent school outside of Philadelphia. The school serves elementary and middle school children with reading problems. Teachers at Benchmark have been actively involved, together with a team of researchers, in the development of transactional strategy instruction. Research on this instruction has involved extensive teacher interviews indicating a high level of enthusiasm and involvement among faculty (Pressley et al. 1991). Pressley makes use of detailed and extensive transcriptions of teacher–student interactions to document this instruction (Pressley et al. 1992).

Both the Palincsar and Brown model and the Pressley model make use of principles believed to be related to effective instruction for children with reading difficulties: carefully sequenced lessons, direct instruction, and opportunity for practice over a long period of time.

Book Clubs

Taffy Raphael's *Book Clubs* are another form of socially mediated learning. These student-led discussions provide a heterogeneous, small group setting within the classroom in which children can share their ideas about what they have read (Raphael and McMahon 1994; McMahon and Goatley 1995; McMahon and Raphael with Goatley and Pardo 1997). Theoretically, the idea of book clubs builds on a foundation of reader response theory and the notion that children construct meaning by discussing what they read in supportive social settings. Once children are taught to engage in productive conversations, the teacher can step back from directing these conversations. Teachers typical circulate and listen in, but make sure that the conversations are student centered. Training in how to engage in these conversations can be carried out through a *fishbowl*, an activity in which one Book Club meets in the middle of the room with other students surrounding it and observing. Observers are encouraged to look for positive features such as turn-taking and being accountable for comments through backing up points of view with text references and joining in a debriefing after the discussion. The fishbowl strategy allows a teacher to set routines for Book Clubs before handing over leadership to the students.

Book clubs are conceptualized as one component of a myriad of reading and writing activities within flexible groupings. Book clubs often are formed around common interests with five to six students participating. If a way can be found for a student with dyslexia to listen to a book (e.g., on tape, with a stronger reading peer, or with a parent), then he or she can participate in the discussion phase of book clubs. This can supplement small group direct instruction in decoding and other skill work usually carried out with reading-level peers, even when the student is reading low reading-level decodable text for decoding instruction. Where children with dyslexia often are isolated from intellectual peers or from friends with common book interests, book clubs provide an opportunity for this valuable sociolinguistic experience. Virginia Goatley, currently teaching at CUNY Albany, has carried out research in which children with reading disabilities have participated successfully in book clubs (Goatley 1996; Goatley, Brock, and Raphael 1995; Goatley and Levine 1997).

Questioning the Author

Isabel Beck and Margaret McKeown have, for many years, carried out research on comprehension instruction, as well as on vocabulary instruction as described in Chapter 9. *Questioning the Author* (QtA) is a comprehension approach that is based on ideas about constructing one's own learning that grew out of the *cognitive revolution*, a rebellion against the notion that learning involves outside reinforcement of "right" answers. Cognitive psychologists like Piaget and Vygotsky believed that learning was constructed internally through a process of constantly adjusting one's schemas in response to new information.

QtA is philosophically aligned with other comprehension programs in which learning is conceptualized as an active process, but learning is not left entirely up to the student. QtA involves very direct instruction of strategies (Beck et al. 1997).

One important QtA strategy invites students to return to the text. In this regard, it is similar to the *clarifying step* in Reciprocal Teaching. However, QtA introduces a new element here. It teaches students to see the author as fallible and themselves as problem-solvers trying to figure out the gist of an idea that has not been well communicated. This removes the burden of not being able to understand content easily from the student and places it on the author. Students are supported by the teacher as they learn to return to the text to try to puzzle out the author's intent.

In order to do this, a second QtA strategy is utilized. This involves segmenting the text into small units of meaning. For very young readers, this can be as small as a sentence or two. Paragraphs work well with older readers. The teacher can model this during a read aloud, or can ask the students to read themselves, but to stop at a designated point for discussion.

Discussion involves a third strategy characteristic of QtA: the use of *queries* rather than traditional questions. Where questions, in Beck's view, tend to be used to evaluate a student's understanding *after* reading, queries are used *during* reading in order to help in the process of building meaning. Queries are used to generate discussions among students and tend to be more open-ended than questions and to involve higher-level thinking. Like reciprocal teaching, query-generated discussion provides an external scaffold for later internalization of the questioning process. As with Beck and McKeown's vocabulary instruction, QtA requires the teacher to know the students well and to be tuned in to nuances of meaning during discussions, but it also involves withdrawing at times to encourage students to talk directly with each other. This promotes more active student participation (Beck et al. 1997).

Computer Assisted Instruction (CAI) for Comprehension

According to information processing theory, the working memory of students with dyslexia is overtaxed by decoding, leaving little processing space for understanding (LaBerge and Samuels 1974). As stated in Chapter 7, decoding that is both accurate and fluent frees processing space for comprehension. One solution for students with dyslexia is to use computers that can "read" difficult text aloud.

Bookwise, a Xerox Corporation computer-delivered literature program, is an example of *computer assisted instruction* (CAI) that takes advantage of current technology, presenting print on a screen while "speaking" the words. Speed is adjustable, the vocalized sentence is highlighted, and text can be scrolled backward and forward. In one study, Jerome Elkind and his colleagues used Bookwise with middle school students in a California school for children with dyslexia (Elkind, Cohen, and Murray 1993). These children were already engaged in multisensory decoding instruction using the Slingerland method. Not all of the 28 subjects had deficits in reading comprehension, but 70 percent were at least a grade level below grade placement in this skill. Treatment involved half an hour using the computer and half an hour discussing the literature each day. Controls read the same books and discussed them within a comparable time frame. Each of the two classes served as control to the other during the two semesters of treatment, so that each child's and each class' gains could be compared with and without CAI. Results were mixed: 70 percent of the students made a year's worth of growth in the CAI semester, and 40 percent made as much as five grade-levels of growth. A few subjects actually lost ground, probably because of kinesthetic-motor problems with the computer.

Comprehension through Imagery

The National Reading Panel Report lists *Mental Imagery* as an effective reading comprehension instructional strategy for improving memory of text. While not in the NRP's top strategies list, the technique is considered an effective alternative, and the NRP Report lists five studies demonstrating effectiveness. Sheikh and Sheikh's (1985) book, *Imagery in Education*, reviews research on comprehension retention through imagery and provides one of these studies as an example of controlled research on the technique in low achieving students. Ellen Peters asked eighth graders to read 12 short biographical passages and to try to create associative images linking the names and accomplishments of the persons in the biographies. Controls were asked, simply, to try to remember the persons' accomplishments. In each instructional condition, there were participants who read two years below grade level and two years above grade level. For both high and low achieving students, the imagery technique provided a strong advantage in ability to remember information from the passages. In fact, the low achieving students with instruction in imagery performed at least as well as the high achieving students in the no-imagery instruction condition (Peters and Levin 1986).

One rationale for using imagery as a mnemonic device in dyslexic students is a claim made, for example, by Aylett Cox (see Alphabetic Phonics in Chapter 20) that some children with dyslexia are believed to have better-than-usual spatial ability or ability with imagery. Advocates of Howard Gardner's (1983) theory of multiple intelligences suggest using imaging techniques with these children because the techniques build on what may be areas of strength. Keep in mind that we have no scientific evidence of superior imaging in children with dyslexia, only evidence that imagery training has been found to improve comprehension.

In a literature review of research on teaching imagery to increase comprehension, Linda Gambrell and Patricia Koskinen summarize implications for teaching (2002). They suggest that teachers can model the imaging strategy by sharing what they see in their heads as they read, much as they do with other strategies modeled during shared readings. They also suggest a sequence of instructional activities that includes the following: creating mental images after looking at an object carefully, creating images in response to the teacher's oral descriptions, recalling familiar scenes as images and then drawing them, creating mental images as the teacher reads descriptions aloud, and guiding students to create images as they read to themselves.

Mark Sadoski and Allan Paivio, in their book *Imagery and Text: A Dual Coding Theory of Reading and Writing* (2001), suggest that reading is aligned with other aspects of cognition in that it involves both verbal and nonverbal components. This link between the verbal, linguistic aspects of reading and the nonverbal images it invokes are at the heart of reading for meaning. The authors provide examples of reading-based Dual Coding Theory (DCT) such as Linnea Ehri's use of mnemonic pictures for teaching letter names (Ehri, Deffner, and Wilce 1984) and mnemonic pictures for vocabulary training (Levin 1985; Pressley, Levin, and McDaniel 1987). They also mention a program designed by Nanci Bell in which induced imagery is used as a support for understanding text in students with reading difficulties.

Nanci Bell, who works with Patricia and Phyllis Lindamood at Lindamood-Bell Learning Processes in San Luis Obispo, California, has developed a program called Visualizing and Verbalizing for Language Comprehension and Thinking (V/V) for use with individuals with comprehension problems (Bell 1986). Bell uses this program to correct what she believes is a cognitive processing disorder that she calls *Concept Imagery Disorder* (CID). Note that many of Bell's subjects have adequate word reading and phonemic segmentation skills, and thus cannot be considered dyslexic. The program, however, is a good example of a highly structured and explicit comprehension model. There are specific, sequenced steps to V/V in which students move from describing pictures with feedback to developing images for increasingly complex language, beginning at the word level, and moving to sentences, paragraphs, and finally, pages of text. Text, level of questioning, and feedback become more abstract as the V/V Program progresses. Evaluation of Bell's program with reading-impaired children has focused on pretest-posttest improvements in individuals in a remedial laboratory setting; these gains have reached statistically significant levels on a number of measures of oral directions and reading comprehension (Bell 1991).

All of these strategies are highly complex. Students need to learn and internalize the components over a period a time. Expertise in using the strategies is cumulative. Use of the vocabulary of instruction needs time to become automatic. Our point is that these strategies require a long-term commitment on the part of the teacher. For additional material on reading comprehension, there are a number of research reviews, edited collections of articles, and "how to" books available (e.g., Blachowicz and Ogle 2001; Block and Pressley 2002; Cornoldi and Oakhill 1996; Maria 1990; Oakhill and Garnham 1988; French, Ellsworth, and Amoruso 1995; Pearson and Fielding 1991; Pressley 2003; Sadoski and Paivio 2001).

11

Spelling Instruction

The word *orthography* comes from the Greek roots *ortho* meaning correct and *graph* meaning write. It means correct or conventional units of written letters. Spelling tends to be an area of weakness for individuals with dyslexia, and weak spelling tends to persist into adulthood, even when reading has been remediated successfully. Keeping Uta Frith's stage model of reading and spelling development in mind, we can conceptualize children with deficits in phonemic awareness as struggling during the alphabetic stage to acquire a phonological representation of spoken words, and continuing to struggle in making the transition to recognizing and remembering units of letters that are used to spell at the orthographic stage.

As mentioned in Chapter 3, *Assessment*, systematic spelling instruction is critical for students with dyslexia. This chapter raises questions related to spelling instructional systems and outlines principles of spelling instruction.

IS ENGLISH REGULAR ENOUGH TO TEACH ITS REGULARITES?

English is a relatively irregular language because its roots come from so many different languages. Words with Celtic origins, like the name *Cian*, do not follow the rule that says that *c* makes its soft sound (i.e., /s/) when it comes before *e*, *i*, and *y* (e.g., ceiling, city, cycle).

Words with Greek roots spell /f/ as *ph* rather than *f*. Richard Venezky provides an informative view into the histories of words in *The American Way of Spelling: The Structure and Origins of American English Orthography* (1999). Children with a gift for the complexities of languages may be fascinated. For children with dyslexia, these inconsistencies and variations make spelling very hard.

The most common way that spelling is taught is through a word list presented on Monday and tested on Friday. Sometimes these words are thematically related (e.g., *ghost, Halloween, pumpkin*) and simply need to be memorized. Sometimes the words have orthographic similarities (e.g., boat, coat, cloak) and are taught by drawing attention to their common pattern. Pattern seeking is a metacognitive strategy and encourages the learner to generalize to other words.

Edmund Henderson has suggested that teacher knowledge of the history of the English language makes it easier to teach English spelling. He pointed out that the historical path of English is recreated in the developmental path taken by young spellers. Children's earliest spellings are alphabetic with correspondence between individual phonemes and letters, as was the case with Old English or Anglo-Saxon spellings. The more complex orthographic patterns that are learned later come from later forms of English (Henderson 1990). This is an idea proposed by Marcia Henry as well (1990). Both Henderson and Henry believe that teachers need this knowledge to help their students make sense out of the complexity of English.

Not everyone agrees with Henderson and Henry however. Some important pedagogical issues related to spelling instruction were brought to light 25 years ago by Margaret Stanback and Marylee Hansen in a review of the literature (Stanback and Hansen 1980). The "generalization controversy" (Yee 1966) is concerned with the question of whether or not the sound–symbol correspondence of English orthography is sufficiently regular to warrant teaching rules and regularities. This question has provoked a number of studies aimed at determining the amount of regularity in the English spelling system. Ernest Horn, the staunchest opponent of teaching generalizations in spelling, states that over a third of the words in a standard English dictionary have more than one pronunciation, that more than half of these contain silent letters, particularly vowels, have more than one sound, and that unstressed syllables are hard to spell (Horn 1960). Horn advocates teaching only those rules that apply to a very large number of words and have few exceptions. In contrast, Paul Hanna and his associates, after conducting a computerized analysis of 17,000 English words, conclude that only 3 percent required rote memorization, falling into the category of "demon" words (Hanna et al. 1966).

Where Horn and Hanna and his colleagues examined words only in terms of their phonemic regularity, Richard Venezky has analyzed 20,000 words, taking into consideration morphemic features as well. As a result of his findings, Venezky recommends three categories of spelling patterns: (a) predictable, (b) unpredictable and frequent, and (c) unpredictable and rare, rather than the standard two-categories classification of words as regular or irregular (Venezky 1970).

Although research on the instructional implications of the generalization controversy has apparently produced ambiguous results, Stanback and Hansen cite two studies that imply that direct instruction in spelling generalization was beneficial to slower learners. They conclude that there may not be one best way to teach spelling, but observe that

> . . . in the light of analyses such as Venezky's, the phonology and orthography are seen to be closely related, especially when certain morphological principles are understood. For example, the past tense marker *-ed* is consistently spelled, no matter that it is pronounced in three different ways (e.g., /id/ in *landed*, /d/ in *planned*, and /t/ in *walked*). In fact, the morphology is highly dependable for spelling, as there are few exceptions. Prefixes and suffixes, inflectional and derivational, are added to roots by fixed and dependable rules (Stanback and Hansen 1980).

These dependable rules are included in the spelling curricula of most of the programs described in Part III of this book.

NATURALISTIC SPELLING METHODS

There has been worry among practitioners about children with dyslexia in whole language classrooms employing the writing process and basing instruction on invented spelling. English orthography is extraordinarily complex and children with dyslexia do not have a flair for picking up its underlying structures. Practitioners also worry that without direct instruction in spelling patterns, children with dyslexia will retain their own misspellings. Even though researchers such as Rebecca Treiman do not find this to be the case, all children benefit from spelling instruction, both the early ear spelling inherent in invented spelling as well as the more formal introduction of orthographic patterns and spelling rules.

Chapter 15 describes spelling procedures used in the *Reading Recovery* approach. Within the context of writing a story based on interest in a book the child has read, a tutor encourages a child to listen for sounds in words that the child cannot spell. Reading Recovery takes advantage of the connections between phoneme segmentation and spelling with Elkonin-type boxes used for writing letters as these words are sounded out with support from the tutor (see Chapter 5, *Phonemic Awareness*). This is a modification of invented spelling, with a tutor providing cues for a child to use in self-correcting. With words that the child wants to use but that are beyond her developmental spelling level, the tutor simply provides the letters for her to copy. Thus the child has the advantage of sounding out invented spellings that are within what Vygotsky would call the "zone of proximal development" without the perceived disadvantage of seeing her own misspellings later in the lesson when these words are used for reading instruction. Research on Reading Recovery has tended to focus on reading rather than spelling so that we cannot be sure of the effect of this instruction on the spellings of these young children who are at risk for reading failure.

MULTISENSORY REMEDIAL SPELLING INSTRUCTION

Multisensory teaching has probably had its greatest impact in the area of remedial spelling instruction, the two best known approaches being the *Orton-Gillingham* and the *Fernald* methods. As previously described in Chapter 4, the Orton-Gillingham approach teaches spelling as the inverse of, in conjunction with, and as reinforcement for, reading. Learning progresses from small units (phonemes and syllables) to larger units (words and sentences). Enormous emphasis is placed on the alphabetic principle and phonetic regularity of the English spelling system. All learning is carefully sequenced. Inconsistent spelling patterns are only gradually introduced, and optional spelling patterns representing similar sounds are taught as separate units. Irregular spellings are not taught until the student becomes comfortable with phonetic spellings. Although considerable practice with syllables is provided, inflectional endings, as well as prefixes and suffixes, are treated as morphemes and taught by the rule. The technique applied to studying spelling is *Simultaneous Oral Spelling (SOS)* wherein the child pronounces the word, spells it orally, and then writes the word, saying the letter names as he writes.

In contrast to the Orton-Gillingham approach, the Fernald method (Fernald 1943), while also multisensory, teaches spelling with whole words of a student's own choosing rather than word units following an orderly sequence. The Fernald procedure closely resembles the *neurological impress* method described in Chapter 7. It focuses on the student's development of a distinct visual image of the word and automaticity for the motor pattern for writing the word, both processes being mutually reinforcing. The technique involves having the student say the word while looking at it with the teacher underlining each syllable as it is pronounced. The student then repeats the word slowly, tracing each syllable as it is pronounced. The next step requires the student to write each syllable while saying it slowly so that individual letter sounds may be heard. Finally, the student writes the whole word from memory (while pronouncing it) on the reverse side of his paper.

With some students, the tracing stage may be bypassed. However, words are never copied. Fernald's approach is based on the rationale that putting all modalities into play compensates for weaknesses in visual perception and visual memory.

Another multisensory approach to spelling is *Bannatyne's method*, which shares some of the features of the two methods just described while differing from them in several respects (Bannatyne 1971). Alexander Bannatyne is primarily concerned with the sound blending problems demonstrated by many learners and stresses the need for disabled spellers to hear their "phonemic vocal inner language" in order to master the sequencing aspects of spelling. Bannatyne's technique requires a student to:

1. first pronounce the spelling word slowly.
2. pronounce it, separating the phonemes.
3. study the word in print visually, separating the graphemes that represent the phonemes.
4. pronounce each phoneme in sequence as a teacher points to the corresponding grapheme.
5. write the graphemes while articulating the phonemes as a rhythmic sequence.
6. practice this technique until the word is learned.

Tracing and copying may be involved if necessary. Multisyllable words are introduced only when the student can spell at the syllable level; with multisyllable words, the syllable, rather than the individual phoneme, becomes the articulated unit.

The Childs Spelling System (Childs and Childs 1971, 1973) is one of several variations on the Orton-Gillingham approach to remedial spelling instruction. Sally and Ralph Childs, the authors of this method, have reorganized and simplified many of the Orton-Gillingham generalizations and rules, classifying spelling words into three groups: sound-words, which can be sounded out; think-words, which require individual study; and see-words, which require memorization. Multisensory techniques are not applied, however, in the Childs system.

The Slingerland Multisensory Approach to Language Arts for Specific Language Disability Children (Slingerland 1971), which was developed for classroom use, incorporates a *simultaneous auditory-visual-kinesthetic approach* intended "to strengthen inner sensory associations" (Aho 1967) and begins with handwriting instruction (see Chapter 21).

Slingerland classifies spelling words into three categories that are similar to those in the Childs' system. *Green-flag words*, or short vowel, purely phonetic words, are studied by having the teacher dictate the word, the student repeat the word, and then give the vowel sound. The student then names the vowel while forming it in the air, then spells the word orally, writing each letter in the air as he names it, and then says the word. Finally, the student writes the word on paper and traces it with two fingers for further memory reinforcement.

In *red-flag words*, which are nonphonetic or irregularly spelled, the difficult parts are stressed, but the word is studied as a whole, involving primarily the visual and kinesthetic modalities. The student copies the word from a model, the teacher checks spelling and letter formations, the student traces over the word, naming each letter, and then, when ready, closes his eyes and writes the word in the air.

Yellow-flag words are words containing ambiguous spelling patterns, or patterns representing sounds that can be spelled in more than one way (e.g., *ai, ay, a-e, eigh* all pronounced as the long /a/ sound), and are introduced only after vowel digraphs, diphthongs, and phonograms have been taught. By third grade, students should be able to recall all of the possible spellings for phonograms and to select the correct one for particular words (Aho 1967). In the Slingerland program, all learning is reinforced by writing from dictation, first as a letter, then the word, and then the sentence level.

In *Alphabetic Phonics*, Aylett Cox incorporates the Orton-Gillingham principles but has reorganized the Orton-Gillingham spelling generalizations and rules (Cox 1992). She brings spelling instruction to a considerably more complex and sophisticated level, as is reflected in the subtitle ("Formulas and Equations for Spelling the Sounds of Spoken English") of her teaching manual, *Situation Spelling* (Cox 1977). The term "situation spelling" refers to the fact that the spelling of a particular speech sound tends to vary with its position in a particular word. In this manual, Cox states:

> By studying systematically each sound and its most likely symbols in every significant position in monosyllabic and multisyllabic words, the student can eventually incorporate all of his knowledge of spelling the separate sounds in base words into his reflexes (Cox 1977).

Cox's remedial program, which has reportedly been successful with children and adults who are dyslexic in tutoring, clinical, and small class settings, presents a challenge to instructors as well as students because of its level of sophistication. Multisensory techniques are incorporated into teaching at all levels of the program, as in the Orton-Gillingham system, and spelling practice uses the Simultaneous Oral Spelling (SOS) method.

The Lindamoods emphasize that, in order to spell, contrasts in spoken language must be perceived before contrasts in written language can be understood (Lindamood and Lindamood 1975). They maintain that many children do not naturally acquire the degree of phonological knowledge, or auditory-perceptual skills, needed for proficient spelling or reading. After working for many years with dyslexic individuals, Lindamood and Lindamood concluded:

> The one factor common to all these students was their lack of auditory-perceptual skills, with its attendant problem in self-monitoring their production of specific sounds and sequences while pronouncing words, or monitoring and integrating sound-symbol identities and sequences during reading and spelling activities (Lindamood and Lindamood 1975).

Spelling instruction in the Lindamood LiPS program begins with auditory conceptualization. A distinctive and important feature of this program is the attention brought to bear on sound production and the labeling of all letter sounds according to the real movements involved in articulating these sounds. The sounds /b/ and /p/, for example, are called "lip poppers;" /f/ and /v/ are called "lip coolers." A student is taught to discriminate sounds in nonsense words by manipulating cards with pictures representing these sound labels. She then progresses to working with colored blocks that represent the sounds (the colors have no specific relationship to the letters but serve only to differentiate one sound from another). Once she can perform this task proficiently with single syllables, the student is given letter symbols to manipulate in spelling activities. Spelling instruction progresses from single to multisyllable words, starting in each case with nonsense words and moving to real words.

Chapters in Section III describe spelling instruction in several multisensory programs (e.g., Alphabetic Phonics, LiPS, Slingerland). These chapters include research on their success in teaching both reading and spelling. Although there is substantial evidence that these and other multisensory programs work with children with learning disabilities, additional research is needed to determine what aspects of these programs are most influential and why. Research on multisensory programs have collected end measures on reading and spelling, but have not attempted to control for the possible contributions of various components of the programs.

British researchers Lynette Bradley and Charles Hulme have been interested in issues of multisensory instruction (Bradley 1981; Hulme 1981). They have used the Orton-Gillingham Simultaneous Oral Spelling or SOS technique in which children choose a word that interests them and practice spelling it by saying each letter as they copy it. Handwritten spellings were contrasted with practice in which subjects chose plastic letters for spellings. Multisensory instruction with handwritten spellings of irregular words was more effective than instruction with plastic letters (Hulme and Bradley 1984).

Anne Cunningham and Keith Stanovich replicated this study with first graders but added a keyboard condition. They found that handwritten spellings were more effective for teaching both reading and spelling, but wondered if the results were affected by the children's unfamiliarity with the keyboard (Cunningham and Stanovich 1990). Sharon Vaughn responded to this work with a training study involving writing, tracing, and typing spellings into a computer. Vaughn found that all three methods worked equally well with children with and without learning disabilities (Vaughn, Schumm, and Gordon 1993).

PRINCIPLES OF SPELLING INSTRUCTION

The *frequency of testing* in spelling instruction, the *type of practice* provided (distributed versus massed), and the *number of spelling words* presented in a lesson have been found to have differing effects on good and poor spellers. According to Stanback and Hansen (1980), these variables have only minimal influence on good spellers who seem to do well under any instructional conditions, but poor spellers do better with frequent testing, with distributed rather than massed practice, and with fewer numbers of words per lesson. This point is made, as well, in a more recent research review that suggests as few as three new words in any single lesson for struggling spellers (Gordon, Vaughn, and Schumm 1993).

In her book, *Spelling Development, Disability, and Instruction* (1995), Louisa Moats provides a comprehensive overview of teaching spelling and of using misspellings to shed light on students' linguistic development. She provides the following principles of instruction:

1. Systematic, direct instruction should involve carefully chosen materials designed not to overwhelm the student in terms of either volume or difficulty.
2. The teacher should model performance and then provide opportunities for immediate feedback. Moats recommends what she calls "spelling pronunciation" in which the teacher exaggerates sounds in a syllable-by-syllable rendition of the target word.
3. Instruction should be multisensory and should focus on the phonemic properties of the word being spelled.
4. Instruction should be well organized and sequential. The teacher should clarify the systematic properties of language, and help the student see these patterns and relate new material to old.

Additional material about teaching spelling can be found in Edmund Henderson's *Teaching Spelling* (1990). It is helpful for teachers within a school to collaborate on a sequence, to agree to teach a few rules at each grade level over time, and to review rules from the preceding years. Teachers working with children who need more intensive help will want to find a spelling program that is embedded in a more complete multisensory program.

12

Handwriting Instruction

The development of handwriting involves the acquisition of both legibility and fluency, which are analogs of reading accuracy and reading fluency. Handwriting is more complex than reading, though, because it involves recognizing letter shapes, names, and sounds, as well as integrating spelling and motor planning in order to produce formations that can be read by others. And it involves being able to do this fairly quickly so that ideas can be generated at the same time. Poor handwriting is not one of the defining characteristics of children with dyslexia, but some individuals do have difficulties in this area, and all children benefit from handwriting instruction.

This chapter describes the handwriting difficulties typical of many young writers. It provides a rationale for handwriting instruction, and presents issues around methodology with examples of instructional approaches.

HANDWRITING DIFFICULTIES

Handwriting difficulties can be analyzed using characteristics of the written letters as well as the underlying processes. Doris Johnson and Joanne Carlisle, in a comparison of the handwriting of learning disabled and typically developing children in Grades 1 to 3, looked at features that contribute to *legibility*: (a) letter formations, (b) letter size, (c) alignment and spacing, and (d) control. They also looked at fluency using a measure of productivity or the quantity of written words (Johnson and Carlisle 1996).

Regina Cicci, in addressing the writing problems of students with dyslexia, listed seven possible underlying difficulties that could lead to poor handwriting: (a) incorrect pencil grasp, (b) excessive tension in pencil grasp, (c) incorrect position of paper, (d) inappropriate size and spacing of letters and words, (e) poor visual memory for letter formations, (f) slow rate, and (g) poor fine-motor coordination or dysgraphia[13] (Cicci 1983). Not all children with dyslexia have handwriting difficulties and not all children with handwriting difficulties are dyslexic. Some handwriting difficulties may be due to lack of instruction and others to underlying processes such as weak eye-hand coordination, small-motor coordination, motor planning, or visual memory.

Johnson and Carlisle (1996) report that poor handwriting in children with learning disabilities has been linked, historically, with deficits in perceptual motor abilities (Frostig 1967). Remedial handwriting programs once focused on matching, tracing, and copying patterns as a precursor to learning letter formations. When research during the 1970s failed to link this perceptual training to growth in literacy skills (Arter and Jenkins 1979), there was a movement away from this approach.

Handwriting, once one of several valued components of the language arts curriculum, seems to have lost its traditional place in many schools (Berninger 1999; Graham and Weintraub 1996). Several explanations for this come to mind. First is the increased pressure on teachers to provide as much instruction in reading as possible because reading is the area through which the language arts program is evaluated. In planning the daily literacy block, schools tend to choose to spend time on whatever aspects of literacy will be tested at the end of the year. Another influence on decreased time spent on handwriting is the whole language movement with its devaluing of basic skills such as spelling and handwriting, and increased emphasis on the content and process of writing. In classrooms that I visit, Writers' Workshop focuses on multiple drafts with revisions for clarity and content, with spelling and handwriting a focus only at the final step. A third influence is the enormous increase in availability of computers in schools and the future prospect of computers in the workplace for this generation of students.

---

[13]The term "dysgraphia" is used by Cicci to denote handwriting difficulty associated with poor fine-motor control. There is little agreement as to a single meaning for this word. Others in the field use it to mean a range of problems from generalized writing difficulty to the very specific spelling problems that are symptomatic of dyslexia (Uhry and Shepherd 1993b).

A RATIONALE FOR HANDWRITING INSTRUCTION

Does handwriting instruction matter for children with dyslexia? To my mind, handwriting is still important as a curriculum component for all children.

Developing Legible and Fluent Handwriting

While computers are more apt to provide a substitute for handwriting than in the past, most students do not have unrestricted use of computers for composing text, nor do they have laptop computers for note-taking. For most students, class notes continue to be written by hand. Being fluent and automatic in handwriting, preferably in cursive handwriting because it is faster than using printed letters, frees the mind for thinking and organizing during the taking of notes as well as for composing stories.

Students are also asked to copy material such as homework assignments. There is evidence that many students with learning disabilities, while able to adjust to the demand for greater speed, remain considerably slower at copying than nondisabled peers, and that legibility suffers when speed is demanded (Weintraub and Graham 1998). Instruction can increase both legibility and speed.

Handwriting as a Component of Multisensory Literacy Instruction

A second argument for teaching handwriting to children with dyslexia comes from the thinking behind multisensory instruction. This argument says that experiencing letters and words kinesthetically supports visual and auditory learning. Handwriting is part of the Orton-Gillingham package. Linkages between visual, auditory, kinesthetic, and tactile experiences are believed to contribute to progress in learning to read and write.

Support for the use of multisensory experiences involving handwriting as a method of teaching other literacy skills comes, for example, from a study carried out by Anne Cunningham and Keith Stanovich in 1990. They taught spelling words to Grade 1 children by displaying a printed word on a card, saying the word aloud, asking the children to spell the word aloud, and then to spell it with lettered tiles, with a computer keyboard, or through writing it. Children who wrote by hand had a significant advantage in spelling the words at posttest. The authors interpreted this finding as support for multisensory instruction. They mention the work of Montessori (1915) and Fernald (1943), both of whom valued the role of motoric activities in learning. The idea is that through motoric experiences, the brain is somehow conditioned to associate the shape of the letter with its name and sound, and the sequence of several letters in a word with the spoken and written forms of the word.

Steve Graham and his colleagues found that Grade 1 children who were taught handwriting were superior to controls at letter knowledge (Graham, Harris, and Fink 2000). In other words, hand-writing practice is valuable because it contributes to the internalization of phonics instruction.

INSTRUCTIONAL ISSUES
CURSIVE VERSUS MANUSCRIPT

The issue of whether to teach manuscript or cursive writing initially to dyslexic children is controversial. According to a history of school handwriting by Joanne Phelps and Lynn Stempel (1987), both cursive and manuscript forms can be traced as far back as ancient Rome, and both have been in continuous use since then.

Cursive Writing

Cox (1992) and King (1985) insist that cursive writing be used exclusively by students with dyslexia. According to Cox, cursive writing reinforces left-right directionality, reduces reversals because the pencil is not raised off the paper, promotes rhythm and flow in letter formation, and eliminates the need to learn two writing systems. Furthermore, she contends that cursive letters are unique letter shapes and not mirror images of other letters. Inexperienced readers can have problems differentiating mirror-image "ball and stick" letters such as *b* and *d*.

There is a precedent for teaching cursive early for typically developing children. All children learned cursive first in the early 20th Century, with manuscript introduced later on for purposes such as labeling maps. Montessori schools typically use cursive writing as early as kindergarten.

Manuscript

The movement away from the early teaching of cursive writing was part of the focus on making reading meaningful in the 1930s. It was deemed important for children's own written words to resemble the words they were learning to read. In this tradition, Beth Slingerland (1971) and Romalda Spalding (Spalding and Spalding 1986) advocate manuscript or print writing in order to conform to general school practices, as well as to avoid confusion with the type face in the child's readers. Cursive writing, in their programs, is not introduced until late second or third grade.

According to Phelps and Stempel (1987), the manuscript writing used today in schools is derived from a system of "balls and sticks" or combinations of circles and straight lines designed in 1924 by a British teacher named Margaret Wise. The system is intuitively appealing. Circles and straight lines are the earliest scribbles of toddlers. These components are easy to form. However, the formations invite directional confusions, and because of the simplicity of the sans serif formations, letters such as *b* and *d* are easily confused (Wise 1924).

Handwriting programs such as the D'Nealian System avoid ball and stick formations with their typical *b/d* confusions by forming letters without lifting the pencil and by adding a follow-through stroke. For example, lower case *a* is drawn as a single stroke starting at the 2 o'clock position, circling counterclockwise back around to 2 o'clock, reversing the stroke down toward the line, and then curving up. This has the advantage of being similar to cursive formations and makes learning cursive easier later on. There are benefits to both the manuscript and cursive points of view, which teachers and clinicians need to weigh before deciding which form of writing to teach.

TRACING VERSUS COPYING

Research on optimal methods for handwriting instruction has explored the question of copying versus tracing, as well as issues of active engagement in learning. Beatrice Furner characterized handwriting development as a perceptual learning process in which the learner must actively participate in order to internalize the procedures for letter formations (Furner 1983). An important aspect of perceptual learning is the ability to discriminate characteristic features. Furner criticizes most existing instructional programs for placing too much emphasis on tracing and copying procedures and not enough on active learning. Although there is a place for these procedures in early writing instruction, in and of themselves they do not force children to discriminate between letter shapes and to note the distinguishing characteristics of each letter.

When compared with tracing, copying seems to promote better learning (Askov and Greff 1975; Hirsch and Niedermeyer 1973). The explanation has been that copying involves a greater degree of visualization and attention to detail. Joanna Williams (1975) found that both copying and letter discrimination training contribute to handwriting development but in different ways. Discrimination training, as in a matching-to-sample procedure, tends to generalize to new letters, whereas copying does not (each letter has to be learned individually). However, when compared to demonstration of letter formations or verbal description of rules for these formations or a combination of these two techniques, copying is found to be the least effective technique (Kirk 1981).

Furner maintained that both discrimination and production are important processes in handwriting development, though they are useful for different reasons, and urges that demonstration and verbalization of letter formations replace the copying and tracing that predominates in handwriting instruction. In her own work, Furner combines perceptual learning principles with problem-solving methods, using questioning and discovery techniques, and she reports data supporting this approach (Furner 1983). Although her research, as well as the research she reviews, deals with normal kindergarten and first grade children, there is no reason to believe that it should not apply to learners with dyslexia.

MULTISENSORY LINKAGES THROUGH HANDWRITING

Many of the instructional principles advocated by Furner may be found in remedial handwriting programs for children with dyslexia, most particularly those programs based on the Orton-Gillingham approach. For example, Alphabetic Phonics (Cox 1992) and Slingerland (1971) include teacher demonstration combined with verbal directions for particular letter strokes that a student repeats while forming the letters.

The Cox and Slingerland programs, as well as that of Diana King (1985), which is designed specifically to teach writing skills to adolescents, all require extensive tracing and copying. However, the inclusion of such practice is not arbitrary, as Furner implied it may be in some classrooms, but rather is considered an essential component of the multisensory training espoused by the authors of these programs. King includes a multisensory prewriting exercise called the *wind tunnel*, a series of circular scribbles that are done with eyes closed to develop rhythm and relaxation. Cox and Slingerland use *sky writing*, a technique using the whole arm for movements in the air prior to forming letters on paper. Correct sitting posture and correct position of the paper are stressed in these programs, with the latter differing for left- and right-handed students. Left-handers are not allowed to hook their wrists in writing.

CAN HANDWRITING BE IMPROVED?

Handwriting is not one of the areas investigated by the National Reading Panel (2000), but both clinicians and researchers who carry out training studies suggest that instruction in this area is worthwhile. Handwriting instruction can improve both legibility and automaticity.

Cox (1992) claims that handwriting retraining for dyslexic students who are not identified early is more difficult and time-consuming than reading remediation. However, King (1985) states that true dysgraphia is extremely rare, despite the fact that the diagnosis is frequently made. She maintains that it is always worth the effort to develop good handwriting, and that with intensive retraining, older

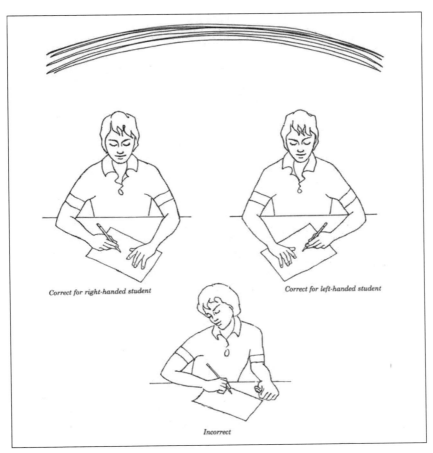

Correct for right-handed student

Correct for left-handed student

Incorrect

From Writing Skills for the Adolescent *by Diana Hanbury King. Reproduced with permission from Educators Publishing Service, Inc., Cambridge, MA. (800) 225-5750, www.epsbooks.com. Copyright 1985.)*

students often make remarkable progress in a relatively short period of time. King and Cox both urge that students with dyslexia learn to type, in addition to, but not in lieu of, developing handwriting skills.

Steve Graham and his colleagues at the University of Maryland have carried out research in which they found that handwriting instruction made a significant contribution to both handwriting itself and to compositional fluency for Grade 1 children, with and without disabilities, who were weak in writing letters. They found that this advantage was present at posttest and that it persisted at least six months after the instruction ended. Their treatment involved tracing, discussing formations, copying, and writing three lowercase letters during each of 27 lessons. Letters with similar formations were taught together. Examples are "slant letters" (e.g., v, w, y) and "backward circle letters" (e.g., c, d, g). This method is typical of Orton-Gillingham writing programs. The Orton-Gillingham approach tends to focus on the accuracy of formations, and Graham added another dimension to the treatment. Fluency was developed through writing letters, once learned, as quickly as possible, and copying sentences as well (Graham, Harris, and Fink 2000).

SUGGESTIONS FOR HANDWRITING INSTRUCTION

The following suggestions are taken from a variety of sources and programs and tend to represent best practice.

1. Begin early. It is difficult to change a child's awkward pencil grip once it has become a habit. Begin encouraging the three-finger grip in kindergarten.
2. Look for fat pencils or soft pencil grips to accommodate individual needs. Some children do well with thin-tip colored markers for handwriting practice because they flow much more easily than pencils.
3. Make handwriting instruction multisensory. Trace, copy, and use words to describe strokes (Furner 1983). Write letters from memory and say the sound as the letter is formed. Use tactile materials. For example, *Recipe for Reading* (Chapter 19) suggests practicing *p* in peanut butter and *j* in jelly.
4. Teach letters by similarities in formation.
5. Build sequences of mastered letters into words. With cursive writing, learning the connecting strokes is just as important as the formations.
6. Combine practice in spelling with practice in handwriting. Dictate words in which both formations and letter sounds have been taught.
7. Just as reading practice involves accuracy first and then fluency, practice letters until they are consistently legible and then practice them for speed.
8. Words can be a scaffold for remembering patterns (e.g., the "swing up letters"). Be consistent in your terminology. Adapting a school-wide program ensures consistent terms from year to year.
9. Handwriting usually takes several years to become automatic. For example, if cursive is begun in Grade 3, it will need to be reviewed and made automatic in Grade 4.
10. Some children may become legible writers but may continue to be slow.
11. Johnson and Carlisle (1996) suggest that some children with illegible or dysfluent handwriting may benefit from occupational

therapy, and that the therapist can often make helpful suggestions about pencil grip and motor planning. Invite the occupational therapist into the classroom to observe and make
suggestions before referring the struggling writer for outside
help.

12. Cicci suggests compensatory modifications such as using parents
as scribes and proofreaders, accepting taped or oral reports, and
reducing length of written assignments (Cicci 1983).

13. Use of the computer has become a significant help to children
who struggle with handwriting.

13

Composition Instruction

Where earlier chapters talk about the spelling and handwriting aspects of writing, this chapter considers text production or the composition of written discourse: units of written language longer than sentences. The chapter discusses the relationship between reading and writing, and the new role writing is currently playing in the assessment of reading comprehension on many standardized tests. It talks about the advantages and disadvantages of Orton-Gillingham writing instruction, writer's workshop, and other writing programs for students who are dyslexic.

THE READING/WRITING RELATIONSHIP

Chapter 6 (*Spelling to Read*) talks about the writing/reading relationship for young children learning to master the alphabetic code, first in spelling (encoding) and then in reading words (decoding). Spelling leads to reading because it makes clear the relationships between spoken sounds and the letters used to represent them in alphabetic languages.

FROM READING TO WRITING

The strong reading/writing relationship goes beyond the early stages of word reading, but for more advanced readers, the relationship is bidirectional and much more complex. That is, writing and reading influence each other. In terms of form or style, the relationship tends to move from reading to writing. Wide reading across genres supports writing in specific genres. Children can be asked to notice that things happen in threes in folk tales before writing their own folk tales. They can be encouraged to read mystery stories to learn how to incorporate typical features of this genre into their own writing of mysteries.

Text structure is another example of what can be learned from reading to enrich the writing repertoire of students. Wide reading of multiple text structures (e.g., compare/contrast; problem/solution) in information text, together with direct instruction in noticing the kinds of words used to signal text structure, can support the use of these structures during students' own composition of nonfiction. For example, students are taught to notice "on the other hand," or "by contrast," in reading information text and to use these words to signal the compare/contrast structure in their own writing.

In both genre studies and text structure studies, the text we read becomes a model for the text we write. Where early invented spellings clarify the nature of alphabetic coding, the reading of text clarifies meaning and it models structures for expressing meaning in writing.

FROM READING TO WRITING TO COMPREHENSION

Writing can also serve as a supportive mechanism or scaffold for comprehension. Having to write about what one has read can serve to clarify comprehension. Writing helps us think about meaning. But for a student with language-based reading and writing difficulties, thinking about reading and putting it in writing can be very difficult. In an article about ways to support student thinking, Michael Pressley writes about teachers using oral language scaffolds in class and about their using questioning to figure out just where thinking has broken down (Pressley et al. 1996). Children with dyslexia may need this help in using oral language to think out the meaning of a story or passage before they can use spelling, handwriting, and thinking all at the same time to write down their thoughts.

THE 21ST CENTURY READING/WRITING CLASSROOM

Donald Graves (1978), a leading authority on teaching writing, contended that instruction in expressive writing was given short shrift in the education of American children. For many children in schools where teachers have been encouraged to use Graves' *Writing Process or Writer's Workshop* approach, the picture has changed dramatically in the past 25 years. Teachers encourage students to simulate the process used by adult writers through brainstorming ideas, writing, sharing their work for feedback, revising for content, and correcting mechanics prior to "publication" in a final draft. Substantial time is spent writing in these classrooms (e.g., Calkins 1983, 1986; Dyson 2001; Graves 1983; Graves and Stuart 1985; Hansen 1987; Harwayne 1992). Graves and others have changed the way writing is perceived and the way it is taught.

These new perceptions of reading/writing connections and of the importance of writing in school have even affected the way students are assessed. Joseph Jenkins and his colleagues in Washington State begin a recent article by saying that a "quiet revolution" has taken place in the performance assessment of reading. Where reading comprehension tests used to be made up of multiple choice items, by 1999, in 30 out of 50 states, standardized testing used a combination of multiple choice and constructed response (Jenkins, Johnson, and Hileman 2004). For example, the New York State standardized English language arts test given to all Grade 4 students each year includes the assessment of reading comprehension through short essay questions about the meaning of written passages.

This phenomenon raises very complex instructional issues for children who are still struggling to read words. Should the instructional focus for children with dyslexia be on word reading and spelling first, and later on more holistic understanding and expression in writing? Or should reading, spelling, comprehension, and composition be integrated right from the start?

INSTRUCTIONAL MODELS FOR COMPOSING TEXT
EXPLICIT, SKILLS-BASED WRITING INSTRUCTION

The traditional approach to writing instruction for students with dyslexia is a bottom-up or skills-emphasis approach. As suggested in the preceding chapters on spelling and handwriting, basic skills are taught before generating connected text.

Orton-Gillingham

Samuel Orton (1937) and his associates Anna Gillingham and Bessie Stillman (1960) believed that spelling and other mechanics constituted the major writing difficulty in children with dyslexia. They feared that free writing would reinforce these problems. Just as reading in Orton-Gillingham programs tends to be restricted to decodable text, writing tends to be limited to the dictation of words and short sentences made up of letter sounds that have been mastered for spelling and handwriting. In terms of the expression of meaning, they advocated that students dictate ideas to tutors and wait until high school to begin written composition.

Orton's theory has influenced programs such as Alphabetic Phonics (see Chapter 20) in which early writing instruction focuses on handwriting, spelling, and phonetically controlled, tutor-dictated words and sentences linked to reading instruction. Historically, Orton-Gillingham instruction has attempted to avoid overloading students. While the tutor or teacher provides linkages between, for instance, spelling and handwriting, the student is not expected to integrate these skills in writing on her own. In the first few years of remediation, teachers and tutors using Orton-Gillingham writing instruction tend to limit the student to words using letters and sounds that have been taught.

Writing Skills for the Adolescent

Diana King's program, *Writing Skills for the Adolescent* (1985), which is based on Orton-Gillingham principles, is intended to be used with Orton-Gillingham reading instruction. This is probably the most comprehensive writing program developed to date for older students with dyslexia. It deals with handwriting, spelling, and composition. It is intended as a tutoring program for college-bound adolescents, many of whom have been diagnosed late as having dyslexia. King's approach is exceedingly pragmatic, most likely because time is of the essence with these students. Rebuilding confidence is an important element of this program for older students, with competence achieved through much drill and practice. The program involves extensive retraining in handwriting, as well as remediation of spelling, mechanics, and formulation.

King's curriculum begins with having students write single words, then sentences, paragraphs, and essays. Early composition is linked with spelling instruction. Lists of spelling words are used as the basis of sentence composition. Once simple sentences can be written with some facility, grammar instruction begins. In her guide, King points out that grammar is important for college-bound students and she informs students that they can learn all they need to know about grammar in just a few months. Grammar is taught by having students compose sentences rather than completing workbook exercises, and involves a progression from parts of speech to various types of clauses—to what King calls *verbals*—by which she means participles, gerunds, and infinitives.

King calls paragraph construction "an exercise in logical thinking." Instruction begins with generating ideas and sentences, moves on to composing a topic sentence from this material, and then ends with weaving all of the sentences together. Several paragraph types are taught (e.g., *definition, narrative, process*). Essay writing follows this pattern of instruction. The student is taught to compose an introductory paragraph with a thesis statement, followed by paragraphs each containing a topic sentence, and ending with a concluding paragraph. King supports her method with a series of convincing case histories including before-and-after writing samples (1985).

King's program, and other Orton-Gillingham writing approaches, are examples of a writing instructional model that George Hillocks (1984) described as a *presentational model*. In this model, the teacher presents specific, skills-oriented lessons and assignments, and provides feedback on student performance.

WRITER'S WORKSHOP OR PROCESS WRITING

Another model identified by Hillocks includes the *natural process model* of writing instruction popularized by Graves. This is in the tradition of progressive schooling. In this model, the teacher acts mainly as a facilitator whose primary role, as Hillocks puts it, is "to free the student's imagination and promote growth by sustaining a positive classroom attitude." Sylvia Ashton-Warner, who taught and wrote in the 1960s, viewed children's writing as developmental rather than instruction-driven. In a child-centered, idealized, and romantic vision of the child, she described children's work as follows:

> But I don't call it teaching: I call it creativity since it all comes from them and nothing from me, and because the spelling and composition are no longer separate subjects to be taught but emerge naturally as another medium (Ashton-Warner 1963).

In her words, we see the beginning of the movement toward meaning-based instruction with skills embedded in authentic work rather than taught directly.

This model incorporates many of Graves' interests such as choosing one's own topics of interest, sharing results with peers for feedback, editing, and revising. Note, though, that unlike Ashton-Warner, Graves structured his model on replicating the process that professional adult writers experience as they proceed through a series of steps in writing: brainstorming ideas and planning, writing a series of drafts and revisions, sharing, conferencing with an editor, final revisions, and ultimately publication. These steps can provide a clear outline of what is expected of young writers. The steps are often outlined on the classroom wall with the thought that this makes the children more independent in moving from step to step.

Writing conferences are an important aspect of structuring writer's workshop. The teacher's questions about a story provide a scaffold or support for the child-author's own plans for revising or expanding work. Conferences are also organized around peers listening and providing feedback on what is clear and what is unclear. Lucy Calkins believes that successful teacher-student conferences, in addition to supporting a child's writing, help the child become a good peer mentor (Calkins 1986).

Another aspect of this structured writing process is the use of literature as a model for writing. Shelley Harwayne, once principal of the Manhattan New School in New York City, wrote that children there are routinely referred to books as part of the planning process or when they are "stuck" in writing, to see how another author resolved an issue or incorporated a technique (Harwayne 1992). For example, if they are writing memoirs, children are referred to memoirs by their teacher.

Mini-lessons play a role in writer's workshop. Teachers often use mini-lessons to model how they, themselves, might think through the ending of a story, or how they might work on keeping language fresh rather than using cliches, or how they might proofread for capital letters. Mini-lessons are an opportunity to observe common needs and respond with direct instruction.

COMBINATION MODELS

Hillocks' environmental model combines aspects of both the presentational and process models, and in many ways, appears a compromise between the two methods described above. Objectives are clearly stated and assignments selected by the teacher. A high degree of structure is used as small groups work through an idea together. Later, children work on their own with teacher support. Hillocks comments that the environmental model "brings teacher, student, and materials more nearly into balance and, in effect, takes advantage of all resources of the classroom" (Hillocks 1984).

A Combination Model for Young Children

In a recent review of the literature on programs for kindergarten children with writing difficulties, Lana Edwards (2003) describes the paucity of researched composition instruction for young children with written language disabilities, but she does mention a series of scientific studies carried out by Virginia Berninger. What is unusual about the instruction in these studies is that in a single instructional session, the model combines work on what the authors call *low level transcription skills* such as spelling and handwriting with the higher level thinking required for composing meaningful text. Rather than being concerned about overload, they point out the importance of making low-level skills automatic and then putting them to use (Berninger 1999; Berninger et al. 1995; Brooks, Vaughn, and Berninger 1999).

Transfer has always been an enormous issue in the research on learning disabilities. It is much easier to teach a low level or transcription skill than it is to teach students to transfer this skill to other situations. For example, in many early studies of children with specific phonological awareness difficulty but without difficulty in listening comprehension, children taught PA and decoding improved in the target skills but not in reading comprehension. In more recent studies where the full hierarchy of skills is taught (i.e., PA, decoding, text reading, comprehension), we see growth in comprehension as well.

Cognitive Strategy Instruction in Writing (CSIW)

Carol Sue Englert and her colleagues at Michigan State University have developed a model of writing instruction for use with children with learning disabilities that might be characterized as an example of Hillocks' *environmental model*. Taking a sociocultural perspective, Englert builds on Vygotsky's (1978) ideas on the importance of social interaction as a scaffold when expectations are a little beyond the student's level of mastery (Englert and Mariage 1996).

In a summary of several studies, Englert (1990) describes what she calls Cognitive Strategy Instruction in Writing (CSIW), a process-oriented approach to expository writing that uses many of the strategies found in Graves' model but within a more teacher-directed framework in the early stages. Englert has based CSIW on extensive research, her own and that of others, describing the writing characteristics of children with learning disabilities (e.g., Englert et al. 1989, 1991; Englert and Thomas 1987). This research suggests that children with learning disabilities have deficits in analyzing text structure in reading and in using it effectively in writing expository text. These children have little knowledge of the vocabulary of the writing process and are poor at self-regulating the writing process steps. They tend to see writing as outer-directed and teacher regulated, and they have little sense of purpose for writing or of audience.

Englert's CSIW instructional model uses the acronym POWER (*Plan, Organize, Write, Edit/Editor, Revise*) for a series of structured steps including *think sheets* to fill in at each new stage in the process. The use of these think sheets is one way in which CSIW is more explicit than other forms of process writing. At the *Plan* step, students are encouraged to consider their audience, their purpose for writing, and their own background knowledge of the topic. At the *Organize* step, they categorize and sequence their ideas and consider text structure. At the *Write* step, they write a first draft on colored paper, reserving white paper for the final draft. The teacher models how to make the text "reader friendly" through the explicit use of key phrases to provide cues to the reader about the text structure being used. Teachers encourage students to elaborate on ideas at this stage. At the *Edit/Editor* step, think sheets are available for both the author, who self-edits, and the peer editor, who reads the work and makes suggestions. Note that Hillocks reports that this has benefits for the peer editor as well as the author. The teacher provides *think aloud* conversations during further editing conferences before the student begins to prepare a final draft. The *Revise* think sheet suggests putting a check mark next to any editing suggestions that the students intend to use. Sharing the final product is an integral part of the process and of the life of the classroom. Englert refers to the creation of "a literacy community of writers and readers," using rhetoric familiar to advocates of Graves' writing process.

Englert emphasizes that the POWER steps must be supported by three important contributions from the teacher: (a) *dialogue* during the writing process, which should include the teacher modeling aloud the thinking process she uses when she composes; (b) *scaffolded instruction* with graduated prompts provided by the teacher until the student is successful, as well as *procedural facilitation* in which prompts remind the student to use learned strategies; and (c) *teaching for generalization* during which the teacher provides fewer and fewer dialogues and prompts and encourages increasing amounts of "self-talk" until the student can work independently without even the support of think sheets. Raphael and Englert describe CSIW more fully in a 1990 article.

CSIW is intended for use in either classrooms or resource rooms serving children with learning disabilities. Several studies have demonstrated the effectiveness of CSIW (e.g., Englert et al. 1989). Reports include extensive use of before-and-after writing samples as well as transcriptions of dialogues. One study demonstrated that socially mediated instruction increased ability to talk about writing processes in upper elementary-age children with and without learning disabilities in comparison with controls, and that this ability was related to both reading and writing achievement. This form of writing instruction had a particularly positive effect on the sense of self-regulation in children with learning disabilities (Englert, Raphael, and Anderson 1992).

STOP & LIST

In another study combining explicit, teacher-directed instruction with process writing, Gary Troia and Steve Graham developed a strategy training program for fourth and fifth grade students identified as learning disabled. Instruction for the 10 children, administered in groups of two, involved strategies for the advance planning phase of writing. The method was called STOP & LIST (Stop, Think of Purposes, List Ideas, and Sequence Them). The teacher modeled STOP & LIST, and then the students were encouraged to rehearse the strategies before they wrote a story together with the teacher. A scale was used by the teacher and students to rate the story. Strategy rehearsal, joint writing activity, and feedback through the rating scale were repeated before students were prepared to write on their own. After several independent writing cycles involving feedback and continuing rehearsal of the strategies, these 10 students wrote stories of higher quality than matched controls writing stories in a process writing condition without direct instruction in strategies (Troia and Graham 2002).

WHICH MODEL IS MOST EFFECTIVE?

Hillocks' meta-analysis of the three models indicates that the environmental mode (the combination model) is nearly three times as effective as either the presentational or process models. Furthermore, the most widely used approach, the presentational model, was the least effective group model. Some of the other outcomes from Hillocks' meta-analysis are worth noting:

1. The problem-solving or inquiry approach, in which students are presented with sets of information and asked to take a position or develop an argument, has an extremely positive effect on writing quality.
2. Sentence combining, or the practice of building more complex sentences from simpler ones, has a positive effect.
3. Establishing criteria for peer critiques has a positive effect.
4. Instruction through presentation of grammar does not improve the quality of writing and can actually lower it.

Keep in mind, in thinking about the implications of this meta-analysis, that the subjects in these studies were not dyslexic or even learning disabled. What we do know, though, is that in general, students with learning disabilities are responsive to extra structure in their area of disability. The combination model makes sense because of its structured experiences in low level skills, together with encouragement, to transfer these skills to higher level thinking in composition.

TECHNOLOGY AND COMPOSITION
WORD PROCESSORS IN WRITING INSTRUCTION

The surge of interest in the writing process during the 1980s, with its emphasis on revisions and multiple drafts, has coincided with a surge in the educational use of computers in schools. The computer is an ideal vehicle for the writing process as it eliminates tedious recopying. For students with spelling problems, the computer provides a release from the tedium and uncertainty of proofreading for misspellings and incomplete sentences. The facilitative power of computers in regard to spelling is an especially important advantage for children with dyslexia. This can make a difference in the mechanics of the finished product so that the focus can shift to content. Of equally great importance, it can also make a difference in terms of willingness to write. MacArthur and Schneiderman (1986) noted advantages of computerized word processing for these students as including the following: (a) word processing produces a neat, easy-to-read, printed copy, which may increase motivation; (b) word processing allows numerous drafts without tedious recopying; and (c) typing can compensate for poor handwriting.

Word processing has become the mode over the past 20 years. The issue today is not whether or not the computer helps in composition, but how to be certain that every writer has adequate access to a computer. The role of the teacher remains a key factor. The teacher's choice of whether to employ a skills approach or a process approach to writing will influence the way computers are used for composition. For example, MacArthur and his colleagues at the University of Maryland have designed a writing curriculum that encourages emphasis on "meaningful writing in a social context." The Computers and Writing Instruction Project (CWIP) curriculum combines use of a computer, a writer's workshop or process approach to writing, and metacognitive strategy instruction. Using methods MacArthur describes as similar to those of Lucy Calkins, children write daily and receive regular support and advice from peers. Metacognitive strategy instruction involves detailed and structured steps for planning, writing, and expanding their work, much as Englert does in her curriculum. MacArthur has used the CWIP curriculum with children with learning disabilities in special classes in Grades 4 through 6. He describes several studies indicating that children in CWIP classrooms outperformed controls in overall quality of writing (MacArthur, Schwartz, and Graham 1991).

In the first edition of this book, Diana Clark wrote that there is no single word processing program deemed best for dyslexic students. This continues to be the case, and choices have become even more difficult since 1988 because of the many new options available to support students with writing disabilities. There are word processing programs that have the capability of checking spelling, grammar, and capitalization, and providing mini-lessons on errors. Some can find synonyms to expand a student's vocabulary. Speech synthesis is available to "read" aloud what has been written. Some word processors can suggest topics at the planning stage and then illustrate the finished story. Portable computers can be taken to class for note taking by older students. A recent and thorough review of these features ends with this advice:

The possibilities increase only to the degree that teachers are informed consumers of the technology available and are able to make sound instructional decisions relative to the needs of their students (Hunt-Berg, Rankin, and Beukelman 1994, p. 178).

SUMMARY OF PRINCIPLES FOR WRITING INSTRUCTION

Despite the limited amount of research on teaching writing to children with dyslexia, there are a number of instructional principles and procedures that seem to be important. The first among them is the need to begin this instruction early rather than waiting for reading or spelling skills to reach a certain level (Barenbaum 1983; Silverman et al. 1981). Graves stresses the importance of daily writing and of a working studio atmosphere in which individuals write with the teacher's presence felt as a support. Barenbaum emphasizes the need for a "safe" environment, which is positive and reinforcing. The finished work of all children should be displayed and valued. One-to-one conferences are important in the revision process. Donald Graves makes four suggestions about correcting errors during these conferences:

1. Identify revision elements in order of importance with a meaningful story line or exposition higher up on the hierarchy than mechanics
2. Choose only one point for revision at a given time.
3. Focus on specific writing problems as the need arises.
4. Provide more than one experience to solidify new learning (Graves 1983).

Diana King cautions against discouraging students by focusing on errors. In her program, tutors are prohibited from placing red marks on student papers for at least a year after remediation has begun and are advised never to correct all errors on a page. One method that makes sense involves expecting children to correct only those spelling patterns that have been directly taught. A major hurdle in beginning work with children with dyslexia is simply getting them to write at all.

III

Reading Programs for
Students with Dyslexia

The chapters that follow provide information on instructional programs for early intervention and remediation of dyslexia. Chapter 14, Early Interventions, briefly describes nine programs for use in kindergarten and first grade. These programs are rich in phonemic awareness activities. Most are classroom-based and appropriate for all young readers. Roughly 75% of at-risk children have been found to catch up before failing at reading if provided with intensive, systematic, direct instruction in phonemic awareness and phonics.

Chapters 15 through 18 are system-wide intervention programs for catching children up to grade level. Reading Recovery is systemic in that it routinely provides tutoring for the very lowest achieving first graders. Success for All, and Direct Instruction's DISTAR are school-wide programs providing systematic direct instruction in phonics as a form of universal design. That is, they provide instruction that is appropriate for both students at risk and typically developing readers. Chapter 18 describes Direct Instruction's Correctional Reading, a Grade 4 to 12 extension of DISTAR for older students who need remedial instruction.

Chapters 19 through 23 describe five Orton-Gillingham-based remedial programs: Recipe for Reading, Alphabetic Phonics, Slingerland, The Wilson Reading System, and Enfield and Greene's Project Read.

Chapter 24 describes The Lindmood LiPS Program (formerly Auditory Discrimination in Depth), an intense phonemic awareness program appropriate as both early intervention and remediation for individuals with the most severe phonological processing problems.

Chapter 25 describes the sort of problem-solving that needs to be carried out in planning instruction. It follows the progress of KM through the two years following her initial educational evaluation (see Chapter 3).

14

Early Interventions

Stanovich's *Matthew Effect* theory suggests that children who get a poor start in word reading because of a core phonological deficit become poorer and poorer over time at both word reading and a host of reading-dependent skills such as vocabulary and comprehension (Stanovich 1986b). It is a misconception to think that giving young struggling readers time to develop will solve the problem. We know that the earlier an intervention is carried out, the more successful it will be. According to the National Reading Panel Report (2000), the students who benefit the most from direct instruction in phonemic awareness and beginning phonics are kindergarten and Grade 1 children at risk because of phonemic processing problems.

The critical issue is whether children provided with early intervention can catch up and stay caught up, or whether they continue to need special reading instruction. Michael Coyne and his colleagues describe these possibilities as *inoculation* and *insulin*. They compare effective early intervention in which children catch up to more competent readers as an *inoculation*, with children able to cope on their own once the intervention has taken place. They compare the ongoing need for special services to *insulin*, which must be used on an ongoing basis to control an ongoing condition (Coyne et al. 2004). Their study reports findings consistent with a review of intervention studies by Torgesen (2000) in which roughly 75 percent of children receiving early intervention were successfully inoculated against future need for remediation.

This chapter reports on nine early intervention programs that incorporate elements found to be effective by the National Reading Panel Report. Other early interventions are described in more detail in the chapters that follow (e.g., Reading Recovery, Slingerland). This chapter also discusses factors that provide optimal circumstances for the success of these programs through supportive school environments.

THE INTERVENTION PROGRAMS

The following programs provide a range of early interventions. Some take advantage of *universal design*, a curriculum term indicating instruction that will benefit the most struggling readers but is appropriate for use with all children in the regular classroom. Others were designed as tutorials for the most at-risk children in a school. All nine of the programs are designed to be used before children fail at reading. They all have preschool or primary grade versions of phonemic awareness and letter-sound instruction, although they vary in the point at which letters are introduced into phonemic awareness instruction. The programs are presented below in alphabetical order.

EARLY STEPS

Early Steps is a first grade, one-to-one tutoring program originally designed by Darrell Morris and his colleagues (Morris, Shaw, and Perney 1990; Santa 1998). Early Steps was chosen by the American Federation of Teachers as one of *Five Promising Remedial Reading Intervention Programs* in 1999. It was designed as a balanced or comprehensive program that incorporates features of both meaning-based and skills-based programs. Each 30-minute tutoring session consists of the following four components:

1. *Reading.* The student begins each Early Steps session by rereading a familiar book, an activity based on the structure of Reading Recovery (see Chapter 15). The leveled book collections used in the program consist of what Morris calls "real" books or trade books, and not phonetically decodable text. The purpose of the rereading is to develop accuracy, speed, and fluency.
2. *Word Study.* Phonological awareness, letter-sound patterns, sight words, and meta-cognitive strategies for sounding out new words are taught during word study. Activities include word sorting, an activity that is meant to draw attention to patterns so that learning

can be transferred to new situations. Word families with short and long vowel patterns are taught through this sorting. Multiple strategy systems are used (e.g., letters, patterns, meaning).

3. *Writing.* The student is asked to write a sentence, saying each word aloud and breaking it into segments for spelling. The sentence is copied over by the tutor, and then the words are cut apart to be reassembled and read by the child. This is another Reading Recovery activity.

4. *New Reading.* The final activity during each tutoring session is a first reading of a new book during which the student is encouraged to use meta-cognitive strategies to figure out words on his own.

Early Steps is described in detail in a research article that examines the effectiveness of its replication in Montana (Santa and Høien 1999). In this study, low achieving first-graders who were tutored for a school year in Early Steps were significantly stronger in spelling, word reading, and passage reading than controls who also received extra instruction in guided reading, but without word study. They remained stronger after tutoring ended when tested again in second grade.

FUNDATIONS

Fundations is a new, younger grades version of the Wilson Reading System (see Chapter 22). Designed for K to 2 classrooms, Fundations includes playful materials such as large, colorful letter sound cards with keyword pictures and owl puppets named Echo and Baby Echo. Small readers with mostly decodable text and beautiful color illustrations come with the program. The 30-minute lessons are designed to complement curriculum that utilizes literature and meaning-based instruction. Fundations can be used for 30 minutes a day with whole classes, and includes supplemental small-group extension lessons for the lowest 30 percent of the class. The program can also be used for daily, small-group, 30- to 50-minute intervention lessons taught by, for instance, a Title I teacher to at-risk readers.

There is a curriculum for each grade level, K to 2 (Wilson 2002, 2004), with a kit of materials including sound cards, puppets, magnetic letter tiles with a well-organized teacher's manual and detailed directions for both lessons and units, and a CD-ROM to help teachers understand the program. The grade-level teachers' kits and classroom materials sets are available through the Wilson Language Training Corporation. Fundations is described by its publisher as including the five essential reading instruction components identified by the Reading First Initiative of the No Child Left Behind Act of 2001 as follows:

(a) phonemic awareness, (b) phonics, (c) vocabulary, (d) fluency, and (e) comprehension. Sample activities at the first grade level follow:

1. *Alphabetical Order.* Students arrange magnetic letter tiles in alphabetical order on a small board, matching a model (an Alphabet Overlay or alphabet matrix with consonants in yellow and vowels in orange), then saying the alphabet.

2. *Drill Sounds.* Students respond to the Large Sound Cards by saying the letter name, naming the keyword picture, and saying the letter sound (e.g., "a," apple, /a/)

3. *Echo/Find Letters.* The teacher says a sound, the students echo it, and then identify the letter associated with the sound on their Alphabet Overlay and find the matching magnetic Letter Tile which is placed on the Overlay letter.

4. *Sky Write/Letter Formation.* Students stand, facing the board, writing arm stretched out straight toward the board, two fingers extended as they follow the teacher's verbalization of letter formations and echo the name, keyword, and sound. The *Wilson Writing Grid* is used both on the board and on paper, and consists of named lines, similar to *Recipe for Reading*'s "little red house." In this system, pictures of a cloud, a plane, grass, and an underground worm provide mnemonics for remembering the various line locations and subsequent positions of the various parts of letters. For example, for a manuscript *t*, the verbalization is as follows:

   > *t* is a skyline letter.
   > It starts on the skyline.
   > Point to the skyline.
   > Go down to the grass line.
   > Cross it on the plane line.

5. *Dictation/Sounds.* Students write letters in response to the teacher's pronunciation of a sound using the program's Dry Erase Writing Tablets.

6. *Dictation/Words.* The teacher says a word aloud and indicates with Echo, the owl puppet, that the students are to echo the word. Students segment by "finger tapping" the phonemes with thumb and first finger, and then write the letters.

7. *Word of the Day.* Construct a word using Sound Cards and discuss its meaning.

In combination, these activities provide direct instruction in systematic, multisensory phonological awareness, and phonics appropriate for beginning readers.

LADDERS TO LITERACY

Ladders to Literacy (Notari-Syverson, O'Connor, 1998; O'Connor, Notari-Syverson, and Vadasy 1998a) wa~ classroom instruction for preschool and kindergarten children alrea~, classified as having special needs, but the program's effectiveness is well researched with both regular and special education students (O'Connor, Jenkins, and Slocum 1995; O'Connor, Notari-Syverson, and Vadasy 1996, 1998b). It is designed for group work, with modifications included for making all lessons meet the needs of children who benefit from higher levels of support. An *Activity Book* for teacher at both preschool and kindergarten level outlines the theoretical base (i.e., Vygotskian scaffolding[14]) as well as a sequence of lessons.

Preschool Activities

The preschool level focuses on play and on acquiring the ability to understand representation through drawing and through symbols such as signs in the block area. Book conventions are taught through listening to stories. Early phonemic awareness activities include listening for the initial sound in the names of play objects, generating rhymes, and inventing spellings for words while writing stories.

Kindergarten Activities

In kindergarten, the focus of Ladders to Literacy is on print awareness, phonological awareness, and oral language. Letter sounds are taught in kindergarten and children are encouraged to sound out words. Instruction is highly explicit. Suggestions for directly teaching and modeling are suggested as follows:

> Here's how I know this word is apple. (Point to the *a*). It starts with *a*, and that says /*aaa*/. Here's a *p*, and it says /p/. /AAAp/. Now see the *l*? That says /lll/. Now we have /aaaplll/—apple. Do that with me.

This program has particularly clear directions for what to do when group instruction is not a good match for a particular child's needs.

OPEN COURT

Marilyn Adams and her colleagues revised this phonics-based, basal-reading series that has a strong phonemic awareness and phonics

---

[14]The term *scaffolding* here means supporting a child's learning so that she can perform on a level that would not be possible in an independent learning situation. The idea is to provide this scaffold with new or difficult material, then slowly withdraw the scaffold as the child becomes more independent. The trick, of course, is understanding exactly where the child is on a continuum and providing just the right instruction with just the right modifications.

component at the K-1 levels (Adams et al. 1995). *Open Court* is designed to use with entire classes of children.

Phonemic Awareness

Phonemic awareness and phonics are taught separately in Open Court. Phonemic awareness is taught first, in kindergarten, and is limited to oral language instruction. Letters are not paired with phonemes until first grade. Kindergarten activities are playful and game-like such as alliterative songs, talking to puppets that speak only in segments rather than words, and clapping the syllables in classmates' names.

Phonics

By the time letter sounds are taught, each target sound has been long-mastered in phonological awareness activities. As suggested by the National Reading Panel Report, phonics instruction is highly explicit. Each letter-sound association has a card with the letter and a key word (i.e., a picture of a monkey for the letter *m*.) Each letter-sound also has a mnemonic rhyme to go with the card, such as the following:

> For Muzzy the Monkey, bananas are yummy.
> She munches so many they fill up her tummy.
> When she eats, she says /m/ /m/ /m/ /m/ /m/.

Note that the sound is not taught as the first sound in monkey, but rather as the sound that the monkey makes. Using naturally occurring phonemes, such as the /t/-/t/-/t/ sound that an egg timer makes, avoids, for example, the schwa-clouded /tuh/ sound that can make blending very difficult for beginning readers. Once a letter-sound has been taught, words composed of the new letters are read in very simple decodable text.

PHONEMIC AWARENESS IN YOUNG CHILDREN

Marilyn Adams and her colleagues designed this classroom-based phonemic awareness program for kindergarten and first grade children as a collaboration among experts (Adams et al. 1998). It was based on the training used in an oft-cited study of the development of phonemic awareness in Danish kindergarten children (Lundberg, Frost, and Petersen 1988). The program is well researched and there is strong evidence of its effectiveness; it was used in Barbara Foorman's NIH-funded, large-scale longitudinal study of kindergarten literacy in Houston, Texas (Foorman, Francis, Beeler et al. 1997).

The teacher's guide includes an informative rationale for the program, and then a sequence of seven chapters, each with a more advanced developmental level of games and activities as follows: (a) listening games, (b) rhyming, (c) segmenting sentences into words,

(d) segmenting words into syllables and blending syllables into words, (e) segmenting and blending initial and final sounds, (f) segmenting and blending all sounds in words, and (g) representing phonemes with letters. This final section is new to this version of the program. Lundberg's version dealt with speech sounds but not with letters. Keep in mind that the research tells us that phonemic awareness instruction is more effective when letters are used along with sounds.

The progression of activities in each chapter provides opportunity for what Adams et al. describe as "the accepted teaching methodology of introducing, practicing, extending, and revisiting" (Adams et al. 1998, p. 5). The activities are well organized and provide clear directions and generous lists of words to use in carrying out instruction. One game that originated in Denmark involves "Troll Talk." This begins with a story about a troll who gives away gifts, but only if the child can guess the name of the gift from the troll's funny way of talking in sound segments. If the troll says /d/-/o/-/g/, the child needs to say "dog."

While the activities are clearly presented, the program is not scripted and teachers are expected to be able to make decisions about how fast to move diverse children through the levels. There is an extensive section with materials for assessment to help with making instructional decisions.

PHONOLOGICAL AWARENESS TRAINING FOR READING

Joseph Torgesen developed this phonemic awareness program as one of the instructional components of his NIH-funded, large-scale study of instructional methods for young children at risk (Torgesen and Bryant 1994a). Its effectiveness with children at risk is well documented by research (e.g., Torgesen, Morgan, and Davis 1992; Torgesen and Davis 1993).

The program is designed for K-2 children to use either as a kindergarten precursor to phonics instruction, or concomitant to first and second grade phonics instruction. The ideal time would be during the second half of kindergarten. It is designed for small groups or for tutoring, and can be completed in a semester if instruction is delivered four times a week for 20- to 25-minute sessions.

Lesson Components

Each session has four components. Warm-up Activities include listening for sounds and listening for rhymes. Blending Activities are carried out with colored squares that are used later for segmenting. Segmenting Activities are designed to take apart phonemic segments that have just been blended. Reading and Spelling Activities use letters to generalize blending and spelling skills to written literacy.

The Program Sequence

Eight wordsets are provided to use in a sequence involving three instructional phases.

1. *Wordset 1* is composed of short and long vowels in CVC structures (e.g., *pan*, *peek*) and are used for onset/rime blending, full phoneme blending, and the segmenting of initial phonemes, but not for instruction using letters.
2. *Wordsets 2 through 5* are composed of similar word structures and include additional phonemes. They are used for full phoneme blending and segmenting.
3. *Wordsets 6 through 8* are composed of 10 consonants and four short vowels, and are used for segmenting and blending with letter cards.

Not all phoneme-grapheme combinations are taught. The program is designed to teach the alphabetic principle and to prepare children for ongoing phonics instruction.

The program comes with a clearly written *Training Manual* with step-by-step instructions for each activity, an audio tape for pronunciation, letter cards, and a set of materials for playing games and for blending and segmenting. The activities are repeated across lessons as new phonemes are introduced, a suggestion of the Report of the National Reading Panel (2000). The program is relatively short. Keep in mind that the National Reading Panel found that PA training could be accomplished fairly quickly if effective instruction was used.

READING READINESS

Reading Readiness is an Orton-Gillingham based early intervention program that was developed by Suzanne Carreker, Director of Teacher Development at the Neuhaus Education Center in Houston, Texas (Carreker 2002). It is derived from Alphabetic Phonics (see Chapter 20) and from the work of Benita Blachman. The Neuhaus Education Center provides training to teachers in both Reading Readiness and Alphabetic Phonics.

Reading Readiness begins with daily lessons in letter recognition and sequencing, phonological awareness, and oral language skills. Once letter recognition and phonological awareness are mastered, the lesson is extended from 20 to 30 minutes through the addition of handwriting and multisensory sound/symbol activities. Activities such as the following examples are presented in a sequence based on research.

Letter Recognition

- Letter recognition begins with a discrimination activity in which plastic letters are matched with letters printed on cards.

- Plastic letters are matched with written letters arranged in an arc from A to Z in order to reinforce letter names and teach the alphabet sequence.
- *Alphabet Bingo* reinforces letter knowledge.

Phonemic Awareness

Rhyme awareness is taught at the program's introductory level. Note that this is consistent with Adams' hierarchy of phonemic awareness levels (1990). Clapping and counting activities are used to teach awareness of words in sentences. Instruction in awareness of initial sounds is facilitated through drawing attention to changes in the lips, teeth, and tongue as various phonemes are articulated. Note that this is similar to the articulatory gestures used in the Lindamood Program (see Chapter 24). Phoneme segmentation is based on Blachman's *Say It and Move It* technique with tiles moved from a picture to a line below in left-to-right order.

Letter-Sound Instruction

Letters are used for phoneme segmentation once letter-sound associations are firm, providing early experiences with stretching out spoken words for spelling. Multisensory methods are used to teach the characteristics of letter sounds (e.g., voiced versus unvoiced sounds, the position of teeth, tongue, lips).

Handwriting

Descriptions of the manuscript letter strokes are used in teaching handwriting (e.g., the letter *a* is described as "around, down" and *p* is "down, up, around"). Multisensory techniques such as skywriting, tracing, and copying are all used to teach letter formations.

ROAD TO THE CODE

Benita Blachman's *Road to the Code* (Blachman et al. 2000) is the program used in several of her intervention studies with young children in high-needs urban schools. Three of these studies are included in the National Reading Panel's meta-analysis (e.g. Ball and Blachman 1991; Blachman et al. 1994; Tangel and Blachman 1992). This 11-week sequence is focused on phonemic awareness and the learning of letter sounds. It targets children at risk but is designed to be used in heterogeneous classrooms with modifications for children who move through the program at different rates. It is appropriate for all young readers, making it a good example of universal design.

The spiral bound teacher's manual includes notes for teachers, lesson plans, and materials that can be photocopied. The 44 lessons are structured around the following instructional activities.

Phonological Awareness Practice

1. *Say It and Move It* is based on Elkonin's phoneme segmentation activities in which the sounds in a word are stretched out and segmented, then represented with small disks or tiles or blocks (Elkonin 1963, 1973). In this version, the disks are placed on a picture representing the word and are moved from the picture onto an arrow pointing from left to right. Toward the end of the 11-week program, lettered disks are used, as recommended by the National Reading Panel Report.

2. *Sound Categorization Games* are based on an "odd–man–out" task developed by Bradley and Bryant (1983, 1985). Sets of pictures are prepared to include three that are alike in, for example, initial sound, and a fourth that differs (i.e., ham, hat, hot, cab). Children name the four pictures and then identify the one that "does not belong." The same game is played with rhyme (i.e., mop, hop, top, cut).

3. *Games, Songs, and Storybooks* are also used to teach children to listen to phonemes in oral language.

Letter Names and Sounds

Letter Name and Sound Cards can be photocopied from the book. These cards are typical of Orton-Gillingham programs, with keyword pictures used as mnemonic devices to help children remember the names and sounds of letters. For example, the short /i/ sound has a picture of iguanas in an igloo, and a vampire playing a violin reclines across the top of the letter *v*.

SOUNDS ABOUND

Hugh Catts, an expert in language disorders who teaches in the Department of Speech, Language, and Hearing at the University of Kansas, and Tina Vartiainen, a speech-language pathologist, developed *Sounds Abound* to help beginning readers age 4 to 9 become aware of speech sounds. Their program provides a five-section sequence of activities for young children (Catts and Vartiainen 1993).

Sound Awareness Books

This section is an extensive bibliography of read-aloud books that lend themselves to developing sensitivity to the sounds in oral language. Genres include nursery rhymes, picture books with rhyme and alliteration such as the Ahlbergs' *Each Peach, Pear, Plum*, poetry collections including Shel Silverstein's *A Light in the Attic*, song books, and books of fingerplay games involving rhyme such as *This Little Pig Went to Market*. Focus on nursery rhymes is consistent with research reporting sensitivity to nursery rhymes (Maclean, Bryant, and Bradley 1987).

Rhyme

This section includes rhyme judgment games structured around matching spoken words by rhyme and finding the "odd-one-out" in triplets (hat, deer, cat). These activities are based on Bradley and Bryant's (1983) study of PA. Reproducible worksheets for circling rhyming pairs are included. This section includes a pretest and posttest.

Beginnings and Endings

This section includes beginning and ending sound judgment games and activities. Spoken words are matched on the basis of alliteration (same initial sound) and ending sounds. Reproducible games are included such as *Go Fish* (matching cards picture the sun, soap, and a seal) and *The Name Game* ("Say your name and then say a food that starts with the same sound"). This section includes a pretest and posttest.

Blending and Segmenting

Once children can match spoken words on the basis of initial and ending phonemes, they are taught to blend and segment each phoneme in words. This section begins with segmenting syllables (e.g., *cow-boy*, *bi-cy-cle*). Game boards are provided for segmenting by pulling tokens down into, for example, each of three squares for *banana*. A picture of a zebra is cut in two for blending together the two syllables in *ze-bra*. Eventually, two- and three-phoneme words are segmented by representing phonemes with tokens in Elkonin boxes. Beginning instruction with two-phoneme words is consistent with the research (Uhry and Ehri 1999). This section includes pretests and posttests.

Putting Sounds Together

The final step involves teaching a few letter-sound associations, then using them to spell words, first by building onto the *at* and *in* word families, and eventually by spelling all phonemes in a word. As with Torgesen's program (see above), not all letter-sounds are introduced. Sounds Abound is meant to teach PA and the alphabetic principle in preparation for phonics instruction.

SCHOOLS AS SUPPORT SYSTEMS

Richard Allington, a critic of what he believes to be the too-narrow focus of the current Bush administration's school reform plans, proposes that we need to change more in schools than the inclusion of specific, scientifically researched phonemic awareness and phonics programs. These programs are important but not sufficient. He makes the valid point that without improving the quality of teachers and the quality of classroom instruction, early interventions will not be enough to reform schools (Allington 2001). Others agree with Allington. Robert Slavin designed *Success for All* (see Chapter 16) as a systemic program and not just as a reading block. Allington proposes proponents of a strong school and a strong reading program that go beyond arguments about the "best" early interventions.

PROFESSINAL DEVELOPMENT FOR TEACHERS

The first of Allington's suggestions is the only one that is at least somewhat under the control of classroom teachers, although the culture of a school determines this to some degree. A positive school culture is usually influenced by a supportive and encouraging principal who provides time and resources for professional development.

One of Allington's suggestions is called TAPER (Teachers as Professional Education Readers). In this model, teachers choose, read, and discuss a book together. Another structure is TIP (Teacher Inquiry Projects). Allington suggests that teams of teachers with common interests work together to understand both curriculum and policy, to research modifications, and to make changes.

To my mind, the best teachers do more than just follow even the best scripted programs. They talk to their colleagues, read, join study groups, take courses, and make every effort to understand not only what to do but why their instruction might or might not be working. They use feedback from children, from conversations with parents and other teachers, and from their readings to make improvements in what they do and in what the school provides to support instruction. While the carefully crafted intervention programs described above are useful for new teachers, reflective practitioners need to move beyond the script as they gain knowledge and experience.

In a study of exemplary Grade 1 classrooms, Michael Pressley and his colleagues report the following influences on these gifted teachers:

1. Teachers benefit from working with a child one-to-one in order to inform themselves of children's needs and to develop a repertoire of responses. Often, this was reported as a highlight of university courses requiring practica. A structure for careful observations of children in their own classes was also reported as a mechanism for growth.

2. Working together with colleagues in structures such as grade-level meetings, school-based study groups, and university courses provides a valued mechanism for reflecting on theory and practice.

3. Playing a leadership role and sharing one's own expertise with other teachers helps to internalize new learning.

4. It is important to find professional development that supports the understanding of basic processes and rationales for instruction rather than just exposure to a new activity (Pressley et al. 2001).

Teachers participating in *Young Readers at Risk*, a professional development collaboration between Fordham University and the Hello Friend/Ennis William Cosby Foundation, report similar influences on their growth. By and large, these Cosby scholars are in underresourced schools, but develop new strengths as teachers through collaboration with peers and through the program practica (Uhry 2003).

SMALL CLASS SIZE

Allington sites Achilles (1999) in indicating that, by and large, schools with smaller class sizes have higher achievement levels. Smaller class sizes are typical of better funded school districts and these districts tend to have better trained teachers. This is a difficult cycle to break. Children who are at risk need a well-trained teacher and a small enough group of classmates so that their teacher can spend time with several small reading groups every day.

I have watched a first grade teacher in a high-needs New York City school as she taught several groups of three or four children, one group after the next, and supervised a student teacher who did the same, within a relatively short period of time during the morning literacy block. The student teacher worked with guided reading groups composed of the stronger readers. The teacher worked with the struggling readers and actually found time to listen and instruct individuals by pairing other group members during short periods of buddy reading during this group time. I have also watched a rural first grade teacher teach large and small group lessons while a parent volunteer read for five minutes with each child in the class using a prepared baggie of appropriate books and a note about the current instructional focus for each child. In both of these classrooms, there were about 22 children and this instruction took place every day of the week. Both of these teachers were enormously skilled and extremely well organized. Both participated endlessly in professional development by reading, going to workshops, and taking classes.

ADEQUATE RESOURCES

Finding funding for resources for all children can be difficult. As Allington points out, all classrooms need books and other literacy materials at many reading levels. Classrooms with diverse learners need multiple resources. Some of urban teachers I work with run out of paper and pencils by the end of the year. They buy books and photocopy them for their reading groups. However, this is not just a funding issue. Teachers need to develop the expertise to know about "just right" materials at each child's level for both independent reading and for instruction.

INSTRUCTIONAL TIME

Uninterrupted instructional time is another of Allington's recommendations. In my experience, some school schedules pull children in and out of the classroom all morning for "specials" such as physical education, library, special pull-out instruction, and science classes. This out-of-classroom schedule drives the teacher's control over instructional time. In other schools, a literacy block of up to two hours or even the entire morning is set aside each day with time for large and small group instruction in both reading and writing. Again, how this time is used is dependent on the expertise of the teacher, the size of the class, and the supply of appropriate materials.

All of these topics play a major role in early intervention. There are a number of good early instructional programs that teach letter names, phonemic awareness, and phonics, and that provide guidance to teachers about teaching directly and systematically. I do not believe, however, that there is such a thing as a "teacher-proof" program. Our best teachers won't stay in teaching just to follow a script. Teachers need to understand what they are doing on a deeper level in order to be engaged by the challenge of making instruction just right for every child. To do this, they need access to well-designed programs, but they also need access to professional development and to system-wide support in terms of class size, resources, and time to teach.

15

Reading Recovery

BACKGROUND AND RATIONALE

Reading Recovery was first developed by Marie Clay in New Zealand during the mid 1970s. The program was conceived as an early intervention program for the lowest achieving children at the time of entry into what is called first grade in the United States. It is closely linked, both philosophically and systemically, with New Zealand's national reading scheme. After a year of a kindergarten program that focuses on early literacy skills, children are screened individually by their teachers who select approximately the lowest 20 percent for Reading Recovery at the beginning of first grade. This intervention involves reading in a one-to-one setting for half an hour a day with a master teacher who has received a year of additional training in Reading Recovery methods. The aim is to provide help before reading failure is established, and then to discontinue this special help and return these children to their regular classroom reading groups as quickly as possible, with 12 weeks as the goal. Children who have not been discontinued after 20 weeks are usually referred for a more intensive kind of help and represent roughly 1 percent of all of the children in a particular grade.

During the 1984–1985 school year, Marie Clay and her New Zealand colleague, Barbara Watson, together with a group headed by

Gay Sue Pinnell at Ohio State University, brought Reading Recovery to the Columbus, Ohio, public schools. Ohio schools have played a leadership role in the American whole language movement, which is philosophically linked to the New Zealand national reading scheme in some (but not all) characteristics, and thus Ohio provided a receptive site for this program. State funding was available for the project very early, and by 1987, it had been selected for federal funding as part of the U.S. Department of Education's National Diffusion Network. By 1993, there were Reading Recovery training sites in 44 states (Lyons, Pinnell, and DeFord 1993) and by 1999, there were 9,000 schools using the program in the United States.

Reading Recovery views reading as the act of constructing meaning. While this is a sensible view, the emphasis on meaning can be provocative to some advocates of phonics instruction who see children with dyslexia as already overrelying on meaning and needing direct instruction in phonics. However, Reading Recovery is a highly complex early intervention system involving structural changes in a school as well as training in the particulars of the teaching method. It assumes a philosophical stance in which children are provided with strategies for self-monitoring with the thought that training will be discontinued once they have internalized these strategies and are reading at the level of their classroom's middle reading group. Marie Clay talks at length about inner controls; one of her books is titled *Becoming Literate: The Construction of Inner Control* (1991). The rhetoric will sound familiar to those of us who remember the late 1960s and its emphasis on the child as learner, except that there is great rigor in the Reading Recovery teacher training and in the expectations placed on the child as an independent learner.

CURRICULUM AND INSTRUCTION

Reading Recovery tutoring involves an entry phase for observing what the child already knows prior to implementation of the teaching program. During this "roaming around the known" phase, the teacher works daily to build the child's confidence in strategies that are already in place, and observes carefully in order to plan instruction based on the child's strengths.

After this two-week period, instruction begins. Each half hour lesson is structured around five steps: (a) rereading familiar books, (b) rereading the most recent book with a "running record" of observed strategies and miscues jotted down by the teacher, (c) a letter-oriented lesson based on a pattern observed to be difficult for the student during the previous day's lesson, (d) a writing lesson based on this book, and finally, (e) introduction of a new book.

There is no standard sequence of reading materials in Reading Recovery, and this represents a radical difference between Reading Recovery and other programs described in this book. The reading materials are small readers called "little books," each with a complete story, profusely illustrated in color, and with short, repetitive, predictable text. The approximately 600 "little books" used by Reading Recovery are organized into a sequence of 20 increasingly more difficult beginning reading levels. There is no particular sequence for reading books within each level; tutors choose books within a level based on each child's interests or instructional needs.

Ideally, similar books are used in the classroom as well. According to Trika Smith-Burke, Reading Recovery has been used in schools using other classroom reading schemes. For example, the Ginn Readers were used in classrooms in the early days of Reading Recovery in Ohio, and phonetically based texts are used in classrooms in the Greenwich, Connecticut, public schools, which use both Reading Recovery and Enfield and Green's Project Read. Smith-Burke feels that the optimal situation involves consistency between the classroom and Reading Recovery in regard to both books and teaching philosophy.

A new book is introduced at the end of a lesson and then reread during the next lesson. Before a child reads a new book, the tutor invites the child to make sense of the story from the title and pictures, and in this conversation, the tutor uses words that the child will be reading. Once the child begins to read, the teacher steps back, encouraging the child to practice strategies for figuring out new words independently. Both letter cues and context cues are encouraged. When the teacher does help, he or she directs the child's attention in a way that encourages successful problem-solving rather than simply providing the answer. The child is encouraged to "cross-check" to see that information from different sources is in agreement (e.g., "If the word is *meanies,* what letter would you expect to see at the beginning?").

During the two Reading Recovery tutoring lessons observed within a training session at New York University, the child, in each case, began by choosing two books that were old favorites to read aloud. Then the child was asked to read the new book from the last lesson. During this reading, the tutor kept a running record of those strategies and letter patterns that were mastered as well as those that needed work. The scheme for observing a child's reading strategies is highly elaborated in both the Reading Recovery literature (Clay 1993a, 1993b) and during training. Observational records provide information to be used in making decisions about instruction. Unlike the traditional error analysis, running records involve observations of effective strategies as well as miscues. Help from the tutor during oral reading tended to involve encouraging the child to try a particular strategy, and this occurred only after the child had tried to solve the problem independently.

This running record was followed by a short lesson (less than two minutes) using plastic letters to teach a strategy for reading a letter pattern that had been misread in a previous lesson. In one case, this involved the *all* word family. The tutor made a point of linking the unknown *all* words (e.g., *fall*, *call*) to those which were already known by the child (e.g., *all*, *ball*). During earlier phases in the development of Reading Recovery, these short "teaching points" were incorporated into reading sessions and presented spontaneously when the child seemed ready for new learning. They are now provided separately so as not to interrupt the focus on comprehension during book reading.

This lesson was followed by a short writing lesson that involved what is called "joint problem-solving" (Lyons, Pinnell, and DeFord 1993). The child composed a sentence aloud based on interest in a recent book, and then wrote it down. Several words were spelled by having the child segment phonemes aloud. The tutor asked, "What letter would you expect to see?" and then wrote each letter in a series of Elkonin-type boxes she had prepared for this word (Elkonin 1963, 1973). Hard words were simply spelled out for the child. The completed sentence was cut up into words, scrambled, and then reassembled by the child as the tutor said the sentence aloud. Marie Clay (1992) built this writing activity into the program in order to capitalize on the reciprocal relationship between reading and writing, and to strengthen phonological awareness skills through the segmenting and spelling boxes. Clay calls this "invented spelling," but notes that the child does not actually misspell words as in many American classrooms using this technique. In Reading Recovery, the child receives teacher support in building words correctly from patterns that have been internalized, and the teacher simply spells out others or parts of others that are, as yet, too difficult for the child.

The final activity in these observed lessons was the introduction of a new book. Prior to reading the new book, the child was engaged in conversation about the pictures, and was encouraged to discuss background knowledge of the content and to make predictions about the story. At this point in the lesson, some children in Reading Recovery tutoring have read as many as five short books during the half hour lesson. The ratio of time actually spent reading text to time engaged in reading-related activities is higher in Reading Recovery than in other programs described here. The efficiency of the lessons was striking. Almost all of the time was spent with the child actually engaged in reading. The books were so carefully chosen and the tutor so in touch with the child's reading that the direct instruction, while minimal, was highly focused and seemed to be quite effective.

TEACHER TRAINING

To enter a Reading Recovery training program in the United States, teachers must be certified and must have at least three years of classroom experience. They must be nominated by their school districts, with only about half of the nominated teachers accepted for training. Teachers in training (and ultimately, Reading Recovery teachers) work with four children for half an hour each during the morning, then return to their old jobs as classroom or resource room teachers in the afternoon.

During the year-long training period, teachers attend weekly sessions at a Reading Recovery training center. These centers are university-based such as the ones at Ohio State University and New York University. Trainees take turns bringing a child for a demonstration lesson, which takes place "behind the glass" or one-way mirror. The other trainees watch and are guided in their observations by a teacher trainer who holds a doctoral degree, is affiliated with a university, and has been trained as a Reading Recovery teacher trainer. The emphasis during these observations is on decision-making for a particular situation rather than simply learning standard techniques. Trainers focus on the reading process and on the impact of a particular teaching point. Careful observation of the child is a major focus.

EVALUATION AND IMPLEMENTATION

Reading Recovery was chosen by the American Federation of Teachers to feature in a 1999 article subtitled *Five Promising Remedial Reading Intervention Programs*. The article states,

> Research on Reading Recovery has been uneven and results have been mixed. At least two careful studies, however, show that, when properly implemented, the program can have significant positive effects on some measures of reading achievement, with effect sizes ranging from +.57 to +.78. A small study of the Spanish-language version of the program—*Descubriendo La Lectura*—also showed positive effects (American Federation of Teachers 1999).

Reading Recovery was one of four, Grade 1 early interventions chosen for analysis in Elfreida Heibert and Barbara Taylor's chapter on beginning reading interventions in the *Handbook of Reading Research, Vol. 3* (2000). They concluded that all four interventions were successful when compared to controls representing status quo instruction.

A number of large-scale research studies have been carried out to evaluate Reading Recovery in the United States (see DeFord, Lyons, and Pinnell 1991). The consensus is that roughly 65 to 85 percent of Reading Recovery children are successfully returned to regular classroom reading groups (Center et al. 1995; DeFord, Lyons, and Pinnell

1991). Several of these studies seem particularly thorough and illuminating. The first teased apart the effective components of this highly complex teaching model. An evaluation team led by Ohio Reading Recovery trainer Gay Su Pinnell (Pinnell et al. 1994) analyzed the effective characteristics of Reading Recovery through a comparison of other interventions with some but not all of its attributes. There were five groups in the experiment: (a) Reading Recovery, (b) Reading Recovery with a shorter teacher training period, (c) another one-to-one tutoring program using direct instruction, (d) Reading Recovery instructional techniques used by trained teachers with small groups rather than with individuals, and (e) controls in existing Chapter One pullout classes. This study used 324 of the lowest achieving first grade children from 10 Ohio school districts. In addition to pre- and posttest measures of reading and writing, extensive analyses of videotaped lessons were carried out. Data from all of these sources suggested that Reading Recovery worked better than any of the other models. Its effectiveness was the apparent result of several key factors: (a) working one-to-one with students, (b) the framework of the lessons, and (c) the teacher training model with an expectation of ongoing learning in a supportive atmosphere. Timothy Rasinski comments, in regard to this study, that the lengthy training of Reading Recovery's already skilled teachers and the intensity of the one-to-one instruction may account for at least some of its effectiveness. The composition of the lesson itself may not be the only factor in considering the program's effectiveness (Rasinski 1995).

A second study with similarly positive conclusions about Reading Recovery was carried out by researchers who are not directly involved with this program (Wasik and Slavin 1993). Note that Robert Slavin is one of the developers of *Success for All*, a multifaceted program for urban at-risk children in the primary grades. They compared five programs designed for at-risk children in the primary grades: (a) Reading Recovery, (b) Success for All, (c) Prevention of Learning Disabilities, (d) The Wallach Tutoring Program, and (e) Programmed Tutorial Reading. Wasik and Slavin compared effect sizes for the five programs as reported by independent researchers. Effect sizes were largest for Reading Recovery and Success for All, which the researchers attribute to use of certified teachers, one-to-one delivery of the programs, and well-articulated models of the reading process. This last point is an important one: understanding basic reading processes is an important feature of Reading Recovery teacher-training; trainees are not taught to teach from scripts, but rather to observe for signs of processes and strategies, and to use these observations in planning instruction. Wasik and Slavin also address the issue of cost effectiveness: both Success for All and Reading Recovery are often criticized as being expensive. Wasik and Slavin make the point that using special education funds for early prevention can save money over the long term (Dyer 1992; Slavin et al. 1992).

In an article describing volunteer tutoring programs, Wasik describes a project involving AmeriCorps volunteers who are trained in the Reading Recovery method and work with young readers whose achievement is low but not low enough to qualify for Reading Recovery services. Wasik describes their training as markedly less than certified Reading Recovery teachers receive but as "very sophisticated" compared to the training that most volunteers receive (Wasik 1998). Research carried out by Reading Recovery on this project did not include controls but demonstrated strong gains on word reading skills but not on comprehension (DeFord, Pinnell, and Lyons 1997). The authors suggest that it is easier to teach word reading that the complexities of comprehension.

A fourth study was carried out in Rhode Island by a Reading Recovery trainer and a university researcher, both from New Zealand (Iverson and Tunmer 1993). It attempted to answer questions about a common criticism of Reading Recovery, which is perceived by many special educators to be a lack of direct instruction in phonemic awareness and phonics. Two groups of Reading Recovery teachers were trained, one in the usual Reading Recovery training program and the other in the usual program with the addition of phonics and phonemic awareness instruction. Both programs were found to be effective, but children in the Reading-Recovery-plus-phonics program were discontinued from tutoring sooner than those in the regular Reading Recovery program.

Unlike many of the other remedial programs described here, there is systematic research to describe characteristics of those children who have not been successfully discontinued from Reading Recovery and to document what the eventual outcome was for them. Marie Clay attempts to answer these questions with preliminary results from a New Zealand study (Clay 1992). Most of the highest functioning of the unsuccessful children in this study did eventually read within the average range after about two years. About a third of the unsuccessful children had low intelligence and were provided with other forms of support. A small number had psychological problems believed to be interfering with learning to read.

One criticism of the Reading Recovery research that has been carried out by Clay and others directly associated with the program is that these researchers have failed to include the reading scores of children who have not been successfully discontinued in follow-up studies of ability to maintain gains (Center et al. 1995). Yola Center states that as many as 30 percent of children are removed from Reading Recovery programs because of failure to make progress. This would tend to skew the success-rate statistics. Center and her colleagues report data from a study carried out in Australia in which Reading Recovery children were compared to controls receiving group-based extra instruction. Reading Recovery children were significantly stronger than controls at the time that the Reading Recovery children were discontinued from one-to-one help, but this advantage faded over the subsequent weeks and months.

Another criticism of Reading Recovery is the high cost. The American Federation of Teachers, in an article on promising interventions, states that estimates of start-up costs range from $2,500 to $10,000 per student (American Federation of Teachers 1999).

Because Reading Recovery is so widely used and is, thus, in the public eye to a greater degree than many of the other programs described here, the quality of the research has been more rigorously controlled. The research is characterized by larger studies and by studies with control groups. Even critics of Reading Recovery (e.g., Center et al. 1995; Rasinski 1995) agree that this individual instruction is effective. Overall, the research carried out on Reading Recovery appears to be both thorough and positive. To date, there is no research on the success rate of Reading Recovery instruction with children screened in kindergarten as being specifically at risk for dyslexia.

16

Success for All

BACKGROUND AND RATIONALE

Success for All was developed by Robert Slavin and his colleagues at Johns Hopkins University in Baltimore, and is one of a number of projects co-directed by Slavin at the Johns Hopkins Center for Research on the Education of Students Placed at Risk (CRESPAR). It is a classroom-based program designed as a type of system-wide school reform. The original goal of Success for All was that every child would be reading at grade level by Grade 3. Its basic premise is that all children can learn if provided with intensive early intervention.

Success for All was first developed in 1986 at the request of Baltimore's school superintendent and school board president who were concerned about the school failure rate among Baltimore's many economically disadvantaged students. A successful pilot program was implemented in 1987, resulting in higher reading scores and lower rates of retention and special education referrals in comparison to controls. The following year, the program was expanded to five Baltimore schools and a school in Philadelphia. By 1995, the program was in 300 schools across 23 states, and a November 2002 newsletter, *Success Story*, celebrated the 15th anniversary of Success for All, stating that the program is currently in 1,500 schools with 480 training staff serving almost a million children (Slavin et al. 1996).

Success for All takes somewhat different forms in its many implementations but the central organizing focus is the reading program for Grades K–3. Other curriculum components for Grades 1 to 5 include *Roots and Wings*, a 1991 reading instruction expansion funded by the New American Schools Development Corporation. The reading component of Roots is used for the end of Kindergarten and Grade 1, while Wings is for students at the end of Grade 1 up through Grade 5. Roots and Wings also includes Math Wings, a curriculum that is based on the standards of the National Council of Teachers of Mathematics and uses Slavin's cooperative learning structures. WorldLab is the science and social studies component. It is organized around interdisciplinary theme units and provides contextualized practice in reading and writing. There is a Spanish-language program, *Lee Conmigo*, which is available for schools opting to provide reading instruction in Spanish. It uses the same reading strategies as Roots and Wings. Other Success for All/Roots and Wings components include reading assessments at eight-week intervals, reading tutors, and preschool and kindergarten readiness programs. An on-site program facilitator works with the principals and teachers, and coordinates a Family Support Team. This Team works with community service agencies that are often located on-site in Success for All/Roots and Wings schools. The Family Support Team also trains parents to support literacy at home, to provide volunteer help in classrooms, and to be part of school-based governance. The facilitator is seen as the critical element in the program and carries out three important jobs: (a) ongoing professional development for teachers, (b) coordination of the many components of the program including their interconnections, and (c) organization of the eight-week assessments. Early intervention and prevention are perceived as systemic, and as involving far more than the presence of exemplary early reading instruction. One important goal of Success for All is meeting special needs in the regular classroom.

CURRICULUM AND INSTRUCTION

The Success for All/Roots and Wings reading curriculum is research-based and draws widely from research findings synthesized by Marilyn Adams in her seminal 1990 book, *Beginning to Read*, as well as from Slavin's earlier program, *Cooperative Integrated Reading and Composition* (CIRC; Stevens et al. 1987).

Early intervention is an important component of Success for All. The preschool and kindergarten curriculum revolves around interdisciplinary theme units that utilize learning centers (e.g., art, dramatic play, water/sand, hands-on science, and so on), as well as a broad spectrum of language arts experiences. The *Peabody Language Development Kit* is used in the classroom by push-in experts such as language specialists who work with small groups. *Story Telling and Retelling* (STaR; Karweit et al. 1990) involves 30 minutes of daily large-group listening comprehension activities focused on literature (e.g., interactive listening using prediction, comprehension monitoring, summarizing, group retelling, and story structure review). These literature activities are carried out to prepare children for later reading comprehension and are connected to the current theme unit. For example, the book *Nobody Listens to Andrew* is used as part of a unit on community helpers. *Emergent Writing* is encouraged as children begin to understand the purposes of written communication, and takes multiple forms such as journal writing and shared writing. *Rhyme with Reason* is a sequence of phonological awareness activities, moving from rhyme recognition to initial phoneme segmentation, carried out three times a week in half-day preschool and kindergarten, and every day in all-day kindergarten. *Shared Book Experiences* use big books to model print conventions as well as comprehension. *Alphabet Activities* involve reading and writing letters, and are integrated into both thematic units and language arts activities throughout the day.

Reading instruction for Roots and Wings takes place in daily 90-minute blocks with children grouped by reading level. While classrooms are heterogeneously grouped, children are regrouped for reading instruction by reading level across both classrooms and grades. Reading groups are small because many staff members (e.g., tutors, reading specialists, ESL teachers, special education teachers), as well as the classroom teachers, take a reading group. Lessons are scripted and skills are introduced sequentially. Eight-week assessments are used to check the progress of every child on a routine basis and to restructure the reading groups depending on changes in reading status. This assessment also provides information about which children need to be provided with tutoring, an important component of the program for the children who are struggling the most with reading. The role of the facilitator is critical here with tutoring decisions to be made and hundreds of children's schedules to be reworked every eight weeks.

Reading Roots is designed to begin in either late kindergarten or early first grade, at the discretion of the school. Reading Roots provides a complete package for beginning reading instruction. It includes preprimer- and primer-level readers and all accompanying materials. Reading Roots continues work on listening comprehension through the STaR program while providing instruction for the transition to using letters to decode words independently. It introduces phoneme blending and full phoneme segmentation, as well as systematic, sequential phonics instruction. Letter-sound associations, phonemic awareness, and the alphabetic principle are taught through a series of short, integrated activities including the following for each new letter-sound:

1. Listen for a new sound in a series of words (e.g., "Fang found five fat fish by the fence").
2. Stretch out the /f/ in these words.
3. Sort pictures of initial-/f/ and non-/f/ words in a yes/no game.
4. Produce the sound /f/ in response to both pictures and later, the written letter.
5. Write the letter f using verbal cueing (i.e., "Curve left, straight down, lift and cross. The sound of f is /f/.").
6. Play a game called *Quick Erase* in which Elkonin-like word-change sequences such as fat - fast - fist - fit - fin - fun - sun are collaboratively developed on the blackboard.
7. Stretch and spell phonetically regular words.
8. Stretch and read phonetically regular words starting with the target letter-sound.
9. Read phonetically regular decodable text using the target letter-sound.

While the term *multisensory* is not used, both the activities themselves and the accumulation of links among the various senses are consistent with the Orton-Gillingham principle and practice of linkages using multisensory instruction. My Fordham colleague, Dr. Valerie Rowe, who was at one time a reading specialist and Success for All facilitator in the South Bronx, described the program as fast-paced, with activities changing every few minutes. In comparison with the language arts program formerly used by her school, she felt that children were less apt to tune-out and more apt to stay actively engaged.

Reading Roots is a balanced literacy program in that word study is linked to meaningful activities in books and literacy is linked to other subject areas right from the start (Madden 1995). *Fast Track Phonics*, slated for 2003 publication, is an updated, systematic introduction to letter sounds and blending for Grades K and 1. *Shared Stories* are designed with portions to be read aloud by the teacher and other, simpler, phonetically regular text portions that children are encouraged to read themselves. *Scaffolding*, provided by the teacher and by the illustrations, is gradually removed until children are reading on their own. These stories are interconnected and the concepts in them are related to theme units. New editions of the stories, with color pictures, will be in publication soon. Listening strategies from STaR such as monitoring for meaning and summarizing are expanded into reading comprehension strategies. *Reading Rehearsal* involves rereadings for fluency. Writing activities focus on sound-based spelling, personal narratives, and writing about theme-unit learning.

Reading Wings carries children from the late first or early second grade reading level through fifth or sixth grade. Materials supplement existing basal readers and replace other materials in a school's basal reading series. Teachers' guides, called Treasure Hunts (Madden et al. 1996), are provided for many of the basal series in current use.

Reading instruction, as outlined in the guides, is focused on solidifying word attack skills, on fluency, on pleasure in reading, and on reading comprehension. Instruction is an adaptation of Slavin's effective CIRC program (Stevens et al. 1987). The guide for a CIRC lesson using a version of the trade book *Jumanji* by Chris Van Allsburg from a Houghton-Mifflin reader is included in the program guide *Every Child, Every School* by Slavin et al. (1996).

Cooperative learning is a major component of CIRC. Students practice and use language arts skills in heterogeneous learning teams for all academic learning outside of the homogeneous reading groups. These cooperative teams also participate in language arts activities such as the following:

- *Partner Reading* involves partners prereading a story silently and then supporting each other's oral reading.
- *Words Aloud* involves supporting team members as they practice reading words aloud introduced in reading groups.
- *Partner Checking* involves signing off on an assignment sheet indicating completion of assigned activities by a reading partner.

The integration of work done in reading groups and in these team-based work groups is complex. Teamwork between the classroom and reading group teachers is critical.

Writing instruction is also carried out in the classroom with children working in cooperative teams. *Writing from the Heart* (Madden, Wasik, and Petza 1989) is the writing program for Grades 1 and 2. Its goals include pleasure in communicating and the fluency that comes with automaticity in skill use. Teachers model both enjoyment and new skills for children. Invented or sound spelling is encouraged in the first draft or "sloppy copy." Writers share with peers, revise, edit, and publish, as in other versions of process writing. *CIRC Writing*, the program for Grades 1 to 3, also uses process-writing principles but is somewhat more formal in nature. Team members provide feedback for revisions.

One-to-one tutoring is an important feature of Success for All with priority given to the lowest achieving children in Grades 1 to 3. The percentage of children who receive tutoring differs from school to school and depends on local resources. In Valerie Rowe's school in the South Bronx, roughly the lowest 30 percent of children in Grade 1 were tutored, and 10 percent in Grades 2 and 3. Tutors are certified teachers with extra training. Tutors work one-to-one for 20 minutes with a number of students each day, and also teach a reading group each day. Tutoring is carefully scheduled to preserve time for both the child's regular reading group and his classroom language arts instruction. Tutoring focuses on learning to read by reading, and includes short periods of related skill work. A typical tutoring session begins with the reading of a familiar book for fluency, confidence, and self-monitoring of comprehension. Then comes the introduction and reading of a new story that uses a letter pattern that is being taught in the regular reading group or classroom. Oral reading is used to assess and plan brief periods of drill in letter, sound, or sight word skills. The final activity during each session is writing with a focus on meaning.

New curriculum materials will be introduced soon with more focus in Reading Wings (Grades 2–6) on vocabulary and comprehension. New support materials for students and teachers will include videos/DVDs designed to supplement curriculum in a wide range of areas including cooperative learning, partner reading, summarizing, and test taking.

What distinguishes the curriculum of Success for All/Roots and Wings from any exemplary preschool or elementary program that embeds skills in meaningful interdisciplinary work? Slavin acknowledges that many components of SFA have been borrowed from other effective programs. He states that the program's strength lies in its comprehensive collection of well-researched and well-integrated components, and in the "relentlessness" with which these components are used in a series of system-wide back-up strategies (Slavin et al. 1996, p. 229).

TEACHER TRAINING

Training in Success for All and Roots and Wings is provided to teachers through schools in which the principal, other key personnel, and 80 percent of the teachers have made a commitment to the program. Trainers at Johns Hopkins provide a five-day workshop for new facilitators who then participate, together with the Johns Hopkins trainers, in school-based initial summer training of teachers in new Success for All schools. Training is extensive and often includes simulations in which instruction is acted out through role-playing. Teachers who have never used cooperative learning before are instructed in cooperative learning teams.

Training sessions are extended over a period of months in terms of Johns Hopkins trainers or regional staff providing workshops as the program components are added a few at a time. These trainers typically visit new schools for about six days during the initial year of the new program. This provides opportunities for maintaining the integrity of the program, but schools are encouraged to work out unique solutions to problems at the local level. Successful local schools are also encouraged to work with new Success for All schools.

Teacher training is seen as the beginning of a professional development program that is ongoing. The facilitator acts as a mentor and coach on a day-to-day basis, and continues to provide on-site teacher training with classroom visits for observation and facilitation of peer observations and peer planning groups. Facilitators also teach demonstration lessons for teachers in their schools. Training includes classroom management strategies as well as strategies for teaching specific subject areas or the interdisciplinary units.

Valerie Rowe described the program as so complex, and with so many components to learn, that the teachers she trained in the South Bronx often had initial difficulty moving quickly enough to stay on the suggested schedule. As the better teachers became more experienced, they were able to maintain the fast pace and put creativity and personality into instruction as well. Her experience was with a school under review by the state education department because of its low reading scores. Many of its teachers were uncertified or inexperienced, or both. Despite this discouraging school history, she reports that there was dramatic improvement in most teachers' effectiveness following training.

EVALUATION AND IMPLEMENTATION

From the beginning, Success for All/Roots and Wings has used a rigorous program of well-controlled research to assess and refine its efforts. Longitudinal evaluations were carried out in the initial six Baltimore and Philadelphia schools using a research model that the program continues to use. Every Success for All school is matched with a comparable local control school. Because Success for All is an early intervention program, only data from children beginning the program at Grade 1 or earlier are reported. Children are evaluated over time using multiple, standardized measures of oral reading and comprehension. Results are reported in grade cohorts rather than in terms of individual students. Data have been analyzed across schools in a series of meta-analyses involving thousands of children, and much of this research has been published in prestigious peer-reviewed journals. The findings have been positive; children in Success for All schools have had significantly higher scores in decoding and comprehension at every grade level in comparison with children in control schools.

One question asked in this research was whether there would be a positive change in effect size if a school continued its teacher training year after year. Effect sizes do tend to rise over a period of years of implementation of Success for All. Another question is whether effects last over time. Students from the first Baltimore cohorts have continued to outperform controls after the program ended when they entered middle schools. Slavin and Madden (1999) cited 14 technical reports from CRESPAR indicating that this trend continues. Effect sizes are largest in schools that have continued the program over a number of years and have utilized all components of the program. Comparisons with Reading Recovery suggest that both programs are effective for at-risk first graders. However, children with special needs in Success for All schools appear to have a more positive outcome in comparison with controls in Reading Recovery schools where these children are not provided with one-to-one tutoring.

The most critical question in evaluating Success for All is whether *all* students really succeed in reading. This has been a difficult goal to meet. In one study, while groups of SFA students outperformed groups of comparable controls, even when only the lowest 25 percent in each group was compared, not all children in the Success for All schools could be considered successful readers (Madden et al. 1993). Fifteen percent of these SFA third graders were a year behind grade level and 3.9 percent were two years behind.

Another important question is how effective SFA is for children with special needs. Research comparing Reading Recovery schools with SFA schools (Ross et al. in press) found both types of schools to be highly effective with most children, but SFA schools outperformed Reading Recovery Schools in terms of first graders classified as having special needs. The special-needs children in SFA schools were in SFA classes, whereas the special-needs first graders in Reading Recovery schools were in special education classes rather than in the Reading Recovery program. SFA schools outperformed Reading Recovery schools but there were no children requiring special services in Reading Recovery tutorials. This is an important point. In this district, Success for All targets all children and provides better services for the lowest performing children than other existing services.

It is hard to evaluate, directly, the effectiveness of Success for All as a program for children at risk for dyslexia. It is hard to identify children with dyslexia in settings where large numbers of disadvantaged kindergarten children have weak phonological awareness and know few, if any, letter names. Slavin has not provided information about individual differences. However, SFA does sound like an ideal environment for minimizing dyslexia's symptoms because it has so many of the features suggested for children with dyslexia (e.g., one-to-one or small-group help, phonological processing instruction, systematic sequential phonics, multisensory linkages, coordination between classrooms and tutoring programs).

What do teachers have to say about the program? The SFA teachers I've visited were enthusiastic about results but had reservations about using a scripted program. They said they liked the script when they started, either because they were new to teaching or because the system was new to them, but that as they became skilled with SFA, they found that the script restricted their ability to individualize. Several experienced and talented SFA teachers whom I observed in a relatively high-achieving school in a low SES neighborhood did deviate from the script but said that this was not encouraged. Valerie Rowe reported another troublesome issue. In an age of accountability, teachers are held responsible for their classroom children's test scores, but much of their children's language arts program in Success for All schools is often administered by another teacher. These are difficult issues for SFA and for other well-researched, effective programs. Our best teachers need to be able to feel ownership of their classroom curriculum and classroom successes or we will lose them, but many, many children in high-needs schools do not have our best teachers.

17

Direct Instruction: DISTAR

BACKGROUND AND RATIONALE

Wesley Becker and Siegfried Engelmann developed the Direct Instruction Model, which became known as *DISTAR* (Direct Instructional System of Teaching Arithmetic and Reading) at the University of Oregon. DISTAR Reading was designed for beginning readers and Corrective Reading is a Direct Instruction curriculum for older struggling readers (see Chapter 18). DISTAR was officially launched in 1968 as one of nine instructional models to be used in Project Follow-Through, a U.S. Government-sponsored project to evaluate the effectiveness of promising educational programs for disadvantaged children in the first three grades.

Four basic assumptions form the theoretical rationale for the DISTAR model (Becker 1977; Carnine et al. 2004). First, all children, regardless of background and developmental readiness, can be taught, and teachers must be held accountable for student failure. Second, acquisition of basic skills underlies all successful learning; for children who are socioeconomically deprived, direct teaching of these skills is essential. Third, disadvantaged children generally lag behind advantaged students in basic skills due to the existing academic structure in most schools. The fourth assumption is that in order to catch up, economically disadvantaged youngsters must be taught more within an allotted instructional time in comparison with advantaged children.

Though originally designed for disadvantaged children, DIS-TAR has been used to teach children with a variety of constitutional disabilities including learning disabilities. Norris Haring, Barbara Bateman, and Douglas Carnine describe DISTAR as follows:

> DISTAR's conceptualization encompasses all essential aspects of the teaching process—analyzing concepts, programming, teaching per se, classroom management, educational materials, and evaluation. It has developed a way of analyzing tasks that isolates the general concept or skill to be taught, and a way to program in which this general case is presented so impeccably that every child can learn it (Haring, Bateman, and Carnine 1977).

CURRICULUM AND INSTRUCTION

Becker (1977) outlined seven essential instructional components of the DISTAR model:

1. Teaching general cases in order that learning can be generalized from selected examples to broader instances.
2. Higher teacher-student ratio.
3. Carefully structured daily curriculum.
4. Rapid-paced, teacher-directed, small-group instruction with a high number of teacher/student interactions.
5. Positive reinforcement.
6. Carefully trained and supervised teaching staff.
7. Biweekly performance monitoring by means of criterion-referenced tests.

One special feature of DISTAR is that all instruction follows a script. The presentation books (flip-books) provide exact wording and precise directions for everything the teacher says and does in each lesson. Instruction is conducted in small groups with students seated in a semicircle close to the teacher in order to be able to see the one-inch printed letters and words in the teacher presentation books. The proximity additionally helps the teacher monitor student response, much of which is done in unison. Teachers use hand signals such as a hand drop, a clap, a point, or other cue to indicate the type and timing of the responses required. The presentation books ensure that all concepts deemed relevant by the program's developers are taught and practiced by the students. They include correction procedures and scripts for anticipated student errors.

DISTAR (Engelmann and Bruner 1983) is published by Science Research Associates, Inc. and is now formally referred to as SRA's Direct Instruction Programs. The programs provide instruction in reading, language, spelling, and arithmetic, and cover grade levels one through six.

The language program has three levels. The first level is for preschool and primary students and focuses on teaching the language of instruction used in school, building vocabulary, developing oral language skills, and establishing the foundation for logical thinking. The second level builds a language foundation for reading comprehension, emphasizing reasoning skills, and teaches following directions and the meanings of words and sentences. The third level focuses on sentence analysis, both spoken and written, and deals with mechanics as well as informational content.

The reading program (Reading Mastery) has six levels; only Levels I and II, which extend from preschool through second grade, will be discussed here. Both decoding and comprehension are taught from the very beginning. In Reading Mastery I, letters are referred to as sounds; in Reading Mastery II, letter names are taught. Prereading activities start with teaching the pronunciations of letter sounds. Diagrams are presented to teach the distinction between continuous sounds (e.g., /s/, /m/, /r/, certain digraphs, and all vowels) and stop sounds (e.g., /b/, /d/, /t/). Games are played to promote sequencing skills and to teach understanding of cue words such as "first" and "next." Oral blending activities begin in the first lesson and continue through the prereading lessons. Children are taught the difference between sounding out words (saying the letter sounds slowly) and pronouncing the words (saying them fast); the teacher uses hand signals in directing other activities. Rhyming activities are introduced to help children learn to blend initial sounds with word endings. Association between sounds and letter symbols is reinforced in take-home activities.

Letter sounds are introduced slowly in Reading Mastery I, about one every three to four lessons. Reading begins when six sounds have been learned. Each new sound to be taught is presented in a word; this word is used throughout the remainder of the program as a mnemonic device to cue the letter sound.

When new words are introduced, children are instructed first to sound out each word and then say it fast. Irregular words—for example, *is, was*—also are taught in this way initially, with the teacher providing the correct pronunciation. It is felt that treating irregular words in this manner, rather than teaching them as "sight" words, emphasizes their stable spellings. All words learned become part of the students' reading vocabulary, and are incorporated first in simple sentences and later in stories.

A modified orthography is used in the early stages of the DISTAR reading program and phased out by the middle of Reading Mastery II. The modification is meant to compensate for the unbalanced ratio of sounds to symbols in the English language, and to increase the number of words that can be read as "regular" words, as

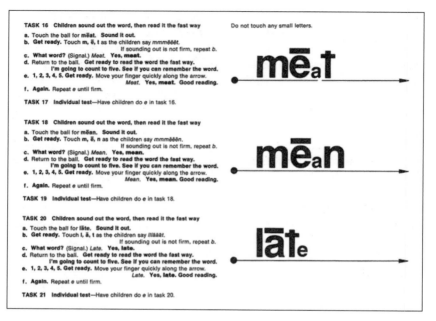

"Teacher's Lesson Script from Reading Mastery I"

well as to highlight differences between visually similar letters. The major features of this orthography include printing silent letters (e.g., *e* in *made*, *i* in *maid*) smaller, placing a heavy macron over letters representing long vowel sounds, printing consonant blends as joined letters, slightly changing the configuration of *d* to distinguish it from *b*, and omitting upper case formations except for *I*.

Comprehension activities at the prereading level include interpreting pictures and ordering events in sequence. At the reading level, comprehension skills are taught first in simple sentences and then in stories. In the early stages, children are asked to predict something about the content of pictures by first reading words related to the picture but presented on a preceding page. Once children are reading stories, oral comprehension questions, such as *wh-* questions, are posed during the reading. In addition, the teacher summarizes the story and asks students to predict what will happen next.

In later stages, children answer written questions about the story. For explicit questions, the group is called upon to respond in unison, but for questions asking for divergent responses such as giving opinions, individual response is requested. When students are able to read stories "the fast way" on first reading, each student's speed and accuracy are checked every fifth lesson. In addition, mastery tests are administered approximately every fifth lesson from the beginning of the program. Spelling instruction is optional in this program, though strongly encouraged. It is suggested that spelling be taught to the entire class if time does not allow small-group practice. The spelling curriculum follows the sequence of the reading curriculum. Spelling activities begin with children writing letters for dictated letter sounds and move on to their writing words and sentences. The Spelling Mastery program begins in second grade and continues through sixth grade level. It starts with teaching basic phonemic spelling strategies and memorization of high-frequency irregular spelling, and later teaches morphographs (word parts that have meaning such as the ending *-tion*) and spelling rules.

Handwriting instruction is included in the reading curriculum and begins in Lesson 7 when children first are asked to write letter sounds (letter names are not yet introduced). Students are taught manuscript letter formations through tracing exercises with faded prompts (the amount of the model letters shown is gradually diminished). Minimal emphasis is placed on handwriting or on written expression in the DISTAR curriculum.

The recommended time for reading lessons is 25 to 30 minutes of group instruction, followed by 15 to 20 minutes of independent work, five minutes of work check for each group and 10 minutes of group spelling practice. Students are given take-home assignments from the first day of the program. Scheduling for DISTAR may vary among schools. In one inner-city school, for example, approximately 60 percent of the school day is allocated to DISTAR reading, math, and language in the first three grades, with one hour per subject area (Meyer, Gersten, and Gutkin 1983).

TEACHER TRAINING

According to Becker (1977), a one-week preservice workshop, followed by one or two hours of inservice training a week is usually adequate for teachers to learn DISTAR. Manuals are provided for trainers, just as scripts are provided for teachers. The training procedure involves demonstration, guided practice, and feedback. In the case of the schools that participated in Project Follow-Through, a project manager (university staff member) trained teachers individually or in groups (Meyer, Gersten, and Gutkin 1983). After initial training, skilled teachers often supervise apprentice teachers within the classroom (Becker 1977).

EVALUATION AND IMPLEMENTATION

Direct Instruction has a history of well-documented effectiveness. DISTAR gained prominence as the only one of the nine instructional models in Project Follow-Through to produce significant gains in basic skills as compared to a traditional instructional approach that was administered to a control group of economically disadvantaged children. Pre- and posttests on the Wide Range Achievement Test (WRAT) indicated that DISTAR students had moved, on average, from the 18th to the 84th percentile in reading (word decoding) on national norms, and from 8th to the 49th percentile in spelling (Becker 1977). DISTAR students did not show the same degree of advantage in reading comprehension on the Metropolitan Achievement Test (MAT), averaging 10 percentile points below the national average, but they still scored significantly higher than students in the other model programs in this area. In both spelling and language, DISTAR students met the national average on the MAT.

A later study, conducted as a follow-up of original DISTAR participants from one inner-city school in New York, looked at the progress of nine cohorts (classes) of those students who had completed three levels of the program (Meyer, Gersten, and Gutkin 1983). The researchers found that DISTAR students continued to score at or above grade level on standardized reading tests in Grades 4 and 5, and that they scored notably above a comparison group of disadvantaged students from the same school district who had not received DISTAR instruction.

Tracing the progress of these same students into high school, Linda Meyer (1984) found that their advantage over the comparison group in reading persisted into ninth grade. Even more impressive was the finding that 34 percent of the DISTAR students had applied and been accepted to college, whereas only 18 percent of the non-DISTAR comparison students applied and 17 percent of these students were accepted. Furthermore, the dropout rate for DISTAR students was almost half that for comparison subjects.

Maureen Lovett has used an adaptation of DISTAR in a series of studies with children with reading disabilities. In one study, with children roughly 7 to 10 years old, she compared groups trained in the following two methods: (a) Direct Instruction for decodable words and whole word memorization of irregular words, and (b) whole word memorization of both decodable and irregular words. Following 35 hour-long training sessions over a nine-week period, both groups had made substantial progress in the specific words that were taught by both methods, but neither group was very strong in transferring these strategies to new words. Lovett suggested that these severely impaired readers might need additional training in phonological awareness to benefit from phonics instruction, or that they might need longer than nine weeks to learn to use the alphabetic strategy (Lovett et al. 1990).

In another study using an adaptation of DISTAR, Lovett compared reading outcomes across three experimental treatments. She

compared one group that was taught synthetic phonics using the DIS-
TAR approach to another group that was taught strategies involving
identifying letter units within words. This was based on a metacognitive analogy strategy designed for the Benchmark School (Gaskins et al.
1988; Gaskins, Downer, and Gaskins 1998). A third treatment group
received a combination of both of the above. All three treatments
proved to be effective, but the combination treatment was statistically
superior to either DISTAR or the metacognitive analogy strategy
alone. In other words, DISTAR is effective, and it is even more effective
in combination with metacognitive strategy training (Lovett et al. 2000).

The National Reading Panel Report includes several studies
comparing DISTAR to other word reading instructional approaches
(e.g., Gersten, Darch, and Gleason 1988) as well as studies by Maureen
Lovett and her colleagues utilizing her adaptation of the Direct
Instruction method (Lovett et al. 2000; Lovett and Steinbach 1997;
Lovett et al. 1990). Seven phonics programs were included in this
analysis. For each of the seven, the NRP analysis used at least three
studies in which phonics instruction was compared to another instructional approach. Analyses were carried out for two questions:

1. Were there significant effect sizes for each program in compari-
    son with its nonphonics controls?
2. Were any of the phonics programs more effective than any others?

The effect sizes for DISTAR were significant, as was the case for
the other six phonics programs studied. That is, children in DISTAR
programs made more progress than did children in other forms of
instruction. While each of these seven programs was more effective
than comparison programs, none of the phonics programs were significantly more effective than any of the others. Orton-Gillingham based
programs had smaller (but not significantly smaller) effect sizes than
DISTAR. As the National Reading Panel Report points out, this is
most likely because programs like DISTAR, which had higher effect
sizes, focused on children beginning this instruction in kindergarten or
first grade, whereas the Orton-Gillingham studies tended to involve
older elementary school children who were already failing in reading
(National Reading Panel 2000). Keep in mind that it was an overall
finding of the NRP that phonics is most effective in first grade.

Despite its success, DISTAR has its detractors. The American
Federation of Teachers, which chose Direct Instruction as one of its *Five
Promising Remedial Reading Intervention Programs* (1999), states that
DISTAR was criticized as being overly rigid and overly focused on the
basics. A common criticism is that the scripted lessons place too much
restriction on teachers. Becker (1977) counters this complaint with the
argument that scripts increase teacher accountability and help supervisors

track teacher and student progress. Elsa Bartlett (1979), who compared DISTAR with a past version of the Open Court basal program, found that DISTAR's modified orthography was particularly detrimental to disadvantaged children who find it difficult to make the transition to traditional orthography. Bartlett also maintained that DISTAR does not provide enough literacy enrichment. However, Isabel Beck and Ellen McCaslin (1978), in comparing eight reading programs on several dimensions, concluded that DISTAR is the best program for compensatory education.

The implementation of the DISTAR model as part of the federally funded Project Follow-Through may be unique. It entailed several elements worth noting for school change policy making. Another important implementation feature, after the provision of funds, was the sponsorship of each Follow-Through program by the program developer and the assignment of a project manger to train the teachers and install each program. According to Linda Meyer, Russell Gersten, and Joan Gutkin (1983) who studied the implementation of DISTAR at P. S. 137 in New York City, the project manager spent up to 40 days a year at the school, conducting inservice training and acting as coordinator between students, parents, faculty, and administration. The project manager was actively involved in setting up classroom schedules, monitoring teacher and student performance, and assigning students and staff. It would be helpful to know if having an external change agent serve as principal administrator rather than a local school official is relevant to the program's success.

Strong parental involvement and support were an extremely important factor in the P. S. 137 program (Meyer, Gersten, and Gutkin 1983). In fact, parents were largely responsible for the school's selection as a Follow-Through site, as well as for the choice of the Direct Instruction Model. Despite budget cuts and high teacher turnover, parents in this school apparently fought successfully to keep the DISTAR program in place for more than 13 years.

Meyer, Gersten, and Gutkin (1983) assert that one of the major strengths of the DISTAR model that has promoted its longevity is the continuity and consistency from preservice to inservice training sessions to continuous classroom observation and demonstration. They cite the Rand Study (Berman and McLaughlin 1975) finding that hands-on technical assistance to teachers is crucial for bringing about educational change.

18

Direct Instruction: Corrective Reading

BACKGROUND AND RATIONAL

Corrective Reading (Englemann et al. 1980) is an extension of Wesley Becker and Siegfried Englemann's Direct Instruction Model developed for fourth through 12th grade students who have failed to achieve in other reading programs. Corrective Reading instruction is intended to compensate for a wide range of constitutional and environmental deficiencies that contribute to reading failure; these include mild mental retardation, neurological impairment, emotional disturbance, socioeconomic deprivation, and language and cultural differences, as well as dyslexia or learning disabilities. Like DISTAR, the program is designed for group administration, and is intended as a core rather than a supplementary reading program; it has been used in both special and regular education settings.

CURRICULUM AND INSTRUCTION

Direct Instruction's Corrective Reading curriculum is divided into two strands, Decoding and Comprehension, each having three levels of skill development (Levels A, B, and C). Lessons are carefully arranged in a sequence so that the skills taught are cumulative. Students are given a test covering both decoding and comprehension to determine their placement in the program. Special lessons at each curriculum level serve as entry points. Students may be placed in one or both of the curriculum strands; if in both, they must be in the same or a lower comprehension than decoding level because the sequence of reading vocabulary in the comprehension strand corresponds to that in the decoding program.

The objective of the decoding program according to the Series Guide (Englemann et al. 1980) is "to teach the skills required to accurately and fluently identify and pronounce words that appear in written passages." It should be pointed out, however, that the decoding strand also deals with reading comprehension; students are asked comprehension questions about passages they read orally.

Placement level in the decoding strand is determined by a student's speed and accuracy in reading a passage orally. Students not meeting baseline criteria are referred for DISTAR I instruction. Students with only minimal reading skills are placed in Level A: Word Attack Basics, which contains 60 lessons. The major instructional goal at this level is to teach the idea that most words are regularly spelled and can be read by blending the letter sounds. Individual letter sounds are taught, first in isolation and then in words. Words are read first in isolation and then in unrelated sentences to avoid predictable context and discourage guessing, the latter strategy being the one most of these students have relied on unsuccessfully to compensate for their lack of letter-sound knowledge.

Only the most commonly used sound for each letter symbol is introduced at this level. This is the stated rationale for teaching the short sound for the vowel *a* and the long sound for the vowel *e* in Lesson 1. Not until Lesson 23 is the short *e* sound introduced; long *a* is not presented until Level B. The digraph *ee* is presented at the same time as the open syllable for long *e* (as in "me"). This practice represents the principle of instructional economy whereby strategies and rules are kept as simple as possible (Gersten, Woodward, and Darch 1986). For this reason, too, terms such as "vowels," "double consonants," or "final *e* words" are avoided. Practice in discriminating vowel sounds is provided by having students identify medial sounds in one-syllable words as in, "Which word has the middle sound /aaaa/: *bean, ban, ben?*"

As in DISTAR, pronunciation of letters and words is practiced by first sounding them out slowly and then saying them fast. When irregular words are first introduced in Lesson 46, the distinction is made between how they are spelled and how they are said. Students first sound out the words, pronouncing and blending the individual letter sounds, for example "wwwaaasss" for *was*. Then the teacher gives the correct pronunciation (i.e., "wuz").

According to the program's authors, 60 to 80 percent of Corrective Reading students enter at Level B: Decoding Strategies, which comprises 140 lessons. The focus of the curriculum at this level is on long and short vowels, vowel-consonant digraphs, vowel digraphs, diphthongs, and common word endings. Long-short vowel confusion errors are referred to as "same vowel mistakes," and teachers are given specific instructions for correcting these errors. Students are asked to note the presence or absence of a final *e* in the word missed that indicates the pronunciation of the preceding vowel. After pronouncing the word correctly, the students repeat the word. The teacher then writes the word as the students mistakenly pronounced it and has them read it. She changes it back to its correct spelling and asks the students to read it again. This model-test-discriminate-retest approach is used as a correcting procedure throughout the program. For correcting vowel confusion errors in words with endings (e.g, "robe" for "robber"), the teacher underlines the word from the beginning to the second letter after the vowel (robber), and students are told, "If the last letter of the underlined part is *e* or *i*, you hear a letter name in the word" (Englemann et al. 1978). Phonics rules are not taught as spelling rules in Corrective Reading as they are in most remedial approaches. Although Level A includes spelling dictation exercises, the Corrective Reading curriculum includes little direct spelling instruction. Two types of word reading exercises are provided at Level B: similar list presentation, which emphasizes orthographic differences between words that share features (e.g., *hat, hate, hated*) and random list presentation of unrelated words which requires remembering specific features of words.

In addition to word attack exercises, Level B involves group story reading which uses a round-robin format, each student reading a sentence or two. Stories contain words introduced in the lessons. Oral reading errors are corrected on the spot, and the student is asked to reread the sentence. The teacher asks comprehension questions during the story reading, calling on individual students to answer. The questions not only ensure that all students are following the text, but also provide a story grammar framework for comprehending its contents. For example, Who is the story about? What does he or she want to do? What happens when he or she tries to do it? What happens in the end? According to Russell Gersten, John Woodward, and Craig Darch (1986), who are strong proponents of Corrective Reading, students begin to "internalize these four questions and generalize this framework to other narrative material." From Lesson 81 on, students are asked to write answers to additional comprehension questions after the story has been read.

Oral reading checks are conducted at the end of each lesson in Level B. Students read aloud individually the same 100-word passage from the story read in that lesson, as well as a second 100-word passage from the previous lesson. Selected peers may act as checkers, according to the program's authors, but most studies of Corrective Reading application report the use of teacher aides for this purpose. Every fifth lesson requires a timed reading check so that a record of speed as well as accuracy can be kept for each student.

Level C: Skills Applications comprises 140 lessons. This top level of the decoding strand continues instruction in word attack skills, reviewing previously introduced digraphs, diphthongs, less common phonemes and syllables, and teaching new ones. It introduces some of the more common affixes. Exercises for teaching these elements follow the formats used in the lower curriculum levels.

Preparing students to read textbook material is a major objective of the Level C Decoding curriculum. Toward this end, more than 600 new vocabulary words are introduced, defined, and presented in text. The basis for selecting these words, however, is not explained; the selections seem to vary widely in frequency rating (e.g., *prevented* as compared to *prestidigitator*). An effort is made to expose students to "sentence types and conventions that characterize text material" (Englemann et al. 1980) such as the passive voice. Group story reading at this level requires answering both literal and inferential comprehension questions in writing. In addition, students read nonfiction information passages during individual oral reading checks. After Lesson 70, they also read magazine and newspaper articles together on topics of their choice.

The program's authors maintain that students who complete Level C are "fluent decoders who make only occasional decoding errors when reading materials that contain a fairly broad vocabulary and a variety of sentence types" (Englemann et al. 1980). The authors believe that although students may still have comprehension deficits, which limit their overall reading ability, their decoding problems at this point are essentially remediated.

Although reading is involved, Corrective Reading's comprehension strand is devoted primarily to the development of cognitive skills and language skills that relate to academic work. Level A, called Thinking Basics, is geared to students who lack essential concepts underlying school curriculum content, who may have a limited store of background information for processing school material, and may also manifest difficulty repeating orally presented information.

Each lesson has three segments. The first, *Thinking Operations*, teaches the following concepts, which are relevant to content area material: analogies and/or basic evidence, classification, deductions, definitions, description, inductions, opposites, same, statement inference, and true-false. These are taught directly by the teacher to the group through example and repetition. In the second lesson segment, students apply these concepts in workbook exercises. In the third, the *Information Track*, they are taught calendar facts (months, seasons, holidays) and biology facts (animals and their classifications); additionally, they learn to recite short poems.

While somewhat more advanced than Level A students, those entering Level B: Comprehension Skills may still lack basic information such as calendar facts. The major thrust at this level is "to teach and reinforce a substantial amount of information and many operations" (Englemann et al. 1980). Areas covered in this curriculum include Reasoning Skills (deductions, basic evidence, analogies, contradictions, and similes), Information Skills (classification, body systems, body rules, and economic rules), Vocabulary Skills (definition), Sentence Skills (parts of speech, subject/predicate, sentence combinations, and sentence analysis), Comprehension Skills (inference and following directions), and Writing Skills (writing directions, editing, writing paragraphs, and writing stories). Each lesson involves group oral work, oral workbook exercises, and independent workbook exercises. Students check each other's answers to these exercises.

At Level C: Concept Applications, the instructional emphasis is on teaching students to apply independently the skills they have learned. Five categories of application skills are taught in this curriculum:

1. *Organizing Information* (main idea, outlining, specific-general, morals, and visual–spatial information).
2. *Operating on Information* (deductions, basic evidence, argument rules, ought statements, and contradictions).
3. *Using Sources of Information* (basic comprehension passages, words or deductions, maps, pictures and graphs, and supporting evidence).
4. *Communicating Information* (definitions, combining sentences, editing, and getting meaning from context).
5. *Using Information* (writing directions, filling out forms, and identifying contradictory directions).

The first two operational categories are classified as "higher-order skills" and the last three as "basic tools." A major change in instructional procedure tasks place at Level C. Rather than the teacher presenting scripted lessons, students read the lesson scripts in their workbooks. The teacher monitors their processing of the workbook exercises, asking questions to ensure understanding. Increasing demands are placed on writing performances at this level.

All Corrective Reading lessons are designed to be administered daily in 35- to 40-minute periods, although several effectiveness studies report the benefit of somewhat longer periods and often more than one period per day. A lesson is designed to be covered within a single period but may be repeated if mastery is not attained by all students in the class. Individual mastery checks, as well as the monitoring of group responses, provide ongoing information on student performance and allow for repetition or acceleration of lessons if needed.

A point system serves as a behavior management device at all curriculum levels. Students are awarded points for successful performance in both group and individual activities throughout the Corrective Reading curriculum; a point schedule is provided for each lesson. In group activities, all students must meet performance criteria in order for any points to be awarded. Bonus points may be given for success or persistence on especially difficult activities or to encourage positive behaviors such as being on time for lessons. Students keep records of points earned. Weekly summaries of accumulated points are intended to provide positive feedback to further reinforce student learning.

Behavior management also entails having each student who enters the program sign a contract indicating his or her willingness to cooperate and work hard. The teacher explains the point system, the need for daily class attendance, and the penalty for making negative comments about peers. The penalty for making fun of another student is paid by the group as a whole to further discourage this detrimental behavior.

As in DISTAR, the hallmark of Corrective Reading is its unique approach to direct group instruction. All lessons are scripted; teachers are told exactly what to say and do. All student exercises are presented in repeated formats; similar activities follow the same formats, which simplifies the teacher's task and serves as a prompt for students to apply a learned skill to new examples. Correction procedures, both general and specific, are carefully spelled out for all activities. Hand signals are used by teachers to direct student response in unison. These allow for fast paced instruction, which is believed to help sustain student attention, increase student achievement, and reduce auditory memory demands on students. The signals include the hand-drop, which indicates that students should respond in unison in naming items pointed to on the chalkboard or in their workbooks; the audible signal (clapping, finger snapping, foot tapping) to redirect student attention; the sound-out signal (the teacher runs her finger along a line under the letter or word to be pronounced), which controls the pace of blending letter sounds; and the sequential-response signal (the teacher holds up one finger to call for a first response and then two fingers to signal a second response), as when students are asked to name two important facts in a story.

The materials used in Corrective Reading Instruction include the Series Guide, which provides an overview of the entire program; a teacher's manual for each level of a curriculum strand, which provides a curriculum guide for that level and the presentation scripts for each lesson; a student workbook, which contains stories to be read and/or exercises to be carried out; and, at Level C, a student textbook that contains the lesson scripts to be read by the students themselves.

TEACHER TRAINING

Teacher preparation for Corrective Reading has not been formalized as in some other remedial programs, and may vary with schools and school districts, depending on their requirements and their budgets. However, training can be arranged through The Association for Direct Instruction (see Resource and Teacher Training Guide in Appendix). On the east coast, it is provided by the Center for Direct Instruction, which is based in New York City. This training is usually conducted in one, six-hour session, most often in a school, though sometimes in university-sponsored workshops offering graduate credit. Follow-up, on-site supervision in classrooms or further consultation to schools is available for an additional fee.

Reporting on the implementation of Corrective Reading with learning disabled and mildly retarded adolescents in a rural/suburban school district, Edward Polloway and Michael Epstein (1986) indicate that teacher preparation involved two full days of in-service training. The first session provided an overview of the program and the instructional methodology, as well as information about placement testing, grouping, and scheduling. The second session focused specifically on teaching techniques. However, even with two training sessions, considerable variability in teacher competence was noted during program implementation.

Epstein and Cullinan (1981) employed teacher aides in their implementation of Corrective Reading. The aides were trained directly in the classroom and received weekly follow-up supervision alongside the classroom teachers. Cynthia Herr (1984) has found teacher aides to be extremely useful for monitoring oral reading checks and supervising work with adult students in Corrective Reading.

EVALUATION AND IMPLEMENTATION

Studies have investigated the use of Corrective Reading with students having a range of mild handicapping conditions, as well as with students for whom English is a second language (Polloway and Epstein 1986). Several of these adults have examined the program's effectiveness with students classified as learning disabled. Polloway and Epstein (1986), for example, measured the effectiveness of Corrective Reading with a mixed group of educable mentally retarded (EMR) and learning disabled (LD) sixth through 12th grade students by comparing reading gains achieved over a year of Corrective Reading instruction to gains made in the previous year of special education instruction. Using the Peabody Individual Achievement Test (PIAT), they found significantly greater gains after Corrective Reading instruction than in the previous year for EMR as well as LD subjects in both word recognition and reading comprehension. Although the LD subjects had greater gains that the EMR subjects on word recognition scores, no significant differences were found in reading comprehension gain scores between the two subject types. However, Polloway and Epstein suggest that the latter finding may be due to the failure of the PIAT to tap the comprehension skills taught in Corrective Reading. In support of this suggestion, they cite teachers' claims that the PIAT underestimates student achievement in this area.

Epstein and Cullinan (1981) investigated the effects of a federally funded model implementation of Corrective Reading with nine-year-old students classified as learning disabled. (It is worth noting that their Slosson IQ scores ranged only from 76 to 86.) Subjects were randomly assigned to self-contained classrooms, two of which used Corrective Reading. The other classroom used unspecified remedial procedures and served as the control condition. At the end of one school year, reading scores (posttest only) were higher for both groups receiving Corrective Reading than the comparison group. However, John Lloyd, along with Epstein and Cullinan, in reporting on the same study, acknowledge that neither of the experimental groups reached normal reading achievement levels in that year and suggest that more instructional time is needed to reach such a goal (Lloyd, Epstein, and Cullinan 1981). It should also be mentioned that the number of subjects in each group was low (seven to eight), as was the case in the Polloway and Epstein study (four to eight). Though optimal for instructional purposes, such small samples weaken the validity of the outcome analyses.

In terms of program implementation, Epstein and Cullinan (1981) maintain that although the planning, training, and evaluation costs of Corrective Reading are considerably higher than the cost of most basal reading programs, the expense is on a par with that of other learning disability programs. A greater challenge, but one worth meeting they believe, is convincing school personnel of the need for carefully supervised, highly structured, task-oriented, direct instruction with learning disabled children.

19

Recipe for Reading

BACKGROUND AND RATIONALE

Recipe for Reading, with a new, fourth edition published in 2000, is an adaptation of the Orton-Gillingham approach (Gillingham and Stillman 1960) and, like other Orton-Gillingham programs, is designed for one-to-one tutorial use. Its simple design and clear explanations make it an appropriate and useful resource for classroom teachers as well. It was developed in the 1950s by Nina Traub and first used in Ossining, New York, with parents serving as tutors for learning-disabled children in the community. Because of its success, funding was obtained in the early 1970s to place the program in five Ossining elementary schools (Traub 1982). Traub's co-author, Frances Bloom has taken responsibility for the program since Traub's death, and Connie Russo takes responsibility for teacher training.

The Traub method applies a synthetic phonics approach, teaching individual letter sounds in isolation before introducing syllables or words. All teaching follows a part-to-whole progression. Although the term *multisensory* does not appear in the manual, the use of visual, auditory, and kinesthetic reinforcement techniques is encouraged throughout the program. Traub developed a sequence for introducing letter sounds based on their visual, auditory, and kinesthetic characteristics.

CURRICULUM AND INSTRUCTION

The Traub method is designed for first through third grade students to be delivered on a one-to-one basis outside the classroom in half-hour sessions five days a week. In developing Recipe for Reading, Traub simplified the Orton-Gillingham curriculum. The revised teacher's manual (Traub and Bloom 2000) is clearly written, easy to follow, and relatively short. An early chapter discusses the rationale for multisensory instruction and describes the structure of its lessons. This section is followed by a page that is devoted to each letter-sound and that includes hints for teaching the patterns as well as sample words to use in instruction.

A curriculum sequence chart is printed on the inside cover. Instruction begins by introducing seven consonants (hard *c* and *g*, *d*, *m*, *l*, *h*, and *f*) and two vowels (*a* and *o*). Explaining the rationale for her selection of these letters, Traub stated in the manual that some letters are learned and written more easily than others. As examples, she maintained that *c*, *o*, *a*, and *d* have the same basic kinesthetic formations (circle to the left), hard *c* and *g* "seem to be among the easiest sounds perceived by the ear," and *d* and *m* are two of the first sounds made by infants (i.e., "da-da," "ma-ma"). The letters *d* and *b* "are introduced at a considerable distance from each other because they are the pair that are most commonly reversed and confused."

Each letter to be learned is first presented on a large piece of oak tag, written in one-inch thick strokes. The teacher gives the letter sound and then writes the letter. The child traces the letter and then writes it independently. When the child has done this successfully, the teacher says the letter name.

Both manuscript and cursive letter formations are taught in the Traub method. Special lined paper is provided to designate orientation points in letter formation. Each writing line is divided into four parallel lines. Letters with no stems should fill the space between the two middle lines, called "the little red house." Upward letter stems should touch the top line ("the attic") and downward stems should touch the bottom line ("the basement"). Directional cues for letter formations are provided at the top of each page, a bat and a ball for letters such as *b* that turn to the right, and a drum and drumstick for those turning to the left. Many multisensory techniques are suggested for the student who has difficulty with letter formations. For example, several activities involve (a) walking on a letter formed with masking tape on the floor, (b) forming a letter with rolls of clay and then tracing it with the eyes open and eyes shut, and (c) writing in the air ("sky writing").

Spelling precedes reading in the Traub approach. After the student has learned the sound and name for each of the first nine letters and is able to write each of these letters, the student is taught to spell c-v-c words with these letters. The teacher dictates words without the student's having seen the words in print. The student repeats the word, spells it aloud, and then writes it while spelling it aloud (simultaneous oral

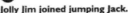

Jolly Jim joined jumping Jack.

Visual – Auditory

The day before this lesson tell the class that tomorrow they are going to learn a new letter with the help of some jam. They are asked to take a vote on the flavor that they wish to have. The next day bring the jam, spread it on a paper plate and have the students trace the letter j with their finger in the jam. They can feel the jam on their hands and are asked to talk about it. The sound becomes j-j-juicy j-j-jam.

Kinesthetic

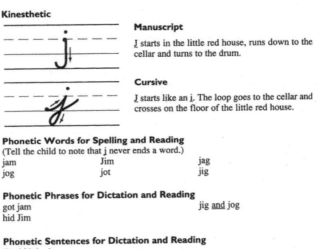

Manuscript

J starts in the little red house, runs down to the cellar and turns to the drum.

Cursive

J starts like an i. The loop goes to the cellar and crosses on the floor of the little red house.

Phonetic Words for Spelling and Reading
(Tell the child to note that j never ends a word.)

jam	Jim	jag
jog	jot	jig

Phonetic Phrases for Dictation and Reading

got jam   jig and jog
hid Jim

Phonetic Sentences for Dictation and Reading

Jim hid the jam.
Did Tim jig and jog?
Mom had a lot of jam.

Phonetic Reader
Alphabet Series I, #3.

Lesson from Recipe for Reading *by Nina Traub with Frances Bloom. (Reproduced with permission from Educators Publishing Service, 625 Mt. Auburn Street, Cambridge, MA. (800)225-5750, www.epsbooks.com Copyright 2000.)*

spelling). If the student has difficulty, he or she is asked to listen for the first sound and give its letter name as the teacher says the word, separating each phoneme. This procedure is repeated with the middle vowel and final consonant. The manual tells the teacher to dictate more naturally "as the child's auditory discrimination improves" (Traub and Bloom 2000).

After the student spells the words, he is asked to read them as printed on "phonetic word cards" (flash cards) rather than in his own writing. If the student has trouble reading a word, the teacher places cards representing each letter ("phonetic sound cards") under the word and has the student say each letter sound. Traub suggested many blending techniques, but like Gillingham and Stillman (1960), she emphasized first blending the initial consonant and following vowel, for example, ba-t, rather than the vowel and final consonant, as in the phonic-linguistic approach (e.g., b-at), which she claimed encourages the wrong directionality.

Once the student can spell several words, the teacher dictates phrases or short sentences for the student to write, and provides the spelling for any nonphonetic word. After writing sentences, the student reads these sentences from "phonetic sentence cards" and when ready, graduates to reading "phonetic storybooks" following the same procedures. In addition to these storybooks, Traub provided a list of phonetic readers from other publishers for supplementary reading. She suggested that teachers alternate oral reading with students to model fluency and expression, and that they discuss the passage. Recognizing the low interest level of most phonetic readers, Traub recommended reading other materials aloud to the student to develop comprehension skills. She suggested asking the student to listen for the answer to a particular question as the text is read.

Having the student dictate his or her own stories is another suggested activity in Recipe for Reading. The teacher types the story, which is then made into a book for the child and others to read, much like the language experience approach. Traub maintained that this activity improves verbal expression and helps build a sight vocabulary. She also recommended using Dolch flash cards[15] (1952) for building sight vocabulary development.

Briefly, the Traub curriculum moves from one-syllable words to two-syllable compound words (e.g., *pigpen*) to two-syllable phonetically regular words (e.g., *dislike*). In the last instance, the student first reads the individual syllables on cards and then puts them together to make words. All letter sounds or groups of letter sounds are introduced one by one: initial consonant blends, three-letter word endings (e.g. *ing, ank*), long vowel words with "magic *e*", vowel digraphs, vowel-consonant combinations, diphthongs, nonphonetic word parts such as *igh*, and common suffix rules such as when to double final consonants before adding vowel suffixes. A special section on affixes and word roots is provided for older students.

Daily lessons begin with a drill on previously learned letter sounds. Then new material is presented and taught as previously described. Depending on the student's ability level, word reading, sentence reading, and story book reading follow in order. Lastly, phonetic word games are played to reinforce learning.

---

[15]The Dolch Basic Sight Vocabulary Cards (Dolch 1952) contain 220 of the words most frequently encountered by beginning readers.

Each student's work is dated and retained in a folder, and his progress is carefully recorded. A count is kept of all words learned. Traub emphasized the importance of making students aware of their progress. For younger children, particularly, she recommended ending lessons with an activity at which they are sure to succeed and acknowledging their success with some sign of approval. By way of additional encouragement, a list of all the books a student has read is included in his folder.

In addition to the teacher's manual, there are Recipe for Reading workbooks, writing paper, sequence pads for keeping records for individual children, and a series of 21 storybooks called the *Alphabet Series* and coordinated with the Recipe for Reading sequence. Clear directions are provided for making materials such as the word and sound cards used in the program. Connie Russo has written a pretest for establishing instructional levels in the new edition.

TEACHER TRAINING

All training for Recipe for Reading teachers or tutors was conducted by Mrs. Traub, the program's author, until her death. Since then, her colleague, Connie Russo, has carried on the program and conducted the teacher training. The following description of the teacher training program was provided by Russo via telephone.

Training is usually done within a public school in daily, five-hour sessions over a two-week period. It is best arranged during the summer when children are attending classes for remedial instruction. The first two hours are devoted to lecture. In the next two hours, each teacher trainee applies the knowledge acquired from the lecture by tutoring two public school students for one hour each under supervision. The last hour involves a sharing and pulling together of all that has been learned that day among the 15 or so teacher trainees.

When training is conducted during the school year, it is usually condensed into six hours of lecture without the tutoring practicum because of problems with classroom pull-out time. However, supervised tutoring experience is arranged individually for each teacher trainee during the year.

EVALUATION AND IMPLEMENTATION

A federally funded validation study, reported by Traub (1982), was carried out in 1976 by the MAGI Educational Service on the initial school implementation of Recipe for Reading in five Ossining, New York, elementary schools. Results of this study indicated that second grade Ossining students who were tutored with Recipe for Reading made significantly greater improvement in reading and spelling, as measured by posttest, than a control group of second grade students from another district tutored using a different remedial method that was not described. Unfortunately, since the tests administered yield only total reading grade equivalents, it is not possible to ascertain which subskills (decoding, vocabulary, or comprehension) are most influenced by the Traub method.

As a result of this validation study, Ossining received a federal IV-C grant to continue and expand the use of Recipe for Reading. Traub (1982) states that subsequent to the program's implementation in Ossining, 26 different school districts had received similar grants to replicate the Ossining program and that she had trained the staff in these schools. She reports positive effects of Recipe for Reading as measured by year to year comparison studies on student achievement conducted in several of these districts. One district cited the program's cost effectiveness, maintaining that personnel was the highest expense and that expense for materials was low. Another district cited enhanced motivation and improved attitude toward reading among students receiving Recipe for Reading instruction.

Recipe for Reading is most often used in self-contained special education classrooms and in resource rooms, or for early intervention with children who are at risk. Though designed for one-to-one instruction, Russo maintains that the method is ideal for groups of as many as five students. Recipe for Reading is also used for whole class and small group lessons in regular education settings. Classroom teachers who like to design their own materials rather than using a basal reading series seem to find Recipe for Reading more valuable than other phonics programs because the structure and sequence are clear but not lockstep or scripted. The program is both linguistically sound and highly creative (e.g., practicing writing *j* in jam and *p* in peanut butter). Cisqua-Rippowam, an independent school for high-achieving children in Bedford, New York, uses Recipe for Reading as a beginning reading program with all students.

20

Alphabetic Phonics

BACKGROUND AND RATIONALE

Alphabetic Phonics is an "organization and expansion" (Cox 1985) of the Orton-Gillingham multisensory approach for teaching children with dyslexia from elementary school through high school. The program was started in the mid 1960s at Texas Scottish Rite Hospital for Children in Dallas as a collaboration between Sally Childs (a colleague of Anna Gillingham), Lucius Waites (a pediatric neurologist who established the Child Development Division at the hospital), and Aylett Royall Cox (a teacher who organized and published the Alphabetic Phonics Curriculum together with the Dyslexia Laboratory staff). The program was developed and revised over a 10-year period during which over 1,000 dyslexic children came daily to Waites' clinic for remedial instruction. In order to meet the needs of the number of children referred, teaching at Scottish Rite was expanded at that point from tutorials to small group remediation.

The Alphabetic Phonics curriculum (Cox 1992) is built upon Samuel Orton's theories, and uses multisensory activities to build linkages between the visual, auditory, and kinesthetic senses. It is an assumption of this curriculum that the majority (80 percent) of the 30,000 most commonly used English words can be considered phonetically regular and, therefore, predictable, once rules have been learned. The term "alphabetic phonics" refers to "a structured system of teaching students the coding patterns of the English language" (Cox 1985). To this theoretical framework, the program has added a discovery approach to learning. Hierarchically sequenced rules for letter sounds are discovered, articulated, practiced toward mastery, and used to build words through a synthetic approach to reading.

CURRICULUM AND INSTRUCTION

The Alphabetic Phonics curriculum is described in a guide for teachers, *Foundations for Literacy: Structures and Techniques for Multisensory Teaching of Basic Written English Language Skills* (Cox 1992), a revision of the earlier guide, which was titled *Structures and Techniques*. In addition, there are two companion guides, *Situation Reading* (Cox 1989) and *Situation Spelling* (Cox 1977), student workbooks, drill cards, and wall cards, all available from Educators Publishing Service.

Progress is documented through use of what Cox calls "Benchmark Measures," or post-instruction measures coordinated with the "schedules" or steps in the sequenced program. These curriculum-based instruments are designed to measure letter knowledge, alphabetizing skills, reading, spelling, and handwriting.

The curriculum is extremely comprehensive in that it covers many aspects of language acquisition including listening skills, and extends from basic skills such as letter recognition to sophisticated levels of linguistic knowledge such as coding polysyllabic words after breaking them into syllables. Students are taught an extensive vocabulary to use in their language learning (e.g., "The word *fight* is a one-syllable base word with the trigraph *igh* in medial position"). Judith Birsh, an Alphabetic Phonics teacher trainer, refers to this terminology as a "meta-language," a language for talking about language (Birsh 1988).

As its name implies, Alphabetic Phonics stresses the unique characteristics of written English, most particularly phonology and letter sequence. The term "situation learning" is applied to both reading and spelling, and refers to the fact that the sound of a letter may vary, depending on the situation. For instance, "one-one-one" words have one syllable and one short vowel followed by one consonant. A striking feature of the program is the time spent teaching students how to code words using diacritical marks as used in *Webster's 2nd edition* for the 68 graphemes that represent 44 sounds in 98 different situations. For example, the digraph *ck* is underlined to indicate that the two letters make a single sound, and the *c* is diagonally slashed to indicate that it is silent. The demands placed on the student are substantial.

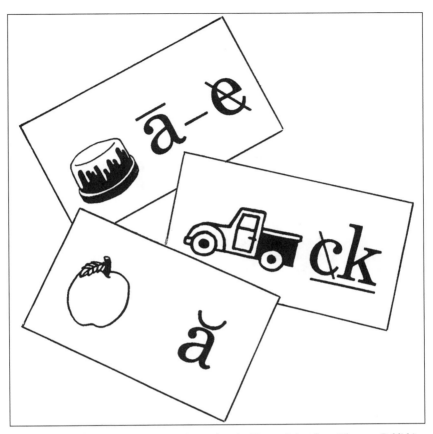

Initial Reading Deck by Aylett R. Cox. (Reproduced with permission from Educators Publishing Service Cambridge, MA. (800) 225-5750, www.epsbooks.com. Copyright 1971.)

The structured daily lesson takes an hour to complete with 11 activities typically lasting three to 10 minutes each. The standard activities with suggested times are outlined below. Each is followed by examples from observations of demonstration lessons by master teachers working with one, two, and three children during training sessions at Teachers College, Columbia University.

1. *Language* (5 minutes). This activity is intended as an orientation to the English language. One teacher showed children a globe and gave a brief lesson on the spread of the alphabet around the shores of the Mediterranean by the Phoenicians.

2. *Alphabet* (5 minutes). This activity emphasizes sequence and directionality, and leads to alphabetizing and dictionary use. During the observed session, two students touched the letters *A* and *Z* on an alphabet strip as they recited "My left hand is my

before hand. My right hand is my *after* hand. *A* is the initial letter of the alphabet. *Z* is the final letter of the alphabet. All the letters between *A* and *Z* are the medial letters." Then they used the left index finger to point at and read each letter *A* to *M*, and with the right hand, finishing up *N* to *Z*.

3. *Reading Decks* (3 minutes). These drill cards (Initial and Advanced Decks) provide practice in responding automatically to letters for reading. A teacher was observed showing beginning students a few Initial Reading Deck cards that had been introduced in prior lessons. Students responded with the name of the letter, the name of the object (key word), and the phoneme or letter sound.

4. *Spelling Decks* (3 minutes). During the observed session, the teacher said the above mentioned phonemes aloud, one at a time, and the students echoed the sounds and then said the letter names. A set of teacher hand signals was used to prompt the student to listen, echo the phoneme, say the letter name, and finally, write the letter. This is a particularly effective technique; trained teachers mentioned spontaneously using the hand signals in other teaching situations as prompts.

5. *New Learning* (5 minutes). In this observation, two students had been taught short *i* in a prior lesson, and were introduced here to the sound of short *a* through the use of a discovery activity. They watched their mouths in a mirror as they said the sound. The teacher asked whether their mouths were open or closed, and whether they could feel vibrations in their throats. One student spontaneously offered, "It's open and voiced so it's a vowel." They practiced coding a written *a* using the term *breve* for the coding mark and were shown a flash card from the Initial Reading Deck with a picture of an apple and an *a* with a breve over it.

6. *Reading Practice* (5 to 10 minutes). Only phonetically controlled text is used in the program, and in the lessons observed there was no use of books at all. The children who were observed in the introductory course had had roughly 10 lessons. They read "instant words" (sight words) on flash cards (e.g., *they, could, people, no*) and they used a left-to-right, letter-by-letter blending strategy to sound out words constructed from letters they had studied. In the advanced training class, an eight-year-old boy, who had been tutored in Alphabetic Phonics for nine months, was given sentences to code prior to reading, but he was not considered ready to read stories yet.

7. *Handwriting Practice* (5 minutes). Cursive writing is taught from the beginning to reinforce left-to-right directionality. Four basic

strokes are taught (see Chapter 10). In one session that was observed, an introductory level student learned to say, "The name of the letter is 's.' Swing up. Stop. Curve out around. Come in to close. Stop and release," while drawing an *s* in the air (a technique called "skywriting"), on the board with chalk, and finally, on lined paper.

8. *Spelling Practice* (10 minutes). Spelling was practiced in the advanced class by asking an eight-year-old to spell two vowel sounds (short *a* and short *u*) using printed letters called "ice tray letters" after the tray used for their display and storage. After this preparation, he spelled *bag*, *bug*, *tag*, and *tug* using "Simultaneous Oral Spelling" (SOS). He listened, echoed the word, "unblended"[16] the word while looking in a mirror, spelled the letters aloud, and then pulled printed letters into place to spell the word. To check himself, he coded the word using a small piece of macaroni for the breve mark and then read the word aloud.

9. *Verbal Expression* (2 to 10 minutes). In a beginning level lesson, the teacher wrote out a sentence and read it aloud, and then used parts-of-speech cards (e.g., *noun*, *article*) from the Winston Grammar Program, asking the child to cover words with them. Parts of speech that had not yet been taught were covered with "mystery cards" or blank cards used as placeholders. These activities differ from teacher to teacher.

10. *Review* (5 minutes). In all sessions, index cards were prepared by the teacher with mnemonic clues for reviewing new learning at the end of a lesson.

11. *Listening or Reading Comprehension* (5 minutes). In an advanced training session, the teacher read four Shel Silverstein food poems aloud and asked the student how the poems were all alike. Material is chosen on the student's intellectual level rather than reading level in order to develop comprehension skills.

Most of the materials either have been designed specifically for the program or are teacher made. Reading materials vary from site to site but are always phonetically controlled (e.g., *Let's Read*, Educators Publishing Service; *J and J Language Readers*, Sopris West; *MTA Readers*, Educators Publishing Service).

---

[16]The term *unblending* in Alphabetic Phonics refers to segmenting, or saying each phoneme in isolation.

TEACHER TRAINING

Training is based on the need to fill three gaps in teacher education: (a) knowledge of the structure and history of written English, (b) knowledge of the science of phonetic spelling, and (c) a carefully structured and hierarchically sequenced curriculum (Cox 1985). Presently, there are at least 14 Alphabetic Phonics teacher training centers in the United States, all listed in the Resource and Teacher Training Guide at the back of this book. This is over twice the number reported in the first edition of this book (Clark 1988). Many of these centers are directed by teacher trainers who originally trained under Aylett Cox or Connie Burkhalter in Texas.

Training for teachers of Alphabetic Phonics is extensive and demanding. It includes a minimum of 150 instructional hours followed by 700 hours of supervised practice with students. Teachers are required to attend a three- to four-week introductory summer course and a two-week advanced course the following summer. During the school year between these summer workshops, they are required to tutor children under supervision and to attend periodic seminars. Daily training sessions during the workshops last for seven hours and include lectures, demonstrations, and practice teaching. In addition, substantial readings and projects are assigned. Trainees become Alphabetic Phonics therapists once they have completed two years of training.

Several introductory and advanced level summer training sessions were observed at Teachers College, Columbia University. The 25 beginners and 12 advanced trainees were classroom and resource room teachers, tutors, and graduate students in special education. They met with master teachers early in the morning in small groups to talk about goals for the tutoring session they were about to view. Trainees then watched through a one-way mirror as a master teacher tutored a child or small group of children for an hour. By the second week of the introductory session, each trainee was assigned a small portion of the lesson. Feedback was provided immediately afterward by the master teacher and by the rest of the group, who then worked together to plan the next day's session. Over the course of training, more and more responsibility for planning and teaching the lesson was assigned to trainees. During the rest of the day, lectures and discussions focused on specific aspects of the program as well as on broader issues such as research. After the day's session, trainees were expected to read assignments and to prepare lessons to teach the next day.

EVALUATION AND IMPLEMENTATION

When this book was first published in 1988, Diana Clark reported that several evaluation studies of Alphabetic Phonics had been conducted during the 1980s (e.g., Brightman 1986; Frankiewicz 1984, 1985; Roy 1986). These four studies indicated gains in reading for children with dyslexia instructed in Alphabetic Phonics in either individual tutorials or small groups. None, however, used control groups, so it could not be claimed that training in Alphabetic Phonics was responsible for the gains.

Since 1988, there have been new studies, most designed, again, to measure gains in standard scores after training, but without the use of controls. For example, Hutcheson, Selig, and Young (1990) describe a collaboration between the Neuhaus Education Center and the Houston public schools in which 126 resource room teachers were trained in Alphabetic Phonics. Later, 252 elementary and secondary students described as learning disabled were tested before and after remediation in resource rooms, and were found to have made significant gains in reading and spelling.

ADAPTATIONS OF ALPHABETIC PHONICS

The *Multisensory Teaching Approach* (*MTA*) is an adaptation of Alphabetic Phonics intended for whole classroom use. It was designed by Margaret Smith and Edith Hogan, both former Alphabetic Phonics teacher trainers, for use in regular classrooms or as a remedial program for dyslexic children. Smith and Hogan have developed a series of kits that contain the essential instructional manuals and materials needed for teaching the program. The manuals provide more specific instruction for teachers than do the original Alphabetic Phonics manuals, and they include actual lesson scripts. The MTA kits are distributed by Educators Publishing Service. The kit is considered an excellent resource for any Alphabetic Phonics teacher. Training is offered by Edmar Educational Services in Dallas, Texas. MTA teachers take a two-week basic course, and academic language therapists take this course plus two years of practicum (four advanced workshops and six individual consultation/demonstrations), followed by an additional two weeks of training.

A four-year evaluation of MTA was conducted in Texas where the program was used in regular public school classrooms as well as in remedial classrooms (Vickery, Reynolds, and Cochran 1987). Children receiving MTA instruction in Grades 3 through 6 were compared with students in the same classrooms in previous years who had received traditional instruction. California Achievement Test (CAT) scores indicated significantly greater gains in reading and spelling for the children instructed in MTA during Grades 3, 5, and 6, but not during Grade 4. Gain sizes tended to increase with additional years in the program.

The Dyslexia Training Program (*DTP*) is another adaptation of the Alphabetic Phonics curriculum. In 1987, DTP introduced videotaped lessons for schools without access to trained therapists. It was developed by Lucius Waites, Anna Ramey, and the staff of the Dyslexia Lab at Texas Scottish Rite Hospital for Children in Dallas, Texas. The tape version of DTP is a two-year program, involving 350 one-hour videotapes for dyslexic students and students at risk for dyslexia. It is currently in use in over 400 school districts in Texas and in over 30 states. The major advantage of the program is that it is relatively cost effective. The classroom teacher, called a *proctor*, learns the program from the teacher's guides and from watching the tapes with the students. A second set of videotapes, the Literacy Program, has been developed at Scottish Rite for adolescents and adults who read poorly for a variety of reasons. This consists of 160 hour-long tapes that can be completed in a school year or in community-based adult literacy programs. Guides, student workbooks, and the Bloomfield-Barnhart Let's Read readers are available from Educators Publishing Service. The videotapes must be ordered directly from the Scottish Rite Hospital.

A report issued by Texas Scottish Rite Hospital for Children and dated 1992 chronicles the progress of 2,037 public school children trained using video tapes in the Dyslexia Training Program. The data was generated by a training project intended as a method of helping classroom teachers provide dyslexic children with appropriate materials as they moved through the program. The children ranged from 2nd grade through middle school. Reading, writing, spelling, and alphabet skill levels are reported in terms of criterion-referenced curriculum levels on the seven schedules (or levels) of the program.

A DTP evaluation study was carried out by a group headed by Jeffrey Black, Medical Director of the Child Development Division of Texas Scottish Rite Hospital for Children (Oakland et al. 1998). The group reported a comparison of progress made over a two-year period by 22 elementary age children with dyslexia in two DTP instructional programs with that of 26 controls who received school-based reading instruction without a phonics emphasis. In comparison with the school-based controls, the two DTP groups made more progress in decoding over two years and more progress in comprehension during the first year. Note, however, that only seven of the 26 school-based controls received any special reading services. Within the two DTP groups, the 12 children receiving taped DTP instruction made as much progress as the 10 children in the live instruction DTP group, which is encouraging in terms of the effectiveness of taped instruction.

21

The Slingerland Approach

BACKGROUND AND RATIONALE

The Slingerland Approach was designed by Beth Slingerland as an Orton-Gillingham adaptation for use with whole classes of students. The program provides an alternative setting for at-risk beginning readers. As with other Orton-Gillingham programs, the Slingerland Approach is based on the premise that language depends on intersensory functioning. Multisensory activities are incorporated into all levels of the program to promote the development of automatic visual, auditory, and kinesthetic associations.

The first teacher education course was developed in 1960 in the Pacific northwest and the program has its headquarters at the Slingerland Institute in Bellevue, Washington. Hundreds of Slingerland classrooms now exist on the west coast and more have sprung up in other parts of the United States.

The program was designed as preventive instruction for children who have been identified by the Slingerland Screening Tests as having "specific language disability" (SLD) and, therefore, are at risk for reading failure. The screening tests are usually administered at the end of kindergarten or the beginning of first grade. Children so identified receive Slingerland instruction in place of the traditional language arts curriculum; most remain in Slingerland classrooms for at least two years. The curriculum can also be used in the upper grades. Older children entering a school using the Slingerland Approach are tested using other versions of the screening tests, which are available up through the high school level and then provided with the Slingerland curriculum where appropriate.

CURRICULUM AND INSTRUCTION

The Slingerland curriculum includes student materials and instructional guides for Grades 1 to 3 and for older students not receiving the curriculum from the start. Books 1 through 3 provide detailed instructions for this multisensory, step-by-step approach.

The Slingerland curriculum has three components: (1) Learning to Write, (2) the Auditory Approach, and (3) the Visual Approach. Training begins with handwriting. Ten consonants and a vowel are taught during the first several months of training. In each case, an individual letter is written on large paper in manuscript (or in cursive beginning in the third year of the program). The students trace the letter with two fingers and then with the blunt end of a pencil before using the sharpened end to trace the letter. The next step is to use paper folded in thirds for tracing, copying, and writing from memory after listening to the teacher say the sound of the letter. This Visual-Auditory-Kinesthetic (V-A-K) association is believed to lead toward automatic recall. After a formation has been mastered, students are given a key word (on a flash card or a wall chart) to go with the letter sound. As they form the letter with an arm swing, they must provide the letter name, the key word, and the letter sound. Both unison and individual responses are used in the Slingerland Approach. In answering individually, the child usually stands up so the rest of the class can observe, as well as hear, the response.

The second component, the Auditory Approach, leads to spelling. Here, too, the stimulus is presented orally and linked with a kinesthetic response. The teacher says each letter sound and asks individual children to name the letter while forming it in the air, then to name its key word and give its sound. The teacher then holds up an alphabet card and has the class repeat the procedure in unison, thus completing the V-A-K linkage for a particular letter.

A technique that Slingerland calls "blending"[17] is introduced with oral activities for beginning readers (very young or severely dyslexic students). The teacher pronounces a c-v-c word, such as *hat*, and the class repeats the word. Then an individual child produces the

---

[17]Note that the term *blending* is used in the Slingerland Approach to refer to what is more often called "segmenting" or the analysis of a spoken word into individual phonemes.

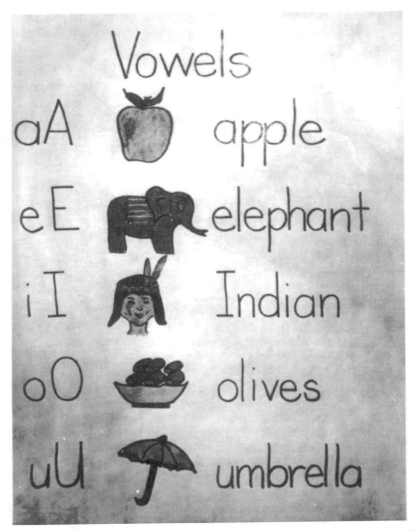

Slingerland Wall Card. Photograph from A Multi-Sensory Approach to Language. Arts for Specific Language Disability Children *by Beth H. Slingerland. (Reproduced with permission from Educators Publishing Service, Cambridge, MA. (800) 225-5750, www.epsbooks.com. Copyright 1971.)*

initial sound /h/, says the name *h*, and places a card with the corresponding letter into a pocket chart. The child repeats the word, pronounces the /a/ sound before naming it, and places the letter *a* next to the *h*, and then repeats this procedure for the final /t/ sound. Eventually, most students are able to approach this task beginning with the vowel sound, as in the following oral response: "Hat - /a/ - *a*; hat - /h/ - *h*; hat - /a/ - *a*; hat - /t/ - *t*; hat - *h - a - t.*" Once students are able to do this and can form the letters correctly on lined paper, writing accompanies the pocket chart activity in "written blending" or spelling. The teacher dictates words, phrases, and sentences, and as the student's proficiency increases, she encourages creative writing.

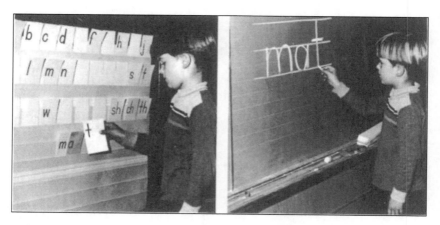

Spelling Activities in the Slingerland Program. Photographs from *A Multi-Sensory Approach to Language Arts for Specific Learning Disability Chidren* by Beth H. Slingerland. (Reproduced with permission from Educators Publishing Service. (800) 225-5750, www.epsbooks.com. Copyright 1971.)

The third component is the Visual Approach, which leads to reading. Here the stimulus is presented in written form. Decoding or "unlocking words" is not taught until the Auditory Approach "blending" skills are in place, usually in the second semester of first grade, as explained in a 1993 supplement provided by Educators Publishing Service with the original materials (Slingerland 1971). Decoding instruction begins with c-v-c words. Beginning readers are asked to pronounce the initial consonant sound, then the vowel sound, to blend the two, pronounce the final consonant sound, and to blend the entire word.

Once older or more competent students are able to "unlock words" letter by letter from left to right, they are taught to look first for the vowel in each word and to say its name, its sound, and then the whole word. One change included in a 1993 supplement to the three 1971 curriculum manuals is that the key word is no longer used to unlock words ("a - apple - /a/ map") as in the earlier version of the program.

Consonant clusters or blends, (e.g., *bl-*, *-lk*) are taught as two distinct letter sounds rather than as units. That is, the word *black* is conceptualized as being made up of four sounds: /b/-/l/-/a/-/ck/. Strings of letters that represent a single sound or "phonogram" (e.g., *th*, *ea*, *tch*) are taught as single units of sound, as are inflectional endings such as *-ed* and *-ing*.

Text reading is taught initially via a whole-word approach, usually with whichever basal reader program is used in the school. It can begin, according to Slingerland, at the same time it is introduced in the other first grade classrooms and is conducted in small groups. A considerable amount of lesson time is spent on "preparation for reading" in which students practice recognizing and reading words and phrases from the text. The teacher writes a new list of words on the chalkboard and the students learn to recognize the words, pronounce the words, and identify their meanings. The teacher might, for example, ask a student to find the word in the list that "tells the name of a girl" (Jill) or "tells what children do" (swim). Phrases are taught in the same way, and fluency and intonation are emphasized, with the teacher modeling by reading aloud. Note that this exposure to words from the text, prior to text reading, is supported by Jenkins' research (Jenkins et al. 2004).

The teacher structures a portion of each day's text reading by breaking several sentences into phrases (e.g., Teacher: "What three words tell where the pony ran?" Student: "to the barn"). The teacher guides comprehension using this technique.

Although the basic Slingerland curriculum is designed for the first two primary grades and is described in corresponding teacher guides (Books 1 and 2), a third-year curriculum has been developed for Slingerland students who need further support after second grade, as well as older reading-disabled students who were not identified earlier (Book 3). Cursive writing is introduced in this curriculum (Slingerland 1971).

The curriculum continues to evolve as new techniques and materials are incorporated. For example, the key word for short *i* has been changed from *Indian* to *inch*. These changes are included in a short addendum available with the 1971 revision of Books 1 through 3. The addendum stresses the importance of ongoing change in response to program usage and states that the changes will be incorporated into the next revisions of the three books.

TEACHER TRAINING

Training as a Slingerland teacher involves participation in a four-week teacher training course. This training usually takes place during the summer within summer school classrooms established for children identified in the Slingerland program as having a specific language disability, and provides graduate credits at an affiliated college or university. Staff members from the Slingerland Institute or Slingerland teachers within the school district serve as teacher trainers. The program is coordinated by a certified Slingerland director who has had two years of Slingerland instruction, plus a third year of classroom supervision, followed by experience as a Slingerland staff teacher.

Dolores Ballesteros and Nancy Royal (1981) describe the organization of a Slingerland summer school training program in a large school district. The program director is responsible for the overall management of the training program, which involves evaluating the training staff. He or she also gives lectures to the teacher-participants on language development, reading, learning disabilities, phonics, and multisensory techniques. Staff teachers must be well versed in the Slingerland techniques and must be approved by the Slingerland Institute. Each staff teacher works with 15 teacher-participants, demonstrating the teaching techniques within a classroom and meeting with teachers for discussion and daily lesson planning. Besides attending lectures and classroom demonstrations, each teacher-participant works daily with an individual child under the supervision of a staff teacher. A clerical staff member is hired when the number of teacher-participants exceeds 45.

School district expenses for a Slingerland summer school training program include staff salaries, minimal supply costs for children's materials, and minimal printing costs, in addition to a teacher-participant service charge to the Slingerland Institute for in-service staff and Slingerland materials. Teacher participants usually pay for teacher's materials and university credit where it is available. Summer schools are held only in districts providing administrative support for teachers interested in Slingerland instruction.

The Slingerland Web site provides information about the following available short courses and modules, which make up the introductory course: (a) Introductory Handwriting, (b) Written Language Expression, (c) Reading Skills, (d) Beginning Reading, and (e) Administering the Slingerland Screening. This is followed by the Second Year Continuum and the Third Year Additional Training

EVALUATION AND IMPLEMENTATION

The Slingerland method has been enthusiastically received in a large number of school districts throughout the country, particularly in the Pacific northwest where it originated, and in California. In many cases, parents have been instrumental in starting Slingerland programs and in some cases, have even threatened to file suit unless their children were provided with this instruction (Lovitt and DeMier 1984). Ballesteros and Royal (1981) describe how the program served as a voluntary magnet for racial integration in schools in southern California. Slingerland classes were established in high minority schools in the San Diego area with two-thirds of the enrollment space reserved for nonminority children from the district that had requested Slingerland instruction. Moreover, through parental petition, Slingerland classes were established here through the 12th grade.

Several studies have demonstrated that the Slingerland Screening Tests, when administered in kindergarten, are significantly correlated with later reading scores. Sears and Keogh have carried out a correlational study in which 104 California children were screened in kindergarten with follow-up testing in Grades 1, 3, and 5 using the Word Study and Reading Comprehension subtests from the Stanford Achievement Tests. The correlation for the Total Score from the kindergarten Slingerland with Grade 1 Word Study Skills was .601, indicating that the Slingerland predicted roughly 36 percent of the variance in Grade 1 Word Study. Subtest correlations with Grade 1 Word Reading varied from .036, which was nonsignificant, to .384 for the Sound-Symbol subtest and .447 for the Sound Identification subtest. The highest subtest correlations with overall Grade 5 reading were for Sound Identification and Sound-Symbol (Sears and Keogh 1993). This is consistent with other sources indicating that kindergarten letter knowledge and phonemic awareness are the best predictors of later reading. The Slingerland correlations were significant but were not as high as those for other available kindergarten measures. For example, kindergarten invented spelling (i.e., sound–symbol knowledge and sound identification) accounted for roughly 50 percent of the variance in later reading in other studies (Mann, Tobin, and Wilson 1987; Morris 1993; Morris and Perney 1984; Uhry 1993a, 1999).

Considerable research has addressed the question of program effectiveness. John Lichter and Leonard Roberge (1979) conducted a three-year study with first grade children receiving Slingerland instruction, comparing their year-end achievement with matched control children in other schools. They reported significantly higher achievement for the Slingerland children. However, because they did not describe the instruction provided to the control subjects, the meaning of the comparison is difficult to interpret.

Beverly Wolf (1985) measured progress on the Metropolitan Achievement Test (MAT) for children in Slingerland classes, some of whom were considered to be language-disabled as determined by the Slingerland Screening Tests, and some of whom were not. She conducted an ex post facto analysis of first to second grade gain scores as compared to the scores of children in traditional classrooms. Instruction in the conventional classrooms, which served as the control treatment, was not described in detail, but appears to have been an eclectic basal reader approach. Thus two experimental groups received Slingerland instruction, those with "specific language disability" (SLD) and those without SLD, and two control groups received conventional instruction, one with SLD and one without. The outcome of the analysis indicated that Slingerland instruction produced significantly greater gains than did conventional instruction on the language section of the

MAT (listening comprehension; punctuation and capitalization; usage, grammar, and syntax; spelling; and study skills) for both SLD and non-SLD students. On the reading section (word and sentence reading; vocabulary; literal, inferential, and evaluative comprehension), the advantage of Slingerland training over conventional instruction approached but did not achieve significance. However, scores of the Slingerland students were less variable than those of the conventionally instructed group. On the other hand, the superiority of Slingerland instruction over conventional instruction was not evidenced in the reading scores for the non-SLD students.

Another ex post facto investigation (McCulloch 1985) compared California Achievement Test (CAT) scores of 15 SLD children who received three years of Slingerland training with 15 SLD children who had been taught in conventional classrooms during the first three grades. Statistical analyses demonstrated significantly higher reading and language scores for the Slingerland trained children. Spelling scores, in contrast, did not reveal significant between-group differences. The study's author, Clara McCulloch (personal communication, May 9, 1994) explains that Slingerland students are taught to spell using an auditory approach consistent with Orton's assertion that a clear-cut auditory pattern of the spelling word must be present. The CAT spelling task is virtually a visual proofreading (orthographic) task, and may not tap phonology, which McCulloch considers more related to spelling.

School-wide and district-wide evaluation studies of the Slingerland Approach have yielded generally positive results. For example, a study conducted in 1980 by the Bureau of Child Educational Services (BOCES; 1980) in South Huntington, New York, determined that by third grade, Slingerland students had achieved reading gains equal to children in regular classrooms although they did not reach the same reading level. The Slingerland Institute has stated emphatically that the achievement levels of SLD students should not be compared to those of normal students, but instead, expected year-to-year gains should be assessed, as in this study.

One observation that was disconcerting to Diana Clark as she visited schools and reviewed research for the first edition of this book (Clark 1988) is the finding that Slingerland instruction has not always been sufficient to meet the needs of all children at risk for reading failure. Clara McCulloch commented (personal communication, May 9, 1994) that the Slingerland Approach was designed for children with Specific Language Disability. Children who are severely dyslexic may require more individualized instruction than a group setting can provide. Children with reading problems because of other handicapping conditions (e.g., children who are mentally retarded or emotionally disturbed) may have their needs met more adequately in other special programs.

22

The Wilson Reading System

BACKGROUND AND RATIONALE

The Wilson Reading System is one of the few remedial programs that was developed especially for adults and adolescents with dyslexia. Recently, a classroom-based early intervention program, *Fundations* (see Chapter 14), was developed for beginning readers. The Wilson Reading System was developed by Barbara A. Wilson who was originally a special educator in the public schools in Massachusetts. When she became concerned about students who had reading difficulty despite average or better cognitive ability, she sought additional training in the Orton-Gillingham approach at the Language Disorders Unit of Massachusetts General Hospital. She remained there for five years once her training was completed, working with adults with dyslexia. The Wilson Reading System was based on this training and was developed through Wilson's private tutoring practice at the Wilson Learning Center. This center was established in 1985 in Hopedale, Massachusetts with her husband, Edward J. Wilson, as business manager. The Wilsons began publishing the Wilson Reading System materials in 1988 and providing teacher training in 1989. By 1991 their focus had changed from tutoring in a private setting to disseminating information about the program to teachers in the public sector through establishment of the Wilson Language Training Corporation (WLT). In 1993, this new center for disseminating materials and training was moved to Millbury, Massachusetts.

The Wilson Reading System is based on Orton-Gillingham principles and is a multisensory, systematic, synthetic approach to teaching reading and writing to students with language-based difficulties in written language. It has many characteristics in common with other Orton-Gillingham based programs such as Alphabetic Phonics (e.g., sounds are taught to automaticity and then used to decode phonetically controlled text; language structure is taught in a systematic, cumulative way; there is constant review and repetition). It is an integrated system for teaching all aspects of decoding and encoding.

Wilson believes that many older poor readers have begun to think of English as so lacking in regularities that it is impossible to learn. Through the introduction of English as a system, students are taught to trust the structure right from the beginning as they learn to be able to count on what they have been taught.

CURRICULUM AND INSTRUCTION

Wilson believes that one-to-one tutoring presents an ideal setting because of the myriad self-esteem issues usually present for the older poor reader. However, her program has also been used successfully in school settings with small groups or even as the spelling curriculum for an entire class.

The program (Wilson 1988a, 1988b) is sequenced in 12 steps that are based on the six syllable types (i.e., closed syllables with short vowels, syllables with long vowels and silent *e*, open syllables ending in long vowels, syllables ending in a consonant -*l*-*e*, syllables with *r*-controlled vowels, and vowel digraph/diphthong syllables). One innovation Wilson brings to the Orton-Gillingham approach is emphasis on these syllable types right from the beginning. Words are coded by the student, as is typical of other Orton-Gillingham programs (e.g., see Alphabetic Phonics, Chapter 21), but complex diacritical marks are not used. Short and long vowel codings and crossing-out of the silent *e* are used together with a code for each of the syllable types.

The traditional Orton-Gillingham "slashing" of syllables is not used (e.g., *con/trast*). Instead, words are "scooped" or underlined by syllables. Wilson points out that this emphasizes the left-to-right movement of reading; she does not "slash" words between syllables because she does not want students moving to the center of the word first as they view it. The underlining mimics the left-to-right movement used during reading.

Steps 1 to 3 of the 12 steps introduce closed syllables with short vowels in single syllable words with three sounds (e.g., *bat*), with four to six sounds (e.g., *shrimp*), and in polysyllabic words (e.g., *consultant*). Step 1 instruction begins with phonemic segmentation in consonant-vowel-consonant (c-v-c) words. Steps 1 and 2 strongly emphasize phonological awareness with segmenting and blending of phonemes up

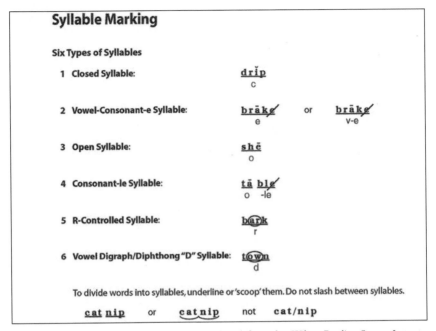

Figure 5   Marking for six syllable types reproduced from the *Wilson Reading System Instructor Manual* by Barbara A. Wilson. (Reproduced with permission from Wilson Language Training, Millbury, MA. Copyright 2004.)

to six sounds. Finger tapping is used for analyzing spoken words into phonemes for spelling. This is similar to the technique called "finger spelling" in Project Read (Enfield and Greene) described in Chapter 24. Wilson also uses finger-to-thumb tapping of phonemes for helping children blend sounds at Steps 1 and 2.

Steps 4 and 5 introduce long vowels in syllables with silent *e* such as in *shine* and in open syllables such as in *program*. Step 6 introduces suffixes in unchanged base words such as *punished* and in consonant -*le* words such as *dribble*. During Steps 1 through 6, the word lists are controlled so that there are no possible alternative pronunciations. Through Step 6, the student reads only phonetically controlled text based on the six word-types that have been introduced, and thus every word can be decoded using phonetic concepts.

Step 7 focuses on what Wilson calls *sound options* for *c* and *g* following *e*, *i*, and *y* (e.g., *decency*, *gigantic*). Step 8 introduces *r*-controlled syllables in words such as *market*. Step 9 introduces diphthong syllables in words such as *plain*, *thyroid*, and *light*. Step 10 introduces suffixes added to changing basewords such as *postponing* and *lagging*. Step 11 includes contractions and advanced suffixes. Step 12 introduces advanced concepts such as the *i* before *e* rule and silent letters. Both real and nonsense words are taught for reading and spelling at each of these steps.

Within each of the 12 steps there are additional substeps, providing 56 in all. Instructors are urged to follow the carefully laid out sequence and to introduce concepts in the suggested order. Lesson plans are consistent in structure and are outlined in the *Instructor Manual* (Wilson 1988a). Detailed directions are provided with each lesson using the following basic plan:

1. *Sound Cards.* A typical lesson begins with sound cards used to introduce a new sound and then to drill old sounds. After a quick drill, the teacher makes words using the phoneme cards to teach and practice the skill being taught. As students advance through the program, syllable and suffix cards are used as well. Wilson believes that the manipulation of these sound cards at every lesson and with every concept is unique to her program. That is, the cards are used first thing in a lesson and then reused at other points (e.g., in preparation for a writing lesson).

2. *Teach/Review Concepts for Reading.* Blank cards, lettered cards, and finger tapping are used to teach phoneme segmentation.

3. *Word Cards.* These cards, each with a printed word, are used to present and practice words using the sounds that were introduced and drilled on the sound cards above.

4. *Word List Reading.* Student readers include word lists that are read and then charted to keep ongoing records of a student's progress in terms of accuracy. Lists of both real and nonsense words are provided for each substep.

5. *Sentence Reading.* The student readers also contain sentences composed of the above words. As with stories in the Student Readers (see below), any words that cannot be decoded using patterns previously taught have been boxed at the top of a page and the instructor simply reads them aloud to the student.

6. *Quick Drill in Reverse.* Spelling is practiced with the teacher saying the sound of the phoneme and the student naming the letter.

7. *Teach/Review Concepts for Spelling.* The student uses finger tapping and the sound cards to segment and spell words said aloud by the teacher.

8. *Written Work.* The student writes sounds, words, and sentences from dictation.

9. *Passage Reading.* The student reads a decodable passage silently, retells it in his or her own words, and then reads it aloud. The 12 phonetically controlled Student Readers are based on the 12 steps of the System. Words that have not yet been covered in the sequence appear in a small box at the top of the page and are read aloud to the student before a reading passage is undertaken.

10. *Listening Comprehension.* The teacher reads aloud at a higher level than the student's reading level and the student retells the story for comprehension practice.

All of the materials used in the program are available from WLT with the exception of the outside reading materials introduced after Step 6. The materials are color coded so that the Student Reader, the Student Workbook, and the Word Cards from a particular step of the system are the same color.

The Sound Cards are also color coded, but not by step. Consonants and consonant units are yellow, vowels are orange, and word families (e.g., *an, ung*) and complex suffixes (e.g., *-tion, -ture*) are pale green. Unlike the Initial Reading Deck cards in Alphabetic Phonics (see Chapter 20), but like that program's Advanced Reading Deck, the Wilson Sound Cards include no diacritical marks or key word pictures on the front. A letter or letters appear on the front for the student to see. The pronunciation, a key word, and the system step at which the sound option is introduced appear on the back for the instructor to see. Instructors are warned to take care not to introduce all sounds at once but to introduce them sequentially and with much review and repetition. Smaller color-coded versions of the Sound Cards, about the size of Scrabble tiles and called Mini Sound Cards, are also available for assembling into words. Consonant clusters are assembled from multiple cards, while the letters in a consonant digraph (e.g., *th*) occur on the same Mini Sound Card, as is the case with the larger Sound Cards. In this regard, the system is like Alphabetic Phonics and unlike Project Read (Enfield and Greene); in the latter method, consonant clusters are taught as single units.

When a new sound is introduced, the student copies information from the Rules Notebook into a personal notebook designed for keeping notes on new concepts. This notebook is used for concepts introduced in other portions of the lesson as well. The emphasis is on the learner's responsibility for taking over management of newly learned concepts. The notebook has sections for sounds, syllables, spelling rules, and sight words.

The content of the Student Readers is geared toward the interests of older readers insofar as possible. As with most phonetically controlled text-based c-v-c words, the earliest stories include instances of the words *cat* and *hat*, but in the Wilson stories, content moves on quickly to the use of words such as *prom, kiss, Red Sox,* and *job.* Many of the stories are about high school activities or about issues related to self-sufficiency such as job hunting or finding a place to live away from home. (See the following sample text from Student Reader Six, which focuses on suffix endings in unchanging basewords.) Supplementary reading materials that follow the 12-step system are also available from WLT. These include student readers and a short novel about a young adult who leaves home to live on his own (Brown 1992; 1994).

Through Step 6 of the program, outside reading is discouraged. The *Instructor Manual* states that this is to discourage guessing and to encourage the reliable use of letter cues in decoding. After mastery of material from the first six steps, noncontrolled text from other sources can be used in the lessons as well as the readers. Instructors are also urged to read aloud to students, with selections made from high interest materials.

Test Forms are available for initial placement in the series and for assessment of mastery of the concepts taught in each of the 12 steps. Instructors are urged to begin with Step 1; the program start-points suggested after initial testing range from Step 1:1 through Step 1:3. For students who can learn the concepts quickly, an accelerated version is available in the form of a Program Overview that is really designed for use in teacher training sessions. In other words, for relatively proficient readers, steps should be reviewed quickly, but never skipped. Progression through all of the steps can take anywhere from six months to three years.

It was a hot, spring day in Alabama. Cathy Jones suddenly had a call. The man on the line had a job for her singing in a local establishment! She had been recommended by a friend. She strongly wanted to be a big-time singer. She shyly responded, "Yes."

Cathy was ready for the risky job. It would be thrilling with so many people witnessing her! Cathy was a great singer, and this club was one of the best in Alabama. An accomplishment here could develop into a limitless future. Cathy had the ability to do quite well as a singer. She was thankful to her friends.

Text from "Cathy Gets a Job" in Student Reader Six in the Wilson Reading System by Barbara A. Wilson. (Reproduced with permission from Wilson Language Training, Millbury, MA. Copyright 1988.)

TEACHER TRAINING

Training and certification in the Wilson Reading System are carried out by the Wilson Language Training Corporation (WLT) in Millbury, Massachusetts. WLT offers an initial two-day Overview Workshop that prepares teachers to begin work with students, but not to consider themselves "Wilson trained." This Overview is a prerequisite to further training. Level I Certified Training involves a year's training and supervision, and prepares teachers to work with individual children in need of multisensory, structured language training. Some of the training at this level can be carried out on the Internet. Level II Certified Training prepares teachers to work with groups (Level II A) and with individuals at advanced reading levels (Level II B). The workshop and courses can be taken for graduate credit through Endicott College, or, in Massachusetts and New Jersey, for professional development points. In a recent look at the Wilson Web site, a three-month schedule for overview training included numerous New England sites as well as New Jersey, Pennsylvania, Tennessee, Virginia, and Colorado. One thousand teachers earned their Level I training in 2002 from states including Arizona and Oregon. Advanced coursework is available online or in intensive four-week summer courses with follow-up school observation visits during the school year. School districts with a number of interested teachers can arrange for onsite training. Barbara Wilson is currently coordinating training in her method to all special education teachers in New York City where The Wilson Reading System is mandated for children receiving special services in reading. Wilson Academy, an online resource, is available for teachers who already have initial training in the system. It provides print materials such as lesson plans and decodable text, together with demonstrations presented in video clips. Additional information about training can be found on the Web site (www.wilsonlanguage.org).

EVALUATION AND IMPLEMENTATION

Research has played an ongoing role in the development of the Wilson Reading system. A well-controlled study (Guyer, Banks, and Guyer 1993) was carried out with 30 students with dyslexia enrolled in the Higher Education for Learning Problems (HELP) program at Marshall University in West Virginia. These students ranged in age from 18 to 32, had a mean IQ of 110, and earned reading achievement scores at least one standard deviation below IQ scores. Most had been diagnosed with dyslexia prior to entering college, and all were enrolled in the HELP program in order to receive remedial assistance with a range of academic problems such as study skills and proofreading papers for coursework. The experimental group received spelling instruction using the Wilson System, and was compared with controls receiving instruction in a nonphonetic spelling method and with those receiving no instruction. Both trained groups were tutored by learning-disabilities specialists with prior training in both the Wilson System and in the nonphonetic spelling method. After two hour-long lessons a week for 16 weeks, the group receiving tutoring in the Wilson System was significantly stronger than either control group on spelling skills as measured by the Spelling subtest of the Wide Range Achievement Test (WRAT-R). While not formally documented, the authors note that several professors commented that these students' contextualized spellings improved over the course of the semester as evidenced in papers.

Another report describes a study carried out with 220 student-teacher pairs (O'Conner and Wilson 1995). Most of the students and teachers were from Massachusetts. Ninety-two of the students were in Grades 3 and 4 and 128 in Grades 5 through 12. Criteria for selecting students involved a special education evaluation indicating IQ in the low average to high average range, reading at least two years below grade level, and lack of outstanding emotional factors. In all cases, there was a history of poor progress made with other reading programs in one-to-one or small group settings. About a third had been retained at least one grade. About half were in regular classrooms with at least a third of the day spent in pull-out settings, and most of the other students were in full time special education settings for the entire day. Tutors attended a two-day Wilson training session and monthly seminars from September through June. During this time, they tutored the students two to three times a week, with the number of sessions ranging from 55 to 100. The average growth from pre- to posttest over this nine-month period was 4.5 grade levels on the Word Attack Test of the Woodcock Reading Mastery Tests and 1.5 grade levels on the Reading Comprehension Test. These results are impressive in light of the minimal progress made by these students in other programs.

In an independently conducted study carried out in Illinois, Dickson and Bursack (1999) provided a professional development program introducing three Grade 1, whole-language oriented teachers to phonological awareness and letter-sound instruction. Ongoing assessment provided feedback on the new programs. In Phase 2 of the project, 20 students who failed to make progress after whole-class instruction (the lowest 25 percent) were taught in small groups by the Title 1 teacher using The Wilson Reading System. The authors report use of a statistical procedure for figuring effect sizes adjusting for pretest differences, which allowed them to use typically achieving children as controls during Phase 2. With this method, there were positive effect sizes on five of the six literacy measures for the 20 lowest children who were taught in small groups with The Wilson Reading System.

In another study, reading scores were collected from Wilson tutors-in-training who worked with 374 children deemed in need of remedial help by their school districts. Pre- and posttest data were analyzed by Frank Wood at Wake Forest University School of Medicine (2002). The average age was 10 to 11 years and the average IQ was around 97. The average pre-test Woodcock Reading Mastery composite standard score was around 84 and the average post-test standard score was around 90 with gains reaching significance on word identification, word attack, and reading comprehension. While control groups were not used in this study, additional analyses yielded interesting findings. Subgroups of children, grouped by six levels of IQ (70–120+), three levels of severity of reading disorder (standard scores below 70 through 90+), Grade (3–8), and setting (inner-city versus total sample) all benefited from the program in terms of making significant gains.

In a study reported by the Lynn, MA public schools for the school year 2000–2001, 17 elementary schools used the spelling component of The Wilson Reading System for Grades 1 through 3. Between 88 percent (Grade 3) and 96 percent (Grade 1) of the children scored above grade level in spelling by the end of the year. Seventy-one percent of the children in bilingual and dual immersion classes scored above grade level. For example, the average spelling grade equivalent for first graders was 2.8. Roughly half of the children in this district are entitled to free or reduced lunch. Sixty-six percent are African American, Hispanic, or Asian, and 16 percent are English language learners.

I recently interviewed 15-year-old Brian who was, at last, learning to read using the Wilson Reading System in his rural Massachusetts special education classroom. Until this year, Brian had been virtually a nonreader, despite years of every sort of help imaginable. His family happened to move and his new high school began instructing him in Wilson in a small group setting about a year before I talked with him. I asked him what made the difference. Brian said that memorizing words in his old school did not help because he just forgot most of them. Brian talked about the closed syllables in Wilson. He mentioned that code marks help him recognize where the vowels are, and that, "Sounding it out with our fingers helps hear the word, the syllable, and the vowel." While there are many possible explanations for Brian's success with this system, his perception was that something about the simple structure of the six syllable types seemed to have made reading manageable for him for the first time.

23

Project Read (Enfield and Greene)

BACKGROUND AND RATIONALE

Mary Lee Enfield and Victoria Greene developed *Project Read* in 1969 for the public school district in Bloomington, Minnesota, in response to the growing number of children who did not seem to benefit from the basal reading program used in the district. It began as a three-year experimental program to deliver direct, systematic phonics instruction within regular classrooms to students performing below the 25th percentile in reading and spelling. The program's goals were to provide cost effective reading instruction to students who were not learning in the district's reading program, to increase coordination between regular classroom instruction and remedial instruction, and to avoid the stigma of removal from the mainstream (Enfield 1976). The authors consider the program an alternative as well as a remedial approach to reading instructions (Enfield and Greene 1981).

Project Read is now being used with students in Grades 1 through 6 who are functioning at the lowest reading levels. Though designed for the classroom teacher, the program may be used effectively in a resource center (Arkes 1986). Extensions of the program, covering reading comprehension and written expression, as well as phonology, are appropriate for intermediate and secondary students who are weak in these areas.

CURRICULUM AND INSTRUCTION

Project Read curriculum comprises three phases. Phase I instruction focuses on phonics, Phase II on reading comprehension, and Phase III on written expression. Phase I is essentially a modification of the Gillingham-Stillman model of systematic, multisensory phonics instruction. Originally designed for Grades 1 through 3, Phase I has since been extended through Grade 9. Instruction in basic phonics knowledge for Grades 1 through 3 is outlined in a teacher's guide (Greene and Enfield 1985a). The guide provides a systematic sequence of skills and concepts that are covered in a series of 60 lessons, each of which may span several days or even a week of instruction. Specific techniques, many of which are multisensory, are described for teaching these skills and concepts. These include tracing letters in a sand tray (called the "memory box"), in the air, on a shag rug, a table, or a chalkboard. Raised letters are provided for showing directionality of confusable letters. Mouth positions are stressed in teaching consonant sounds; for example, for *b*, a voiced explosion of air, for *t*, a tongue bounce, for *m*, mouth closed. Finger puppets and key words are mnemonics suggested for teaching vowels, and children are given practice in identifying the vowels from among the other letters in the alphabet sequence. Long and short vowel markings are taught in the first lesson.

Each lesson introduces a new phonic element such as a letter sound, and a particular concept; for instance, the fact that vowels have a significant value for building words. A lesson begins with a review of previously learned material that includes both decoding and encoding practice. Hand signals are used to direct unison response. The teacher flashes letter cards and the students say the letter symbols. Next, new sounds are introduced and reinforced with multisensory techniques. Students then build words or syllables with letter cards and decode them. Various techniques for sound blending are described in the teacher's guide. Spelling practice follows with students saying the letter sound as they write each letter.

Oral reading is the last activity of each lesson. The program has incorporated the *SRA Basic Reading* linguistic series (Rasmussen and Goldberg 1976) for this purpose, although alternative materials are suggested in some of the lessons. Students are taught to follow along with a finger or pencil while reading, and if they have difficulty decoding, to trace over the particular letter or letters "to unlock the sound" (Greene and Enfield 1985a). Oral reading involves both "reinforcement reading," where the material is usually phonetically regular and students are expected to have little decoding difficulty, and "stretch reading," in which the material may include unfamiliar words. Irregular words contained in reinforcement reading material are taught separately. In stretch reading, the teacher supplies any words that may be beyond the students' skill level.

Three categories of words are distinguished in Project Read: "green words," which are phonetically regular for both decoding and encoding (e.g., *cat*); "yellow words," which are regular for decoding but follow spelling generalizations for encoding (e.g., *back*); and "red words," which are irregular for both decoding and encoding (e.g., *the*).

One teaching point that distinguishes Project Read from other Gillingham-Stillman oriented programs involves the teaching of consonant clusters or blends. While other programs teach digraphs such as *-ch* as a single sound and consonant clusters or blends such as *bl* as two sounds for reading and spelling, Project Read teaches both digraphs and clusters as single units. That is, the cluster *bl* is taught as a single sound rather than as two sounds (i.e., /b/-/l/) as in other Orton-Gillingham programs such as Alphabetic Phonics and Slingerland.

A continuation of Phase I for students in fourth through ninth grades focuses on vocabulary development by teaching affixes and common word roots. The curriculum is outlined in a second Phase I teacher guide, referred to as the Affix Guide (Greene and Enfield 1981). The guide presents a unique approach to unlocking word meaning. Rather than drawing attention to word roots, which may be elements too obscure to bear apparent meaning (for example, the syllable *dict* in the word *unpredictable*), students are taught to look for known parts (in this case *predict*), which are referred to as "word foundations." After identifying the known foundation, the attending affixes are isolated and identified.

Another creative aspect of Enfield and Greene's curriculum is their application of the concept of comprehension to the understanding of affixed words. Students learn that these words actually represent phrases; for example, *unpredictable* equals "cannot be predicted." The teacher's guide presents pairs of sentences, one containing such a phrase, the other the corresponding affixed word. It also provides sentences that can be used for demonstration and reinforcement in dictation exercises, using the affixed words in meaningful context. A spelling guide incorporating a structured phonics approach is also included in the Project Read materials (Greene and Enfield 1985a). The guide provides the teacher with valuable information about English spelling patterns and rules. It takes into consideration three relevant aspects of English graphemes: their origin (e.g., Anglo Saxon, Latin), their frequency, and their placement in words. In terms of frequency, Enfield and Greene maintain that teaching the least frequently encountered spellings for a particular phoneme first—for example, *ue* before *ew*—helps students learn to sort and classify words according to spelling patterns.

The syllable is the unit of emphasis in this spelling guide. According to Greene and Enfield, all syllables in the English language fall into one of seven categories: closed, open, vowel team, vowel-consonant-final *e*, diphthong, final consonant *le*, and vowel controlled by *r*. They stress the fact that the type of syllable determines the sound of the vowel or vowels it contains.

Phase II of Project Read focuses on reading comprehension and vocabulary development, and begins when a student has mastered basic decoding skills, usually toward the end of first grade. However, major emphasis on comprehension instruction takes place in Grades 4 through 6. The curriculum is outlined in a teacher's guide (Greene and Enfield 1985b), which has incorporated instructional materials from other publishers for teaching reading comprehension skills such as the Barnell Loft Specific Skills Series (Boning 1990). Most of these materials are nonfiction.

The guide distinguishes two levels of text analysis and presents a sequence of comprehension skills within each level. At the literal level, these skills include identifying the subject of the text, selecting and defining unfamiliar words, noting punctuation and understanding its purpose, and determining whether the text material is fiction, nonfiction, or procedural (telling how to do something). At the interpretive level, the skills include identifying and sequencing the information in the text (either key facts or key procedural steps), finding the supporting details, making inferences, and drawing conclusions. Students also are taught to outline the organizational form of a text.

Multisensory activities are suggested to reinforce the concepts being taught; for example, having students write key facts on paper-cutout keys and pasting the keys in the margins, pointing to the facts as written in the text, or having students feel an object hidden in a paper bag and making assumptions about that object from touch.

The major focus in the inference unit of the curriculum is on teaching students to look for clues in the text that lead to or support assumptions about the context. Toward this end, the teacher may make an inferential statement and ask students to find the clues in the text that lead to this inference, or the teacher may ask an inferential question for the students to answer and indicate the clues that led to their answer.

Phase III of Project Read encompasses instruction in written expression, provided systematically and incorporating multisensory techniques. Handwriting instruction, however, is not included in the program. The focus in this phase is on teaching sentence structure and paragraph development. Instruction moves from basic sentence structure (simple sentences) to complex sentences. Students are taught to diagram sentences; they spend considerable time at this activity.

Concepts are practiced in creative writing experiences. Phase III extends from the end of Grade 1 through Grade 9 and may be used as an alternative to the regular English program in Grades 5 through 9 (Arkes 1986).

A variety of materials are available including teacher guides, classroom posters (e.g., syllable types) to clarify instruction, students copies of report forms, and story charts.

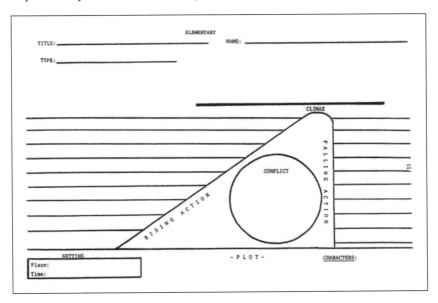

Diagram of Story Form from *There's a Skeleton in Every Closet, Teacher Text* by Victoria E. Greene and Mary Lee Enfield. (Reproduced with permission from the authors. Coyright 1976.)

TEACHER TRAINING

In the early stages of Project Read, training was carried out by 10 former classroom teachers who had learned the program. Using demonstration and observational methods, they, in turn, taught the program in schools to elementary teachers as they worked with groups of low achieving students in their classrooms. At the end of two or three weeks, the classroom teacher took over full responsibility for the program, supported by periodic visits from the project staff for further observation, feedback, and demonstration as needed.

Today, Mary Lee Enfield, Victoria Greene, and the Language Circle staff teach two- to four-day professional development workshops both in Bloomington and on-site in schools across the United States. Workshops focus on one of the three strands of the program: phonology, reading comprehension, or written expression. Recently, Project Read's Web site listed more than 80 national workshops over a 10-month period.

EVALUATION AND IMPLEMENTATION

The first evaluation of Project Read was conducted by Mary Lee Enfield in 1976 as a pilot study. An experimental group of 45 children in Grades 1 through 3, 15 at each grade level, who were reading below the 25th percentile, received Project Read instruction. As compared to a matched control group of children from another school district who did not receive Project Read instruction, the experimental subjects made significantly greater gains on measures of reading and spelling achievement. Because of these favorable results, the Bloomington school board mandated the implementation of Project Read in all first through third grade classrooms in the district.

A second evaluation was conducted on the initial three years of the program as implemented district-wide (Enfield 1976). Data were analyzed from a battery of reading and spelling tests administered to a random sample of 665 students in Grades 1 through 3 who had participated in Project Read. Results of the analyses indicated the following:

1. There were significant gains for Project Read students on most of the tests given.
2. There was a significant reduction in the number of children requiring tutoring services at the end of the three-year period.
3. Project Read students demonstrated greater yearly gains in reading than did the children in previous tutoring programs.
4. There was a significant reduction in teacher cost per pupil for Project Read students as compared to students in tutoring programs.
5. After two years of Project Read implementation, there was a district-wide reduction of students who scored below grade level in reading.

One of the major limitations of the study, as Enfield herself has pointed out, was the lack of a control group. She also acknowledges the possibility of a "Hawthorne effect" or performance enhancement due to the novelty of a program. Following that study, Enfield and Greene evaluated the progress of students in Grades 2, 4, and 6 of the Bloomington public schools who were receiving Project Read instruction (Enfield and Greene 1983). Separate evaluations were conducted on results of district-wide standardized testing in reading and spelling for nonlearning disabled students in the Project Read program and students classified as learning disabled who received Project Read instruction. Both evaluations indicated that Project Read students were performing above 75 percent of their achievement potential (estimated on the basis of IQ). Enfield and Greene maintain that this performance level represents significant improvement for these students who were otherwise functioning in the bottom quartile of their class. Their claim, however, must be regarded as being based on subjective judgment.

Project Read is being used increasingly in public school districts around the country such as Portland, Oregon, Irvine, California, and Tampa, Florida, to name just a few. According to Dr. Enfield (personal communication), an enthusiastic leader is needed to convince the school administration to undertake a pilot study. In some instances, leadership has come from a motivated teacher.

The town of Greenwich, Connecticut, has implemented the program district-wide, without on-site supervision from Project Read staff, through the enthusiastic leadership of teachers and special education administrators. Initially, elementary classroom teachers from one elementary school attended the summer training session in Bloomington and implemented the phonics strand with the lowest achieving students in their classrooms. Subsequently, training has been provided routinely in all schools in the district, and is an expectation for all teachers who teach reading either in the classroom or in special support situations. The Project Read phonics strand has been incorporated into the regular language arts curriculum, and is considered a bridge between the regular education classroom and special education settings. According to Nancy Eberhardt, curriculum coordinator for Special Education in the district (personal communication), Project Read training was used as a vehicle "to help all teachers involved with beginning literacy instruction understand the profile of the learner who needs direct, concept-driven, multisensory education."

24

The Lindamood LiPS Program

BACKGROUND AND RATIONALE

*T*he *Lindamood Phoneme Sequencing Program for Reading, Spelling, and Speech (LiPS)* (Lindamood and Lindamood 1998) was developed by Charles and Patricia Lindamood, the former a linguist and the latter a speech pathologist. In its first (1969) and second (1975) editions, it was called Auditory Discrimination in Depth (ADD) and was described as a preventive, developmental, or remedial program designed to teach auditory conceptualization skills basic to reading, spelling, and speech. The program is intended to complement any reading program. It can be used with kindergarten children to bolster the development of auditory-perceptual awareness of speech sounds as well as with children and adults who fail to read and spell successfully because of failure to acquire phonemic analysis skills.

Of all the programs for intervention and remediation of reading problems, the LiPS Program represents the most intense and thorough training in phonological awareness. Instead of linking phonemes to letters in the early stages, it links phonemes to what the Lindamoods call "articulatory gestures," or movements of tongue, lips, and teeth that are involved in producing speech sounds. Much of the instruction is derived from multisensory techniques used by speech therapists. Instruction in phonological awareness does not use letters and focuses on auditory conceptualization judgment, defined as "the ability to perceive the identity, number, and sequence of speech sounds in spoken patterns, and to perceive *how* and *where* patterns are different" (Lindamood and Lindamood 1980). This component of phonological awareness is referred to as the "comparator function" or the ability to hold two phonological structures in memory for comparison (Lindamood, Bell, and Lindamood 1992). The Lindamood Auditory Conceptualization Test measures this ability by asking the student to use colored blocks to represent nonsense words with items such as, "If this (yellow-red-yellow sequence of blocks) says *pip*, show me *ip* (red-yellow)." The student is expected to make a judgment about how and where the words are different based on this auditory comparison and then to represent the new word by changing the blocks.

This ability has been found to be significantly correlated with word reading in Grades 1 to 12 (Calfee, Lindamood, and Lindamood 1973). The Lindamoods' research led them to conclude that for over half the population, auditory conceptualization matures naturally and is fully developed for single-syllable words by fourth grade, but that for a substantial segment of the population, this skill does not develop spontaneously and remains deficient into adulthood. Regardless of the age of an individual, however, the Lindamoods contend that auditory conceptual function can be developed through direct, multisensory instruction.

CURRICULUM AND INSTRUCTION

The LiPS techniques are designed for classroom use with small, homogeneous groups of students. Historically, the program has been used in clinical settings for one-to-one tutorials. As with the earlier ADD Program, LiPS contains five developmental levels. The first level of LiPS, called *Setting the Climate for Learning*, introduces the concept of auditory perception and how we can aid our learning by making it consciously multisensory. Activities include identifying environmental sounds, comparing sounds, and sequencing sounds. The focus is on awareness of how to monitor one's own learning about sounds.

Identifying and Classifying Speech Sounds at Level 2 involves matching speech sounds with articulatory gestures. Using classifications made by speech therapists and linguists, speech sounds are categorized and labeled within the LiPS Program on the basis of the shape and position of the lips, teeth, and tongue. For example, 16 of the consonant sounds are grouped in unvoiced/voiced pairs as demonstrated in the following figure. Notice that the phonemes /p/ and /b/ are paired, with /p/ as the *quiet brother* and /b/ the *noisy brother*. It is suggested that the reader experience this distinction by saying the sound /p/ and then whispering the sound /b/. When /b/ is whispered, it sounds like /p/. Notice the "explosion" of air that pops between your lips when either phoneme is said. The label *unvoiced and voiced lip poppers* is used by students, rather than the traditional classification used by speech therapists and linguists in which /p/ and /b/ are "unvoiced and voiced bilabial plosives."

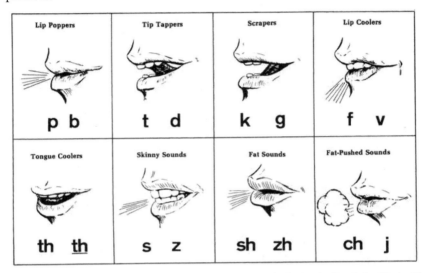

Letter Sound Labels. The A.D.D. Program: Auditory Discrimination in Depth *by Charles H. Lindamood and Patricia C. Lindamood. (Reproduced with permission from PRO-ED. Copyright 1976.)*

Flexible plastic photographs called the *Static Cling Mouth Pictures* have replaced the earlier ADD line drawings for more realistic representation. They involve a photograph of a mouth position with line drawings showing either a puff of air or a stream of air exiting the mouth, for example, across the tongue or onto the lower lip. The photographs provide a clearer illustration of the tongue as can be seen in the photographs reproduced here. I have used these static cling pictures attached to a mirror so that a student could see both the picture and his own mouth at the same time.

For vowels, which have more subtle characteristics in pronunciation, students are taught to "associate the physical sensation of making each sound, the appearance of the mouth when the sound is made, and the sound they hear" (Lindamood and Lindamood 1975). Students are asked to think of the vowels as falling on a half circle moving from the front to the back of the mouth, depending on placement of the tongue when a vowel is pronounced. The short /i/ sound, for instance, is produced with the tongue placed high in the front of the mouth. This concept is called the *Vowel Circle*. Instruction involves asking students to watch as the teacher says, for example, the vowel sounds /ee/ as in *eek*, /i/ as in *it*, /e/ as in *Ed*, and /ae/ as in *ate* while they watch the shape of her mouth change and her chin drop a little lower with each sound. The Vowel Circle comes in a version for American teachers, as well as versions for Australian and Canadian English-speaking teachers. Once the concept of the Vowel Circle has been introduced, the sequence for teaching involves vowels that are nonadjacent in the circle to maximize sound and articulatory gesture differences. This is a principle that is used in most Orton-Gillingham programs, such as Alphabetic Phonics, which introduces short /i/ followed by /a/, but not in Recipe for Reading where short /a/ and /o/ are introduced together.

LiPS uses a Socratic questioning method. Instructional feedback centers on questions drawing attention to sensory input so that the student can self-correct. The example below, called a *discovery dialogue*, is taken from the consonant section of the third edition.

T: What do you feel working when you say /t/?
S: /t/ ... /t/ ... lips.
T: Your lips are open a bit; do they move when you say /t/—check with your mirror. No? How about your tongue—can you see it move on /t/? (Lindamood and Lindamood 1998, p. 14).

This focus on metacognition and sensory feedback is the distinguishing feature of the Lindamood program.

Tracking Speech Sounds, the third level, teaches students to distinguish and name the various sound categories by representing them with colored blocks. This begins in kindergarten with children categorizing speech sounds that have been isolated by the teacher (e.g., the teacher says "/b/-/b/-/b/" and the student produces three blocks that are the same color). Later, the student learns to segment and track sounds in nonsense words (e.g., "If that says *zab* show me *zat*" and the child removes the yellow block in a red-blue-yellow sequence to replace it with any other color). In this way, simple syllables (CV, VC, CVC) and complex syllables (CCV, VCC, CCVC, CVCC, CCVCC) are conceptualized. Not until students have become proficient at encoding nonsense words in this manner are letter symbols applied to spelling and reading.

At the fourth level, *Associating Sounds and Symbols*, students begin to use letters printed on tiles to represent sounds in real words. Students learn to sort out phonetically regular, or dependable, words from nonphonetic words. This allows them to concentrate on the irregular features of the latter type, according to the Lindamoods, and reduces the number of words that must be memorized.

Spelling (Encoding) and Reading (Decoding) are taught at the fifth or highest level of the program. Note that this is consistent with Uta

Given Sound Pattern	Student's Label and Block Pattern*		Given Sound Pattern	Student's Label and Block Pattern
"Show me /b/ /b/ /b/." (one sound repeated three times)	"three lip poppers" (three blocks of the same color)	"Show me /ab/." (two different sounds)	"A smile /a/ and a lip popper" (two blocks of different colors)
"Show me /t/ /m/." (two different sounds)	"a tip tapper and a nose sound" (two blocks of different colors)	"If that says /ab/, show me /zab/." (same two sounds as in original pattern, with the addition of a new and different initial sound)	"A skinny sound came at the beginning." (same two blocks as in original pattern, with the addition of a block of a third color at the beginning)
"Show me /s/ /s/ /g/." (one sound repeated two times, followed by one different sound)	"two skinny sounds and a scraper" (two blocks of the same color, followed by one block of a different color)	"If that says /zab/, show me /zaf/." (same initial and middle sounds as in previous pattern, with the substitution of a different final sound)	"The lip popper is gone and a lip cooler took its place." (same two initial and middle blocks as in previous pattern, with a block of a different color substituted for the final block)

*The block drawings are not intended to represent specific colors. They simply indicate the pattern of sameness or difference within each sequence.

Color-Encoding Isolated Sounds: The ADD Program: Auditor Discrimination in Depth *by Charles H. Lindamood and Patricia C. Lindamood. (Reproduced with permission from PRO-ED. Copyright 1976.)*

Color-Encoding Isolated Sounds in Syllables: The ADD Program: Auditor Discrimination in Depth *by Charles H. Lindamood and Patricia C. Lindamood. (Reproduced with permission from PRO-ED. Copyright 1976.)*

Frith's (1985, 1986) model in which spelling leads into reading (see Chapter 2). As stated in the third edition of the program, spelling precedes reading and "involves the translation of sequences of sounds into sequences of letter symbols" (Lindamood and Lindamood 1998, p. 13). Reading instruction at this level begins with lettered tiles and then moves to printed words. Word units are small, beginning with VC or CV combinations. The program systematically brings into play a three-way sensory feedback system from the ear, eye, and mouth, with emphasis on verbal mediation and self-correction.

There are two routes through these five levels in terms of letter-sound associations. The first involves completing the first three levels for all consonant sounds before introducing letter-sound associations in Level 4, the idea being that a thorough multisensory foundation in sound formations is necessary before using letters and using them to spell and read words. This is phonemic awareness in its pure form. The second route involves becoming really solid on a consonant at Level 2, and then introducing its letter as one more piece of information before moving on to other consonants in Level 2.

The Lindamood materials do not include readers but suggest using the *Poppin Auditory Discrimination Series* (Smith and Stayton 1998), in which the sequence matches the *Vertical Path* of the LiPS sequence, or Level C of the *Barnell Loft Specific Skills Series* (Boning

1990), which is a match for the LiPS *Horizontal Path*. Minimal coverage is given to reading comprehension in the LiPS teacher manual (i.e., nine out of 406 pages). Procedures that promote growth in reading comprehension through visual imagery have been developed by Nanci Bell (1991) for use in the Lindamood clinic, Lindamood-Bell Learning Processes (see Chapter 8).

The Lindamoods have recently revised the test that is used with their curriculum. The Lindamood-Bell Auditory Conceptualization Test–Third Edition (LAC–3; Lindamood and Lindamood 2004) measures an individual's ability to distinguish, conceptualize, and manipulate speech sounds. Tasks are similar to tasks used in the training. This revision includes more items at the upper levels such as five-phoneme syllables and multisyllabic words in comparison with earlier editions of the test. Standard scores are reported for individuals between the ages of 5:0 and 18:11.

TEACHER TRAINING

Teacher training for the Lindamood LiPS program is conducted in two, five-day, nine-hour seminars. The first seminar teaches theory and demonstrates concepts and techniques. The second seminar usually follows immediately after the first and involves practical application of concepts and techniques.

Training is offered at Lindamood-Bell Learning Processes corporate headquarters in San Luis Obispo, California, and at 37 other learning center locations in the United States and at a center in London. The centers offer professional development workshops for teachers and this can be arranged on-site in school locations as well. Demonstration videotapes are available. As the duration of training is much shorter, inservice training costs are considerably less than those offered by Alphabetic Phonics and Slingerland.

EVALUATION AND IMPLEMENTATION

Analyses of data on the effectiveness of the Lindamood program have yielded generally positive results. Marilyn Howard (1982), conducting a 10-year longitudinal study in Arco, Idaho, found that average reading scores for children who had received ADD instruction as first graders rose by more than 30 percentile points over a five-year period. In a second report, Howard (1986) found that both boys and girls, and both kindergarten and first graders trained in ADD made greater gains in word attack and reading skills than did controls.

A two-year study by the Institute for Training and Research in Auditory Conceptualization (INTRAC; 1983) investigated the effects of incorporating the Lindamood program with the Ginn basal reader program in first through fourth grade classrooms in the Santa Monica public schools. INTRAC compared academic progress in these classrooms to progress in classrooms using only the Ginn program. At the end of the first year, superior gains were evidenced in the experimental classrooms as compared to the control classrooms, not only in auditory conceptualization but also on the spelling, reading, and word attack subtests of the Wide Range Achievement Test (WRAT) and Woodcock Reading Mastery Tests (WRMT). At the end of the second year of ADD training, students in the experimental classrooms increased their lead over the control subjects. As a result of the favorable outcome for ADD instruction in the INTRAC study, the Santa Monica school board voted in the third year to provide in-service training for teachers and to include ADD curriculum in all kindergarten through second grade classrooms in the school district.

A group of clinicians and a neurologist working with Joseph Torgesen in Florida (Alexander et al. 1991) used ADD with 10 dyslexic children ranging in age from seven through 12 who were attending an after-school remedial center. Treatment was sustained until all levels of ADD had been completed. Treatment time varied from 38 to 124 hours, with an average of 65 hours. Significant progress was made by the group in terms of standardized reading scores. While there was no control group in this study, an important experimental comparison was made: there was no difference at posttest between Word Identification and Word Attack subtests on the Woodcock Reading Mastery Tests. There was little in the research literature before this study to suggest that dyslexic children could be taught to read nonsense words effectively despite gains in real word reading following remediation.

More recently, the Lindamood Program has been used as one component of a large-scale, NICHD-funded longitudinal intervention study carried out by a research team directed by Joseph Torgesen at Florida State University in Tallahassee (Torgesen et al. 1999). Participants included 138 children with weak letter naming and weak PA who were selected from a pool of 1,436 kindergarten children. Treatment involved 88 hours (four 20-minute sessions a week) of individual instruction from late kindergarten through early Grade 2 and was designed to contrast the intensity of PA training. One PA treatment, which the researchers labeled *Phonological Awareness plus Synthetic Phonics (PASP)*, included the early levels of the 1984 Lindamood ADD program (80 percent of instructional time) and Poppin readers (20 percent of time). The second PA treatment, called *Embedded Phonics (EP)*, included PA and phonics (43 percent of time) using a Harcourt Brace basal series for text reading (57 percent of time). A third condition, used to provide controls and called *Regular Classroom Support* (*RCS*), involved individual instruction in the regular classroom instruction, and varied to include phonics, sight word practice, and story discussions. A fourth group of children received no individual tutoring at all and served as a *No-Treatment Control* (*NTC*).

The PASP treatment that used the Lindamood ADD Program produced the largest gains in word reading with end-of-treatment scores at the average range. The PASP group was significantly stronger than the other groups in what Torgesen calls *phonemic decoding efficiency* (timed word attack skills). In addition, at posttest in Grade 2, there were fewer children in the PASP group who scored below a standard score of 85, and more who scored above 100 on tests of word identification, word attack, and passage comprehension in comparison to the three other groups. This sort of carefully controlled program evaluation is rare and provides evidence for the Lindamood program as an intervention benefiting children with weak kindergarten PA in terms of ability to use letter-sound associations to decode new words.

25

Curriculum Planning: A Case Study

The issue of determining the appropriate instructional treatment for a particular student is crucial. As educators, this should be our principal concern, whether we are school administrators responsible for implementing and funding remedial or preventive curricula, or teachers working directly with students.

This book concludes with an illustration of this process, using the case history of KM. Her end-of-first-grade evaluation was outlined in Chapter 3, and is used here as the starting point in planning an instructional program for her. For this edition of the book, I have added an addendum to this chapter

DECISIONS ABOUT SETTING

Having come to the conclusion that KM was dyslexic because her reading was so poor in relationship to her superior IQ, and because of her unusually slow serial naming rate, our first consideration in formulating an educational plan involved choosing an appropriate setting. We wondered if KM should stay in her present school or if she should move to a school with a more traditionally structured phonics program. Would she do well in a special education setting? In looking at a plan for KM, we wanted to keep in mind that while she appeared to need direct instruction in both reading and spelling, she did extremely well in school in math and in activities involving oral language.

KM attended a school with a whole-language curriculum and without any direct instruction in phonics. This did not present an ideal situation. On the other hand, we did not think KM belonged in a special education setting. There are many wonderful schools in New York City that provide specialized environments, tailored to children with dyslexia and other learning disabilities, and we often recommend them to families of children with dyslexia. However, we thought that KM ought to remain in a regular classroom setting because she functioned very well in areas other than reading and writing. We wanted to keep her with other children who functioned at a high level intellectually because she thrived on the cognitive stimulation.

We would have preferred to see KM receive at least an hour a day of language arts instruction that included direct instruction in letter-sound associations and guided practice using this knowledge in reading. Two of the programs reviewed here offer this in regular classrooms for children KM's age. The Slingerland program and Enfield and Greene's Project Read involve direct instruction in phonics in regular classrooms. Recipe for Reading is also used by some regular classroom teachers to supplement the curriculum. These programs were not available in KM's school.

Another possibility that occurred to us involved a resource room. In cases where a phonics-based classroom program is not available, a resource room is often an appropriate option for children needing direct instruction in phonics but not in need of a full-day special education classroom. This was not available in KM's school. Even in public schools where the option is mandated, the educational approach is not always appropriate. Few resource room teachers have specialized training in the programs reviewed here.

After-school tutoring appeared to be the most workable plan. Even if specialized help had been available in her school, few schools offer this help on a one-to-one basis. Reading Recovery is a notable exception but KM was too old for this program.

KM'S INITIAL CURRICULUM PLAN

KM was tutored by graduate students under our supervision in the Child Study Center for two years. We initially designed her tutoring plan by reviewing remedial programs believed to work well with children with word-reading problems, and by looking at KM's particular profile.

LETTER KNOWLEDGE

We wanted a program in which KM's difficulty responding automatically and rapidly to stimuli would be minimized. A sight word approach would have involved learning thousands of words to the automatic level. In a synthetic phonics approach, there are only 98 letter-sound correspondences to be learned. We knew that KM was relatively strong in blending sounds and we reasoned that automatizing 98 sounds seemed less daunting than memorizing thousands of sight words to the point where they could be retrieved quickly. Learning these 98 sounds would allow her to use letter cues to sound out new words.

For this letter-sound training, we chose the Initial Reading Deck (IRD; Cox 1971) from Alphabetic Phonics, and began each session over the two years of tutoring by asking KM to respond to each letter or unit of letters with its sound. We began with just a few consonants she knew already and worked on speed of response. We added a new card roughly once a week. We also worked on response time for encoding; we said a sound and asked KM to say the letter name as quickly as she could. For KM, only about five minutes per tutoring session were spent on these two activities combined.

SEGMENTING/SPELLING

We knew that KM was able to segment to some degree, but that she struggled with spelling when she needed to retrieve letter names for these segments and to think at the same time while composing. We did some phonological awareness training with KM in the form of segmentation/spelling (see Chapter 5). It is a principle of Orton-Gillingham training to provide practice in isolation before asking a child to juggle several skills or strategies at once. For each new letter-sound pattern KM was taught using the IRD, she was asked to segment words into component phonemes, then to represent each phoneme with a letter or letters, either with tiles or through handwritten spellings. That is, when the digraph *th* was taught, KM was asked to segment the spoken word *with* into the sounds /w/-/i/-/th/, and then to spell it with lettered tiles. Spelling was often extended to written sentences. The spelling dictation portion of this technique can be found in a number of Orton-Gillingham programs such as Alphabetic Phonics and Recipe for Reading.

PHONETICALLY DECODABLE TEXT FOR ORAL READING

It is fairly common practice with children with dyslexia to use text that provides practice in newly learned phonetic patterns and that is limited to patterns that have been introduced already. With KM, we began with *Mac and Tab* from the Primary Phonics series (Makar 1985) available from Educators Publishing Service, but we could have used any number of books limited to short vowels introduced one at a time in a synthetic phonics format. KM read these little books with good accuracy but continued to sound out each word, letter-by-letter. Practice with the IRD helped her sound out each letter with increasing speed, but she failed to increase her retrieval rate for whole words.

Formative assessment at that point indicated rapid growth in nonsense word reading. KM's score on the Word Attack Test of the WRMT jumped from 61 to 94 in about six months while her Word Identification score remained at 78. Because of her poor growth rate in reading real words as sight words, we switched her to the Merrill Linguistic Readers, Books B and C toward the end of her first year of tutoring. We thought that the emphasis on rimes (rather than the phonemic units used in synthetic phonics) would help her retrieve units of letters (e.g., *an*, *itch*) more quickly, and would encourage a switch from letter-by-letter reading to more automatic reading of units of letters in words. By the fall of her second year of tutoring, KM began to read whole words more automatically but her reading rate remained slow. Should we have started with the Merrill Readers earlier rather than with a synthetic program? Linnea Ehri's research indicates not. Her work suggests that phonics knowledge and the letter-by-letter strategy facilitate both the sort of analogy reading that the Merrill readers encourage (Ehri and Robbins 1992) and the acquisition of a sight word vocabulary (Ehri 1992).

NARRATIVELY CONTORLLED OR PREDICTABLE TEXT: TRADE BOOKS

While many of the Orton-Gillingham programs limit early reading to decodable or phonetically controlled text (e.g., Alphabetic Phonics, Wilson Reading System), we saw KM's inability to integrate various cue systems as a problem that we wanted to remediate from the beginning. We tried to chose text that was interesting and that included (but was not limited to) exemplars of phonetic patterns she was practicing in other activities. This provided additional exposure to the pattern introduced with the IRD during a particular lesson, and to words using that pattern introduced in the segmenting/spelling activity and read in the phonetic text. For example, during the end of KM's second grade year (her first year of tutoring) when we worked on consonant digraphs and blends with short vowels, we used the Harper I-Can-Read book, *The Grandma Mix-Up* (McCully 1988). The text is rich in this word type, but it also has a strong and compelling story line and lively illustrations. For many children with dyslexia, this sort of text might be inappropriate, but keep in mind that from the start, KM had at least a marginally developed sense of phonological awareness and of the alphabetic principle. She simply lost this strategy in any sort of applied situation. Focus during the reading of narrative text was similar to that found in Reading Recovery lessons; KM was encouraged to develop strategies for using letter cues as well as context cues, and for checking her own reading by being sure that there was consistency between these cue systems. Roberta, her tutor, took notes during that period indicating that while KM easily read words with blends (e.g., *sled, slip*) in isolated situations such as games, she still over-relied on context and simply guessed when she read them in text. KM's reading during this period was characterized by poor motivation and doggedness about holding on to inefficient and incomplete strategies. She had trouble focusing and was quite resistant to reading. Throughout, she loved to have Roberta read aloud to her.

Note that this lesson outline, with a balance between phonics practice and trade book reading, is similar to one developed by Benita Blachman (Blachman 1987; Blachman et al. 1994).

ONGOING ASSESSMENT

Most preventive and remedial programs include a series of curriculum-based measures designed to tell us if a child has mastered a set of concepts and is ready to move on to new learning (for example, see Chapter 13, *Alphabetic Phonics*). Because KM tended to read more accurately given words out of context, we wanted to keep track of her application of a concept in contextualized reading rather than in isolation. For this reason, we used the Reading Recovery (see Chapter 22) *running record* system of ongoing assessment of reading in trade books to be sure KM had mastered a principle before we introduced new material. Keeping a log of observations allows immediate modifications to even the best laid plan.

KM'S SECOND YEAR OF TUTORING

Tutoring sessions continued to be based on the instructional elements outlined above, beginning with a review of consonant blends and digraphs before moving into long vowels. Her second-year tutor, Sally, proceeded slowly with any new material, knowing that KM was apt to revert to inefficient strategies when overwhelmed. KM began this year reading from simple I-Can-Read trade books at the late first grade level and read from Merrill readers D, E, and F throughout the year. Miscues collected while reading trade books continued to indicate problems in using all available letter cues (e.g., She read *tale* as "talk, *dirt* as "dry," and *calls* as "cries"). We continued to use lettered tiles for segmenting/spelling activities (e.g., "Spell *hid*. Change it to *hide*. Change it to *side*") in order to reinforce letter order and a sequence of particular letter-sound patterns. To encourage more rapid retrieval, some of these words were put on cards for timed reading. KM enjoyed trying to beat her own record, so we kept charts of her time from session to session, and this was a successful activity in terms of motivation.

By the end of this year, her third grade year in school, KM was reading short chapter books (e.g., *Something Queer at the Lemonade Stand*, *The One in the Middle is a Green Kangaroo*) and Random House Step-up Classics at roughly the third grade level (e.g., a retelling of *Peter Pan*). Trade book activities focused on meaning. In her final tutoring report, Sally noted, "KM's confidence in herself as a reader has risen dramatically. She will go back and reread the text or sound out words to make meaning." KM still read quite slowly, but she was beginning to read whole phrases more smoothly.

Writing had become an issue in school; KM became reluctant to invent spellings and became a perfectionist about getting spellings right. Her story content became limited to words she knew how to spell. Her tutor provided structured writing experiences consistent with Orton-Gillingham methods in which sentences were built up from previously practiced words. Cursive handwriting was undertaken and KM enjoyed this. She was less resistant to writing when dictations were approached as practice in cursive writing. Letter formations were taught in groups using terminology and formations from Alphabetic Phonics (e.g., *swing up letters*).

KM'S FINAL EVALUATION

At the end of her second year of tutoring, KM moved to another state. We administered a second formal evaluation to accompany her to her new school where she would enter the fourth grade. Her scores were no longer discrepant from age peers but continued to be lower than predictions based on her superior range IQ. Note that KM's oral language scores, after remediation, continued to be higher than reading comprehension which, in turn, was stronger than word reading and spelling.

KM's Standard Scores over the Course of Two Years of Tutoring			
	1992	1993	1994
PIAT General Information (oral questions)	—	—	138
PPVT (oral vocabulary)	124	—	—
WIAT Listening Comprehension	—	—	120
WIAT Reading Comprehension	—	—	103
WIAT Basic Reading (word lists)	81	87	94
WRMT Word Identification (word lists)	78	78	95
WRMT Word Attack (nonsense words)	61	94	99
WIAT Spelling (dictated words)	84	88	94

KM's time on serial naming on the RAN continued to be several standard deviations slower than age norms. She demonstrated a significant discrepancy between reading accuracy and reading speed when we administered oral passages from the Gray Oral Reading Test (GORT–3). This is consistent with results from Wood and Felton (1994) indicating that rapid naming problems persist into adulthood and inhibit the development of reading rate.

KM's final piece of writing for us described her new home. Note that she over-relied on phonological spelling rather than using conventional orthography. Even in regard to phonics, not all vowel patterns or basic spelling rules for adding suffixes were in place. Her writing was spare in comparison with her gregarious oral style.

> My house is verry cold! But cossy. My room is verry small. I have a farm. there are lots of play gouns in the park. There are 5 Maces. There are 2 J.C. penes. Good by. P.S. I mess my friends.

Writing is often the last skill to fall into place once children with dyslexia have had successful remedial training. KM's final tutoring report listed the following areas for further work: 1) letter-sound training in the remaining vowel digraphs, and in hard and soft *c* and *g*; 2) practice of accuracy and fluency in phonetically controlled text such as Merrill Reader G; 3) practice of accuracy and fluency as well as higher level thinking in interesting trade books; and 4) encouragement of self-initiation of written expression.

No single reading program meets all of the instructional requirements of students with dyslexia. We chose to construct a program for KM from the components of a number of different programs. Had any of the age-appropriate programs described in Part III of this book been available in KM's school from the beginning of first grade, we are confident that she would have learned to read more easily than she did. However, any of these programs would have needed some adjustments to best fit KM's needs.

SUMMARY

The lessons to be learned from watching KM and other children with dyslexia learn to read and write can be summarized as follows:

1. Be sure that all children are screened in kindergarten for early signs of dyslexia.
2. Begin appropriate instruction as early as possible if there is any question of dyslexia. This is especially crucial for children in families with other affected members.

3. Provide direct instruction in phonological awareness and phonics, and teach these children how to integrate these strategies with meaning-based strategies.
4. Read aloud to these children in order to provide intellectual stimulation and a knowledge base ordinarily acquired through reading.
5. Provide ongoing assessment in order to modify and adjust the curriculum.

Tutors and teachers involved with these children need to continue their own professional development through conferences, additional training, and readings from the research. Those of us who work with children and adolescents with dyslexia should take a greater role than we have in the past in planning their language arts curriculum. In addition to using the research results of others to plan curriculum, we should also be documenting and sharing what we ourselves are doing, thereby adding to the research base.

ADDENDUM

Ten years after first writing about KM, I am heartened by the opportunities for children with dyslexia to receive instruction in phonemic awareness and phonics right in their classrooms. In second grade, KM responded so quickly to systematic instruction that I wonder if she would have needed outside tutoring had this instruction begun in kindergarten. Most likely she would have needed extra instruction in fluency. In kindergarten, this would have meant supplementary practice in quickly recognizing letter names. A Title I teacher, aide, or student teacher could have done this for a few minutes a day using letter cards such as those used in Fundations or Alphabetic Phonics. Her classroom teacher might even have been able to find this time. In first grade, KM would have needed this extra time to practice recognizing words quickly, and in reading and rereading these words in connected text. Again, this supplementary instruction could have been planned by her teacher and carried out by a closely supervised student teacher. Working one-to-one in tutoring a child is a valuable experience that ought to be built into all initial teacher education programs.

References

Aaron, P. G., and Phillips, S. 1986. A decade of research with dyslexic college students. *Annals of Dyslexia* 36:44–68.

Achilles, C. M. 1999. *Let's Put Kids First, Finally: Getting Class Size Right.* Thousand Oaks, CA: Corwin Press.

Adams, M. J. 1990. *Beginning to Read: Thinking and Learning about Print.* Cambridge, MA: The MIT Press.

Adams, M. J., Bereiter, C., Hirshberg, J., Anderson, V., and Bernier, S. A. 1995. *Framework for Effective Teaching, Grade 1: Thinking and Learning about Print.* Chicago: Open Court.

Adams, M. J., Foorman, B. R., Lundberg, I., and Beeler, T. 1998. *Phonemic Awareness in Young Children.* Baltimore: Paul H. Brookes Publishing Company.

Aho, M. S. 1967. Teaching spelling to children with specific language disability. *Academic Therapy* 3:45–50.

Alexander, A. W., Andersen, H. G., Heilman, P. C., Voeller, K. K. S., and Torgesen, J. K. 1991. Phonological awareness training and remediation of analytic decoding deficits in a group of severe dyslexics. *Annals of Dyslexia* 41:193–206.

Allington, R. L. 2001. *What Really Matters for Struggling Readers: Designing Research Based Programs.* New York: Longman.

American Federation of Teachers. 1999, July. *Building on the Best, Learning from What Works: Five Promising Remedial Reading Intervention Programs.* Washington, DC: American Federation of Teachers.

Arkes, J. 1986. *The ABCs of Project Read.* Bloomington, MN: Bloomington Public Schools.

Armbruster, B. B., Lehr, F., and Osborn, J. H. 2001. *Put Reading First: The Five Building Blocks for Teaching Children to Read.* Washington, DC: National Institute for Literacy.

Arter, J. A., and Jenkins, J. R. 1979. Differential diagnosis-prescriptive teaching: A critical appraisal. *Review of Educational Research* 49:517-55.

Ashton-Warner, S. 1963. *Teacher.* New York: Simon and Schuster.

Askov, E., and Greff, N. 1975. Handwriting: Copying versus tracing as the most effective type of practice. *Journal of Educational Research* 69:96–98.

Badian, N. A. 1988. *Predicting dyslexia in a preschool population. In Preschool Prevention of Reading Failure,* eds. R. L. Masland and M. W. Masland. Parkton, MD: York Press.

Baker, L., and Brown, A. L. 1984. Metacognitive skills in reading. In *Handbook of Reading Research,* ed. P. D. Pearson. New York: Longman.

Ball, E. W., and Blachman, B. A. 1991. Does phoneme segmentation training in kindergarten make a difference in early word recognition and developmental spelling? *Reading Research Quarterly* 26:49–66.

Ballesteros, D. A., and Royal, N. L. 1981. Slingerland-SLD instruction as a winning voluntary magnet program. *Bulletin of the Orton Society* 31:199–211.

Bandura, A. 1982. Self-efficiency mechanism in human agency. *American Psychologist* 37(2):122–47.

Bannatyne, A. 1971. *Language, Reading, and Learning Disabilities.* Springfield, IL: Charles C Thomas.

Barenbaum, E. M. 1983. Writing in the special class. *Topics in Learning and Learning Disabilities* 3:12–20.

Barker, T., and Torgesen, J. 1995. An evaluation of computer-assisted instruction in phonological awareness with below average readers. *Journal of Educational Computing Research* 13:89–103.

Barron, R. W. 1980. Visual and phonological strategies in reading and spelling. In *Cognitive Processes in Spelling,* ed. U. Frith. New York: Academic Press.

Bartlett, E. J. 1979. Curriculum, concepts of literacy, and social class. In *Theory and Practice of Early Reading, Vol. 2,* eds. L. B. Resnick and P. A. Weaver. Hillsdale, NJ: Lawrence Erlbaum Associates.

Bateman, B. 1979. Teaching reading to learning disabled and other hard-to-teach children. In *Theory and Practice of Early Reading, Vol. 1,* eds. L. B. Resnick and P. A. Weaver. Hillsdale, NJ: Lawrence Erlbaum Associates.

Baumann, J. F., Edwards, E. C., Boland, E. M., Olejnik, S., and Kame'enui, E. J. 2003. Vocabulary tricks: Effects of instruction in morphology and context on fifth-grade students' ability to derive and infer word meanings. *American Educational Research Journal* 40:447–94.

Beck, I. L., and McCaslin, E. S. 1978. An analysis of dimensions that affect the development of code-breaking ability in eight beginning reading programs. Pittsburgh, PA: Learning Research and Development Center, University of Pittsburgh. ERIC Document Reproduction Service No. ED 155 585.

Beck, I., McKeown, M. G., Hamilton, R. L., and Kucan, L. 1997. *Questioning the Author: An Approach for Enhancing Student Engagement with Text.* Newark, DE: International Reading Association.

Beck, I. L., McKeown, M. G., and Kucan, L. 1991. Conditions of vocabulary acquisition. In *Handbook of Reading Research, Vol. II,* eds. R. Barr, M. Kamil, P. Mosenthal, and P. D. Pearson. Mahwah, NJ: Lawrence Erlbaum Associates.

Beck, I. L., McKeown, M. G., and Kucan, L. 2002. *Bringing Words to Life: Robust Vocabulary Development.* New York: Guilford.

Becker, W. C. 1977. Teaching reading and language to the disadvantaged—What we have learned from field research. *Harvard Educational Review* 47:518–43.

Bell, N. 1986. *Visualizing and Verbalizing for Language Comprehension and Thinking.* Paso Robles, CA: Academy of Reading Publications.

Bell, N. 1991. Gestalt imagery: A critical factor in language comprehension. *Annals of Dyslexia* 41:246–60.

Benton, A. L. 1985. Visual factors in dyslexia: An unresolved issue. In *Understanding Learning Disabilities: International and Multidisciplinary Views,* eds. D. Duane and C. K.

Leong. New York: Oxford University Press.

Berlin, D. 1887. *Eine Besondere Art der Wrotblindheit Dyslexie*. Wiesbaden: J. F. Bergman.

Berliner, D. 1981. Academic learning time and reading achievement. In *Comprehension and Teaching*, ed. J. T. Guthrie. Newark, DE: International Reading Association.

Berman, P., and McLaughlin, M. 1975. Federal programs supporting educational change, Vol. 4: The findings in review Report No. R-1589/4. Santa Monica, CA: Rand Corp. ERIC Document Reproduction Service No. ED 108 330.

Berninger, V. W. 1999. Coordinating transcription and text generation in working memory during composing: Automatic and constructive processes. *Learning Disability Quarterly* 22:99–112.

Berninger, V. W., and Abbott, R. D. 1994. Redefining learning disabilities: Moving beyond aptitude-achievement discrepancies to failure to respond to validated treatment protocols. In *Frames of Reference for the Assessment of Learning Disabilities*, ed. G. R. Lyon. Baltimore: Paul H. Brookes Publishing Co.

Berninger, V., Abbott, R., Whitaker, D., Sylvester, L., and Nolen, S. 1995. Integrating low level skills in treatment protocols for writing disabilities. *Learning Disability Quarterly* 18:293–309.

Birch, H. G., and Belmont, L. 1964. Auditory-visual integration in normal and retarded readers. *American Journal of Orthopsychiatry* 34:852–61.

Birsh, J. March 1988. Multisensory teaching and discovery learning in Alphabetic Phonics. Paper presented at the Fifteenth Annual Conference of the New York Branch of the Orton Dyslexia Society.

Bissex, G. L. 1980. *GNYS at WRK: A Child Begins to Write and Read*. Cambridge, MA: Harvard University Press.

Blachman, B. A. 1987. An alternative classroom reading program for learning disabled and other low-achieving children. In *Intimacy with Language: A Forgotten Basic in Teacher Education*, ed. R. Bowler. Baltimore: The Orton Dyslexia Society.

Blachman, B. A., Ball, E. W., Black, R. S., and Tangel, D. M. 1994. Kindergarten teachers develop phoneme awareness in low-income, inner-city classrooms: Does it make a difference? *Reading and Writing: An Interdisciplinary Journal* 6:1–18.

Blachman, B. A., Ball, E. W., Black, R., and Tangel, D. M. 2000. *Road to the Code: A Phonological Awareness Program for Young Children*. Baltimore: Paul H. Brookes Publishing Company.

Blachman, B. A., Schatschneider, C., Fletcher, J. M., and Clonan, S. M. 2003. Early reading intervention: A classroom prevention study and a remediation study. In *Preventing and Remediating Reading Difficulties: Bringing Science to Scale*, ed. B. R. Foorman. Baltimore: York Press.

Blachman, B., Tangel, D., Ball, E., Black, R., and McGraw, D. 1999. Developing phonological awareness and word recognition skills: A two-year intervention with low-income, inner city children. *Reading and Writing: An Interdisciplinary Journal* 11:239–73.

Blachowicz, C., and Ogle, D. 2001. *Reading Comprehension: Strategies for Independent Readers*. New York: The Guilford Press.

Blaskey, P., Scheiman, M., Parisi, M., Ciner, E. B., Gallaway, M., and Selznick, R. 1990. The effectiveness of Irlen filters for improving reading performance: A pilot study. *Journal of Learning Disabilities* 23:604–12.

Block, C. C., and Pressley, M. 2002. Eds. *Comprehension Instruction: Research-based Best Practices*. New York: The Guilford Press.

Bloom, L. 1999. *Language Development from Two to Three*. Cambridge, MA: Cambridge University Press.

Bloom, L., and Lahey, M. 1978. *Language Development and Language Disorders*. New York: Macmillan Publishing Company.

BOCES Regional Office of Planning and Evaluation. 1980. A study of the South Huntington School District Slingerland Program. Suffolk County, NY: Author.

Boder, E. 1971. Developmental dyslexia: A diagnostic screening procedure based on three characteristic patterns of reading and spelling. In *Learning Disorders: Vol. 4*, ed. B. D. Bateman. Seattle, WA: Special Child Publications.

Boettcher, J. V. 1983. Computer-based education: Classroom application and benefits for the learning disabled. *Annals of Dyslexia* 33:203–19.

Boning, R. 1990. *Barnell Loft Specific Skills Series*. DeSoto, TX: SRB/McGraw Hill School Publishing.

Bowers, P. G. 1995. Tracing symbol naming speed's unique contributions to reading disabilities over time. *Reading and Writing: An Interdisciplinary Journal* 7:189-216.

Bowers, P. G. 2001. The nature and extent of time-related deficits in developmental dyslexia. In *Dyslexia, Fluency, and the Brain*, ed. M. Wolf. Baltimore: York Press.

Bowers, P. G., Sunseth, K., and Golden, J. 1999. The route between rapid naming and reading progress. *Scientific Studies of Reading* 3:31–53.

Bowers, P. G., and Swanson, L. B. 1991. Naming speed deficits in reading disability: Multiple measures of a single process. *Journal of Experimental Child Psychology* 51:195–219.

Bowers, P. G., and Wolf, M. 1993. Theoretical links among naming speed, precise timing mechanisms and orthographic skill in dyslexia. *Reading and Writing: An Interdisciplinary Journal* 5:69–85.

Bradley, L. 1981. The organization of motor patterns for spelling: An effective remedial strategy for backward readers. *Developmental Medicine and Child Neurology* 23:83–91.

Bradley, L. 1985. Dissociation of reading and spelling behavior. In *Understanding Learning Disabilities: International and Multidisciplinary Views*, eds. D. Duane and C. K. Leong. New York: Plenum Press.

Bradley, L., and Bryant, P. E. 1979. Independence of reading and spelling in backward and normal readers. *Developmental Medical Child Neurology* 21:504–14.

Bradley, L., and Bryant, P. E. 1983. Categorizing sounds and learning to read—a causal connection. *Nature* 301:419–21.

Bradley, L., and Bryant, P. E. 1985. *Rhyme and Reason in Reading and Spelling*. Ann Arbor, MI: University of Michigan Press.

Brady, S., Fowler, A., Stone, B., and Winbury, N. 1994. Training phonological awareness: A study with inner-city kindergarten children. *Annals of Dyslexia* 44:26–59.

Brady, S., Poggie, E., and Rapala, M. 1989. Speech repetition abilities in children who differ in reading skill. *Language and Speech* 32:109–22.

Brady, S., Shankweiler, D., and Mann, V. 1983. Speech perception and memory coding in relation to reading ability. *Journal of Experimental Child Psychology* 35:345–67.

Breitmeyer, B. G. 1993. Sustained (P) and transient (M) channels in vision: A review and implications for reading. In *Visual Processes in Reading and Reading Disabilities*, eds. D. M. Willows, R. S. Kruk, and E. Corcos. Hillsdale, NJ: Lawrence Erlbaum Associates.

Brigance, A. H. 1977. *Brigance Diagnostic Inventory of Basic Skills*. North Billerica, MA: Curriculum Associates.

Brigance, A. H. 1991. *Brigance Diagnostic Inventory of Early Development*. North Billerica, MA: Curriculum Associates.

Brightman, M. F. 1986. *An Evaluation of the Impact of the Alphabetic Phonics Program in the Kinkaid School from 1983–1985*. Houston, TX: Neuhaus Foundation.

Brooks, A., Vaughn, K., and Berninger, V. W. 1999. Tutorial interventions for writing disabilities: Comparisons of transcription and text generation processes. *Learning Disability Quarterly* 22:113–29.

Brown, A. L., Palincsar, A. S., and Armbruster, B. B. 1984. Instructing comprehension-fostering activities in interactive learning situations. *In Learning and Comprehension of Text*, eds. M. Mandl, N. L. Stein, and T. Trebasso. Hillsdale, NJ: Lawrence Erlbaum Associates.

Brown, J. 1992. *Stories for Older Students*. Millbury, MA: Wilson Language Training.

Brown, J. 1994. *Travels with Ted*. Millbury, MA: Wilson Language Training.

Bruck, M. 1990. Word recognition skills of adults with childhood diagnoses of dyslexia. *Developmental Psychology* 26:439–54.

Bruck, M., and Treiman, R. 1990. Phonological awareness and spelling in normal children and dyslexics: The case of initial consonant clusters. *Journal of Experimental Child Psychology* 50:156–78.

Bryant, N. D., and others. 1980. The effects of some instructional variables on the learning of handicapped and nonhandicapped populations: A review. *Integrative Reviews of Research: Vol. I*, 1–70. New York: Teachers College, Institute for the study of Learning Disabilites.

Bryant, P., and Bradley, L. 1985. *Children's Reading Problems*. New York: Basil Blackwell.

Bryant, P. E., Nunes, T., and Bindman, M. 1997. Children's understanding of the connection between grammar and spelling. In *Foundations of Reading Acquisition and Dyslexia*, ed. B. Blachman. Mahwah, NJ: Erlbaum.

Bryant, S. 1979. Relative effectiveness of visual-auditory versus visual-auditory-kinesthetic-tactile procedures for teaching sight words and letter sounds to young disabled readers. Ed.D. diss., Teachers College, New York.

Burns, M. S., Griffin, P., and Snow, C. E. 1999. *Starting Out Right: A Guide to Promoting Children's Reading Success*. Washington, DC: National Academy Press.

Byrne, B. 1981. Deficient syntactic control in poor readers: Is a weak phonetic memory code responsible? *Applied Psycholinguistics* 2:201–12.

Byrne, B., and Fielding-Barnsley, R. 1991. Evaluation of a program to teach phonemic awareness to young children. *Journal of Educational Psychology* 83:451–55.

Byrne, B., and Fielding-Barnsley, R. 1993. Evaluation of a program to teach phonemic awareness to young children: A 1-year follow-up. *Journal of Educational Psychology* 83:104–11.

Byrne, B., and Fielding-Barnsley, R. 1995. Evaluation of a program to teach phonemic awareness to young children: A 2- and 3-year follow-up and a new preschool trial. *Journal of Educational Psychology* 87:488–503.

Calfee, R., and Associates. 1981–1984. The Book: Components of Reading Instruction. Unpublished manuscript.

Calfee, R., and Henry, M. K., 1985. Project READ: An inservice model for training classroom teachers in effective reading instruction. In *The Effective Teaching of Reading: Theory and Practice*, ed. J. Hoffman. Newark, DE: International Reading Association.

Calfee, R., and Henry, M. K. 1996. Strategy and skill in early reading acquisition. In *Essays in Memory of Dina Feitelson*, ed. J. Shimron. Cresskill, NJ: Hampton Press.

Calfee, R., Henry, M. K., and Funderberg, J. 1988. A model for school change. In *Changing School Reading Programs*, eds. J. Samuels and D. Pearson. Newark, DE: International Reading Association.

Calfee, R., Lindamood, P., and Lindamood, C. 1973. Acoustic-phonetic skills and reading; Kindergarten through twelfth grade. *Journal of Educational Psychology* 64:293–98.

Calkins, L. M. 1983. *Lessons from a Child*. Portsmouth, NH: Heinemann.

Calkins, L. M. 1986. *The Art of Teaching Writing*. Portsmouth, NH: Heinemann.

Cardon, L. R., Smith, S. D., Fulker, D. W., Kimberling, W. J., Pennington, B. F., and DeFries, J. C. 1994. Quantitative trait locus for reading disability on chromosome 6. *Science* 266:276–79.

Carlisle, J. F. 1993. Selecting approaches to vocabulary instruction for the reading disabled. *Learning Disabilities Research and Practice* 8:97–105.

Carnine, D., Silbert, J., Kame'enui, E. J., and Tarver, S. G. 2004. *Direct Instruction Reading.* Columbus, OH: Merrill.

Carpenter, D. 1983. Spelling error profiles of able and disabled readers. *Journal of Learning Disabilities* 16:102–4.

Carreker. S. 2002. *Reading Readiness.* Dallas, TX: Neuhaus Education Center.

Catts, H. W. 1986. Speech production/phonological deficits in reading disordered children. *Journal of Learning Disabilities* 19:504–8.

Catts, H. W. 1989. Defining dyslexia as a developmental language disorder. *Annals of Dyslexia* 39:50–64.

Catts, H., and Vartiainen, T. 1993. *Sounds Abound.* East Moline, IL: LinguiSystems, Inc.

Center, Y., Wheldall, K., Freeman, L., Outhred, L., and McNaught, M. 1995. An evaluation of Reading Recovery. *Reading Research Quarterly* 30:240–63.

Chall, J. S. 1983a. *Learning to Read: The Great Debate.* New York: McGraw-Hill.

Chall, J. S. 1983b. *Stages of Reading Development.* New York: McGraw-Hill.

Chall, J. S. 1987. Two vocabularies for reading: Recognition and meaning. In *The Nature of Vocabulary Instruction*, eds. M. G. McKeown and M. E. Curtis. Hillsdale, NJ: Lawrence Erlbaum Associates.

Chall, J. S., Roswell, F. G., and Blumenthal, S. H. 1963. Auditory blending ability: A factor in success in beginning reading. *The Reading Teacher* 17:113–18.

Chall, J. S., and Stahl, S. 1985. Reading comprehension research in the past decade: Implications for educational publishing. *Book Research Quarterly* 1:95–102.

Childs, S. B., and Childs, R. S. 1971. *Sound Spelling.* Cambridge, MA: Educators Publishing Service.

Childs, S. B., and Childs, R. S. 1973. *The Childs Spelling System: The Rules.* Cambridge, MA: Educators Publishing Service.

Chomsky, C. 1971. Write first, read later. *Childhood Education* 47:296–99.

Chomsky, C. 1979. Approaching reading through invented spelling. In *Theory and Practice of Early Reading, Vol. 2*, eds. L. B. Resnick and P. A. Weaver. Hillsdale, NJ: Lawrence Erlbaum Associates.

Chomsky, N. 1972. *Language and Mind.* San Diego, CA: Harcourt Brace.

Cicci, R. 1983. Disorders of written language. In *Progress in Learning Disabilities: Vol. 5*, ed. H. Myklebust. New York: Grune and Stratton.

Clark, D. B. 1988. *Dyslexia: Theory and Practice of Remedial Instruction.* Parkton, MD: York Press.

Clark, D. B., and Uhry, J. K. 1995. *Dyslexia: Theory and Practice of Remedial Instruction.* Parkton, MD: York Press.

Clarke, L. K. 1988. Invented versus traditional spelling in first graders' writings: Effects on learning to spell and read. *Research in the Teaching of English* 22:281–309.

Clay, M. M. 1991. *Becoming Literate: The Construction of Inner Control.* Portsmouth, NH: Heinemann.

Clay, M. M. 1992. A second chance to learn literacy. In *The Assessment of Special Education Needs: International Perspectives*, ed. T. Cline. London: Routledge.

Clay, M. M. 1993a. *Observation Survey.* Portsmouth, NH: Heinemann.

Clay, M. M. 1993b. *Reading Recovery: A Guidebook for Teachers in Training.* Portsmouth, NH: Heinemann.

Cone, T. E., Wilson, L. R., Bradley, C. M., and Reese, J. H. 1985. Characteristics of LD students in Iowa: An empirical investigation. *Learning Disability Quarterly* 3(3):211–20.

Connors, C. K. 1978. Critical review of "Electroencephalographic and neuropsychological studies in dyslexia." In *Dyslexia: An Appraisal of Current Knowledge*, eds. A. L. Benton and D. Pearl. New York: Oxford University Press.

Cornoldi, C., and Oakhill, J. 1996. Eds. *Reading Comprehension Difficulties: Processes and Intervention*. Mahwah, NJ: Lawrence Erlbaum Associates.

Cowley, J. 1990. *Mrs. Wishy-washy*. Bothell,, WA: The Wright Group.

Cox, A. R. 1971. *Initial Reading Deck*. Cambridge, MA: Educators Publishing Service.

Cox, A. R. 1977. *Situation Spelling*. Cambridge, MA: Educators Publishing Service.

Cox, A. R. 1985. Alphabetic Phonics: An organization and expansion of Orton-Gillingham. *Annals of Dyslexia* 35:187–98.

Cox, A. R. 1989 *Situation Reading*. Cambridge, MA: Educators Publishing Service.

Cox, A. R. 1992. *Foundations for Literacy: Structures and Techniques*. Cambridge, MA: Educators Publishing Service.

Coyne, M. D., Kame'enui, E. J., Simmons, D. C., and Harn, B. A. 2004. Beginning reading intervention as inoculation or insulin: First-grade reading performance of strong responders to kindergarten intervention. *Journal of Learning Disabilities* 37:90–104.

Critchley, M. 1970. *The Dyslexic Child*. Springfield, IL: Thomas Publishing Company.

Cunningham, A., and Stanovich, K. 1990. Early spelling acquisition: Writing beats the computer. *Journal of Educational Psychology* 82:159–62.

Cunningham, P. M., and Cunningham, J. W. 1992. Making words: Enhancing the invented spelling-decoding connection. *The Reading Teacher* 42:106–15.

DeFord, D. E., Lyons, C. A., and Pinnell, G. S. Eds. 1991. *Bridges to Literacy: Learning from Reading Recovery*. Portsmouth, NH: Heinemann.

DeFord, D. E., Pinnell, G. S., and Lyons, C. December 1997. AmeriCorps for literacy and math. Paper presented at the annual meeting of the National Reading Conference, Scottsdale, AZ.

DeFries, J. C., Olson, R. K., Pennington, B. F., and Smith, S. D. 1991. Colorado reading project: An update. In *The Reading Brain: The Biological Basis of Dyslexia*, eds. D. Duane and D. Gray. Parkton, MD: York Press.

Denckla, M. B. 1978. Critical review of "Encephalographic and neuropsychological studies in dyslexia." In *Dyslexia: An Appraisal of Current Knowledge*, eds. A. L. Benton and D. Pearl. New York: Oxford University Press.

Denckla, M. B., and Cutting, L. E. 1999. History and significance of rapid automatized naming. *Annals of Dyslexia* 49:29–42.

Denckla, M. B., and Rudel, R. G. 1974. Rapid "automatized" naming of pictured objects. colors, letters, and numbers by normal children. *Cortex* 10:186–202.

Denckla, M. B., and Rudel, R. G. 1976a. Naming of object-drawings by dyslexic and other learning disabled children. *Brain and Language* 3:1–15.

Denckla, M. B., and Rudel, R. G. 1976b. Rapid automatized naming (RAN): Dyslexia differentiated from other learning disabilities. *Neuropsychologia* 14:471–79.

Denckla, M. B., LeMay, M., and Chapman, C. A. 1985. Few CT scan abnormalities found even in neurologically impaired learning disabled children. *Journal of Learning Disabilities* 18:132–36.

DeVilliers, P. A., and deVilliers, J. G. 1979. *Early Language*. Cambridge, MA: Harvard University Press.

Dickson, S. V., and Bursack, W. D. 1999. Implementing a model for preventing reading failure: A report from the field. *Learning Disabilities Research and Practice* 14:191–202.

Dolch, E. W. 1952. *Basic Sight Vocabulary Cards*. Champaign, IL: Garrard Publishing Co.

Dole, J. A., Duffy, G. G., Roehler, L. R., and Pearson, P. D. 1991. Moving from the old to the new: Research on reading comprehension instruction. *Review of Educational Research* 61:239–64.

Duane, D. D. 1983. Neurobiological correlates of reading disorders. *Journal of Educational Research* 77:5–15.

Durkin, D. 1978–1979. What classroom observations reveal about reading comprehension instruction. *Reading Research Quarterly* 14:481–533.

Dyer, P. 1992. Reading recovery: A cost-effectiveness and educational-outcomes analysis. *Educational Services Research Spectrum* 10:10–19.

Dykman, R. A., and Ackerman, P. T. 1991. Attention deficit disorder and specific reading disability: Separate but often overlapping disorders. *Journal of Learning Disabilities* 24:96–103.

Dyson, A. H. 2001. Writing and children's symbolic repertoires: Development unhinged. *Handbook of Early Literacy Education*, eds. S. B. Neuman and D. K. Dickinson. New York: The Guilford Press.

Eden, G. F., Stein, J. F., Wood, M. H., and Wood, F. B. 1995. Verbal and visual problems in reading disability. *Journal of Learning Disabilities* 28:272–90.

Eden, G. F., Wood, F. B., and Stein, J. F. 2003. Clock drawing in developmental dyslexia. *Journal of Learning Disabilities* 36:216–28.

Edwards, L. 2003. Writing instruction in kindergarten: Examining an emerging area of research for children with writing and reading difficulties. *Journal of Learning Disabilities* 36:136–48.

Ehri, L. C. 1989. Movement into word reading and spelling: How spelling contributes to reading. In *Reading and Writing Connections*, ed. J. M. Mason. Boston: Allyn and Bacon.

Ehri, L. C. 1992. Reconceptualizing the development of sight word reading and its relationship to recoding. In *Reading Acquisition*, eds. P. B. Gough, L. C. Ehri, and R. Treiman. Hillsdale, NJ: Lawrence Erlbaum Associates.

Ehri, L. C. 1995. Teachers need to know how word reading processes develop to teach reading effectively to beginners. In *Thinking and Literacy: The Mind at Work*, eds. C. N. Hedley, P. Antonacci, and M. Rabinowitz. Hillsdale, NJ: Lawrence Erlbaum Associates.

Ehri, L. C., Deffner, N. D., and Wilce, L. S. 1984. Pictorial mnemonics for phonics. *Journal of Educational Psychology* 76:880–93.

Ehri, L. C., and McCormick 1998. Phases of word learning: Implications for instruction with delayed and disabled readers. *Reading and Writing Quarterly: Overcoming Learning Difficulties* 14:135–63.

Ehri, L. C., Nunes, S. R., Stahl, S. A., and Willows, D. M. 2001. Systematic phonics instruction helps students learn to read: Evidence from the National Reading Panel's meta-analysis. *Review of Educational Research* 71:393–447.

Ehri, L. C., Nunes, S. R., Willows, D. M., Schuster, B. V., Yaghoub-Zadeh, Z., and Shanahan, T. 2001. Phonemic awareness instruction helps children learn to read: Evidence from the National Reading Panel's meta-analysis. *Reading Research Quarterly* 36:250–87.

Ehri, L. C., and Robbins, C. 1992. Beginners need some decoding skill to read words by analogy. *Reading Research Quarterly* 27:12–26.

Ehri, L. C., and Saltmarsh, J. 1995. Beginning readers outperform older disabled readers in learning to read words by sight. *Reading and Writing: An Interdisciplinary Journal* 7:295–326.

Ehri, L. C., and Sweet, J. 1991. Fingerpoint-reading of memorized text: What enables beginners to process the print? *Reading Research Quarterly* 26:442–62.

Ehri, L. C., and Wilce, L. S. 1985. Movement into reading: Is the first stage of printed word learning visual or phonetic? *Reading Research Quarterly* 20:163–79.

Ehri, L. C., and Wilce, L. S. 1987a. Cipher versus cue reading: An experiment in decoding acquisition. *Journal of Educational Psychology* 79:3–13.

Ehri, L. C., and Wilce, L. C. 1987b. Does learning to spell help beginners learn to read words? *Reading Research Quarterly* 22:47–65.

Elkind, J., Cohen, K., and Murray, C. 1993. Using computer-based readers to improve reading comprehension of students with dyslexia. *Annals of Dyslexia* 43:238–59.

Elkonin, D. B. 1963. The psychology of mastering the elements of reading. In *Educational Psychology in the U.S.S.R.*, eds. B. Simon and J. Simon. London: Routledge and Kegan Paul.

Elkonin, D. B. 1973. U.S.S.R. In *Comparative Reading*, ed. J. Downing. New York: Macmillan.

Enfield, M. L. 1976. An alternate classroom approach to meeting special learning needs of children with reading problems. Ph.D. diss., University of Minnesota, Minneapolis, MN.

Enfield, M. L., and Greene, V. E. 1981. There is a skeleton in every closet. *Bulletin of the Orton Society* 31:189–98.

Enfield, M. L., and Greene, V. E. 1983. An evaluation of the results of standardized testing of elementary Project Read and SLD students based on district wide tests administered in October, 1983. Bloomington, MN: Bloomington Public Schools.

Engelmann, S., Becker, W. C., Hanner, S., and Johnson, G. 1978. *Corrective Reading: Decoding B*. Chicago: Science Research Associates.

Engelmann, S., Becker, W. C., Hanner, S., and Johson, G. 1980. *Corrective Reading Series Guide*. Chicago: Science Research Associates.

Engelmann, S., and Bruner, E. C. 1983. *Reading Mastery I and II: DISTAR Reading*. Chicago: Science Research Associates.

Englert, C. S. 1990. Unraveling the mysteries of writing through strategy intervention. In *Intervention Research in Learning Disabilities*, eds. T. E. Scruggs and B. Y. L. Wong. New York: Springer-Verlag.

Englert, C. S., and Mariage, T. 1996. A socio-cultural perspective: Teaching ways-of-thinking and ways-of-talking in a literary community. *Learning Disabilities Research and Practice* 11:157–67.

Englert, C. S., Raphael, T. E., and Anderson, L. M. 1992. Socially mediated instruction: Improving students' knowledge and talk about writing. *Elementary School Journal* 92:411–49.

Englert, C. S., Raphael, T. E., Anderson, L. M., Gregg, S. L., and Anthony, H. M. 1989. Exposition: Reading, writing, and the metacognitive knowledge of learning disabled students. *Learning Disabilities Research* 5:5–24.

Englert, C. S., Raphael, T., Anderson, L., Anthony, H., Stevens, D., and Fear, K. 1991. Making strategies and self-talk visible: Cognitive strategy instruction in writing in regular and special education classrooms. *American Educational Research Journal* 28:337–73.

Englert, C. S., and Thomas, C. C. 1987. Sensitivity to text structure in reading and writing: A comparison of learning disabled and nonhandicapped students. *Learning Disability Quarterly* 10:93–105.

Epstein, M. H., and Cullinan, D. 1981. Project EXCEL: A behaviorally-oriented educational program for learning disabled pupils. *Education and Treatment of Children* 4:357–73.

Farnham-Diggory, S. 1986. Introduction to the third revised edition. In *The Writing Road to Reading*, eds. R. B. Spalding and W. T. Spalding. New York: Quill/William Morrow.

Farnham-Diggory, S. 1990. *Schooling*. Cambridge, MA: Harvard University Press.

Farnham-Diggory, S. 1992. *The Learning Disabled Child*. Cambridge, MA: Harvard University Press.

Felton, R., Naylor, C., and Wood, F. 1990. Neuropsychological profile of adult dyslexics. *Brain and Language* 39:485–97.

Felton, R., and Wood, F. 1989. Cognitive deficits in reading disability and attention deficit disorder. *Journal of Learning Disabilities* 22:2–13.

Fernald, G. M. 1943. *Remedial Techniques in Basic School Subjects*. New York: McGraw-Hill.

Fernald, G. M., and Keller, H. 1921. The effect of kinesthetic factors in development of word recognition in the case of non-readers. *Journal of Educational Research* 4:355–77.

Feuerstein, R. 1979. *The Dynamic Assessment of Retarded Performers: The Learning-Potential Assessment Device, Theory, Instruments, and Techniques.* Baltimore: University Park Press.

Fletcher, J. M., Francis, D. J., Shaywitz, S. E., Lyon, A. G. R., Foorman, B. R., Stuebing, K. K., and Shaywitz, B. A. 1998. Intelligent testing and the discrepancy model for children with learning disabilities. *Learning Disabilities Research and Practice* 13:186–203.

Flowers, D. L. 1993. Brain basis for dyslexia: A summary of work in progress. *Journal of Learning Disabilities* 26:575–82.

Foorman, B. R., Chen, D. T., Carlson, C., Moats, L., Francis, D. J., and Fletcher, J. M. 2003. The necessity of the alphabetic principle to phonemic awareness instruction. *Reading and Writing: An Interdisciplinary Journal* 16:289–324.

Foorman, B. R., Francis, D. J., Beeler, T., Winikates, D., and Fletcher, J. M. 1997. Early interventions for children with reading problems: Study designs and preliminary findings. *Learning Disabilities: A Multidisciplinary Journal* 8:63–71.

Foorman, B., Francis, D. J., and Fletcher, J. M. April 1995. Early interventions for children with reading disabilities and at risk for developing reading disabilities. Paper presented at the annual meeting of the American Educational Research Association in San Francisco.

Foorman, B. R., Francis, D. J., Fletcher, J. M., Schatschneider, C., and Mehta, P. 1998. The role of instruction learning to read: Preventing reading failure in at-risk children. *Journal of Educational Psychology* 90:37–55.

Foorman, B., Francis, D., Novy, D., and Liberman, D. 1991. How letter-sound instruction mediates progress in first-grade reading and spelling. *Journal of Educational Psychology* 83:456–69.

Foorman, B., Francis, D., Winikates, D., Mehta, P., Schatschneider, C., and Fletcher, J. 1997. Early interventions for children with reading disabilities. *Scientific Studies of Reading* 1:255–76.

Fountas, I. C., and Pinnell, G. S. 1996. *Guided Reading: Good First Teaching for All Children.* Portsmouth, NH: Heinemann.

Frankiewicz, R. G. 1984. *An Evaluation of the impact of the Alphabetic Phonics Program in Cypress Fairbanks Independent School District from 1981 through 1984.* Houston, TX: Neuhaus Foundation.

Frankiewicz, R. G. 1985. *An Evaluation of the Alphabetic Phonics Program Offered in the On-to-One Mode.* Houston. TX: Neuhaus Education Center.

Frederiksen, J. R., and others. 1983. *A Componential Approach to Training Reading Skills. Final Report.* Cambridge, MA: Bolt, Beranek, and Newman.

French, J., Ellsworth, N. J., and Amoruso, M. Z. 1995. *Reading and Learning Disabilities: Theory and Practice.* New York: Garland.

Frith, U. 1985. Beneath the surface of developmental dyslexia. In *Surface Dyslexia: Neuropsychological and Cognitive Studies of Phonological Reading,* eds. K. E. Patterson, J. C. Marshall, and M. Coltheart. London: Lawrence Erlbaum Associates, Ltd.

Frith, U. 1986. A developmental framework for developmental dyslexia. *Annals of Dyslexia* 36:69–81.

Frostig, M. 1967. Testing as a basis for educational therapy. *Journal of Special Education* 2:15–34.

Frostig, M., Lefever, D. W., and Whittlesey, J. R. B. 1964. *The Marianne Frostig Developmental Test of Visual Perception.* Palo Alto, CA: Consulting Psychologists Press.

Fuchs, D. 2003. On responsiveness-to-intervention as a valid method of identification: Some things we need to know. *Perspectives* 29:28–31.

Fuchs, L. S., and Fuchs, D. 1998. Treatment validity: A unifying concept for reconceptualizing the identification of learning disabilities. *Learning Disabilities Research and Practice* 13:204–19.

Furner, B. A. 1983. Developing handwriting ability: A perceptual learning process. *Topics in Learning and Learning Disabilities* 3:41–54.

Galaburda, A. M. 1983. Developmental dyslexia: Current anatomical research. *Annals of Dyslexia* 33:41–54.

Galaburda, A. M. 1985. Develpmental dyslexia: A review of biological interactions. *Annals of Dyslexia* 35:21–34.

Galaburda, A. M., and Kemper, T. L. 1979. Cytoarchitectonic abnormalities in developmental dyslexia: A case study. *Annals of Neurology* 6:94–100.

Galaburda, A. M., Rosen, G. F., and Sherman, G. D. 1989. The neural origin of developmental dyslexia: Implications for medicine, neurology and cognition. In *From Reading to Neurons*, ed. A. M. Galaburda. Cambridge, MA: The MIT Press.

Gambrell, B., and Koskinen, P. S. 2002. Imagery: A strategy for enhancing comprehension. In *Comprehension Instruction: Research-based Best Practices*, eds. C. C. Block and M. Pressley. New York: The Guilford Press.

Ganschow, L. 1984. Analysis of written language of a language learning disabled dyslexic college student and instructional implications. *Annals of Dyslexia* 34:271–84.

Gardner, H. 1983. *Frames of Mind: The Theory of Multiple Intelligences*. New York: Basic Books.

Gaskins, I. W., Downer, M. A., Anderson, R. C., Cunningham, P. M., Gaskins, R. W., Schommer, M., and Teachers of the Benchmark School. 1988. A metacognitive approach to phonics: Using what you know to decode what you don't know. *Remedial and Special Education* 9:36–41, 66.

Gaskins, I. W., Downer, M. A., and Gaskins, R. W. 1986. *Introduction to the Benchmark School Word Identification/Vocabulary Development Program*. Media, PA: Benchmark School.

Gentry, J. R. 1982. An analysis of developmental spelling in GYNS AT WRK. *The Reading Teacher* 36:192–200.

Gentry, J. R., and Gillet, J. W. 1993. *Teaching Kids to Spell*. Portsmouth, NH: Heinemann.

Gersten, R., Darch, C., and Gleason, M. 1988. Effectiveness of a direct instruction academic kindergarten for low-income students. *The Elementary School Journal* 89:227–40.

Gersten, R., Woodward, J., and Darch, C. 1986. Direct Instruction: A research-based approach to curriculum design and teaching. *Exceptional Children* 53:17–31.

Geschwind, N. 1982. Why Orton was right. *Annals of Dyslexia* 32:13–30.

Geschwind, N. 1983. Biological associations of left-handedness. *Annals of Dyslexia* 33:29–40.

Geschwind, N. 1986. The biology of dyslexia: The unfinished manuscript. In *Biobehavioral Measures of Dyslexia*, eds. D. B. Gray and J. F. Kavanagh. Parkton, MD: York Press.

Geschwind, N., and Behan, P. 1982. Left-handedness: Association with immune disease, migraine, and developmental learning disorder. *Proceedings of the National Academy of Science* 79:5097–100.

Gillingham, A., and Stillman, B. 1960. *Remedial Training for Children with Specific Disability in Reading, Writing, and Penmanship*. Cambridge, MA: Educators Publishing Service.

Gillon, G., and Dodd, B. 1994. A prospective study of the relationship between phonological, semantic and syntactic skills and specific reading disability. *Reading and Writing: An Interdisciplinary Journal* 6:321–45.

Ginsburg, H. P., and Baroody, A. J. 2003. *Test of Early Mathematics Ability*. Austin, TX: PRO-ED.

Gittelman, R. 1983. Treatment of reading disorders. In *Developmental Neuropsychiatry*, ed. M. Rutter. New York: Guilford Press.

Goatley, V. J. 1996. The participation of a student identified as learning disabled in a regular education book club: The case of Stark. *Reading and Writing Quarterly* 12:195–214.

Goatley, V. J., Brock, C. H., and Raphael, T. E. 1995. Diverse learners participating in regular education "book clubs." *Reading Research Quarterly* 30:353–80.

Goatley, V. J., and Levine, J. 1997. Participating in student-led book clubs: The case of Jennifer. *Language and Literacy Spectrum* 7:14–18.

Godfrey, J. J., Syrdal-Lasky, A. K., Millaj, K. K., and Knox, C. M. 1981. Performance of dyslexic children on speech perception tests. *Journal of Experimental Child Psychology* 32:401–24.

Goodman, K. 1967. Reading: A psycholinguistic guessing game. *Journal of the Reading Specialist* 6:126–35.

Goodman, K. 1993. *Phonics Phacts*. Portsmouth, NH: Heinemann.

Gordon, J., Vaughn, S., and Schumm, J. S. 1993. Spelling interventions: A review of literature and implications for instruction for students with learning disabilities. *Learning Disabilities Research and Practice* 8:175–81.

Goswami, U. 1986. Children's use of analogy in learning to read: A developmental study. *Journal of Experimental Child Psychology* 42:73–83.

Goswami, U. 1988. Orthographic analogies and reading development. *Quarterly Journal of Experimental Psychology* 40A:239–68.

Goswami, U., and Mead, F. 1992. Onset and rime awareness and analogies in reading. *Reading Research Quarterly* 27:152–62.

Gough, P., and Hillinger, M. L. 1980. Learning to read: An unnatural act. *Bulletin of The Orton Society* 30:179–96.

Gough, P., and Tunmer, W. E. 1986. Decoding, reading and reading disability. *Remedial and Special Education* 7:6–10.

Goulandris, N. K., and Snowling, M. J. 1991. Visual memory deficits: A plausible cause of developmental dyslexia? Evidence from a single case study. *Cognitive Neuropsychology* 8:127–54.

Graham, S., and Weintraub, N. 1996. A review of handwriting research: Progress and prospects from 1980–1994. *Educational Psychology Review* 8:7–87.

Graham, S., Harris, K. R., and Fink, B. 2000. Is handwriting causally related to learning to write? Treatment of handwriting problems in beginning writers. *Journal of Educational Psychology* 92:620–33.

Graves, D. H. 1978. *Balance the Basics: Let Them Write*. New York: Ford Foundation.

Graves, D. H. 1983. *Writing: Teachers and Children at Work*. Portsmouth, NH: Heinemann.

Graves, D. H., and Stuart, V. 1985. *Write From the Start*. New York: New American Library.

Greenbaum, C. R. 1987. *The Spellmaster Assessment and Teaching System*. Austin, TX: PRO-ED.

Greene, V. E., and Enfield, M. L. 1981. *Project Read Affix Guide*. Bloomington, MN: Bloomington Public Schools.

Greene, V. E., and Enfield, M. L. 1985a. *Project Read Reading Guide: Phase I*. Bloomington, MN: Bloomington Public Schools.

Greene, V. E., and Enfield, M. L. 1985b. *Project Read Reading Guide: Phase II*. Bloomington, MN: Bloomington Public Schools.

Guyer, B. P., Banks, S. R., and Guyer, K. E. 1993. Spelling improvement by college students who are dyslexic. *Annals of Dyslexia* 43:186–93.

Hammill, D. 1998. *Detroit Tests of Learning Aptitude–4*. Austin, TX: PRO-ED.

Hanna, P. R., Hodges, R. E., Hanna, J. L., and Rudolph, E. H. 1966. Phoneme-grapheme correspondence as cues to spelling improvement. Washington, DC: Department of Health, Education, and Welfare, Office of Education.

Hansen, J. 1987. *When Writers Read*. Portsmouth, NH: Heinemann.

Hansen, J. 1998. "Evaluation is all day, noticing what is happening:" Multifaceted evaluation of readers. In *Fragile Evidence: A Critique of Reading Assessment*, eds. S. Murphy, P. Shannon, P. Johnston, and J. Hansen. Mahwah, NJ: Erlbaum.

Hardyck, C., and Petrinovich, L. F. 1977. Left-handedness. *Psychological Bulletin* 84:385–404.

Haring, N. G., and Bateman, B. 1977. *Teaching the Learning Disabled Child*. Englewood Cliffs, NJ: Prentice-Hall.

Haring, N. G., Bateman, B., and Carnine, D. 1977. Direct Instruction—DISTAR. In *Teaching the Learning Disabled Child*, eds. N. G. Haring and B. Bateman. Englewood Cliffs, NJ: Prentice-Hall.

Harris, T. L., and Hodges, R. 1995. *The Literacy Dictionary: The Vocabulary of Reading and Writing*. Newark, DE: International Reading Association.

Harste, J. C. 1985. Becoming a nation of language learners: Beyond risk. In *Toward Practical Theory: A State of Practice Assessment of Reading Comprehension Instruction. Final Report*, eds. J. C. Harste and D. Stevens. Bloomington, IN: Indiana University.

Harwayne, S. 1992. *Lasting Impressions*. Portsmouth, NH: Heinemann.

Heibert, E. H., Colt, J. M., Catto, S. L., and Gary, E. C. 1992. Reading and writing of first-grade students in a restructured chapter 1 program. *American Educational Research Journal* 29:545–72.

Heibert, E., and Taylor, B. 2000. Beginning reading instruction: Research on early interventions. In *Handbook of Reading Research, Vol. III*, eds. M. Kamil, P. Mosenthal, P. D. Pearson, and R. Barr. Mahwah, NJ: Lawrence Erlbaum Associates.

Henderson, E. H. 1990. *Teaching Spelling*. Boston: Houghton-Mifflin.

Henderson, E., and Beers, J. W. 1980. *Developmental and Cognitive Aspects of Learning to Spell*. Newark, DE: International Reading Association.

Henk, W. A., Helfeldt, J. P., and Platt, J. M. 1986. Developing reading fluency in learning disabled students. *Teaching Exceptional Children* 12:202–6.

Henry, M. 1988. Beyond phonics: Integrated decoding and spelling instruction based on word origin and structure. *Annals of Dyslexia* 38:259–77.

Henry, M. 1989. Children's word structure knowledge: Implications for decoding and spelling instruction. *Reading and Writing: An Interdisciplinary Journal* 2:135–52.

Henry, M. 1990. *Words: Integrated Decoding and Spelling Instruction Based on Word Origin and Word Structure*. Los Gatos, CA: Lex Press.

Henry, M., and Redding, N. C. 1990. *Tutor 1, Tutor 2, Tutor 3*. Los Gatos, CA: Lex Press.

Herr, C. M. Spring 1984. Using corrective reading with adults. *Direct Instruction News* 3–4.

Hill, J. R. 1981. *Measurement and Evaluation in the Classroom*. Columbus, OH: Merrill.

Hillocks, G. 1984. What works in teaching composition: A meta-analysis of treatment studies. *American Journal of Education* 93:133–70.

Hinshelwood, J. 1896. A case of dyslexia: A peculiar form of Word Blindness. *Lancet* 2:1451–4.

Hinshelwood, J. 1917. *Congenital Word Blindness*. London: H. K. Lewis.

Hirsch, E., and Niedermeyer, F. C. 1973. The effects of tracing prompts and discrimination training on kindergarten handwriting performance. *Journal of Educational Research* 67:81–83.

Hiscock, M., and Kinsbourne, M. 1982. Laterality and dyslexia: A critical view. *Annals of Dyslexia* 32:177–228.

Hohn, W. E., and Ehri, L. C. 1983. Do alphabet letters help prereaders acquire phonemic segmentation skill? *Journal of Educational Psychology* 75:752–62.

Holdaway, D. 1979. *The Foundations of Literacy*. Portsmouth, NH: Heinemann.

Hook, P. E., Macaruso, P., and Jones, S. 2001. Efficacy of Fast ForWord training on facilitating acquisition of reading skills by children with reading difficulties—A longitudinal study. *Annals of Dyslexia* 51:75–96.

Hooper, S. R., Montgomery, J., Swartz, C., Reed, M. S., Sandler, A.D., Levine, M. D., Watson, T. E., and Wasileski, T. 1994. Measurement of written language expression. In *Frames of Reference for the Assessment of Learning Disabilities*, ed. G. R. Lyon. Baltimore: Paul H. Brookes Publishing Co.

Hoover, W. A. October 1994. The simple view of reading: Analyses based on a monolingual sample. Paper presented at NATO Advanced Study Institute: Cognitive and Linguistic Bases of Reading, Writing, and Spelling, Alvor-Algarve, Portugal.

Horn, E. 1960. Spelling. In *Encyclopedia for Educational Research*, ed. W. S. Monroe. New York: Macmillan.

Howard, M. 1982. Utilizing oral-motor feedback in auditory conceptualization. *Journal of Educational Neuropsychology* 2:24–35.

Howard, M. 1986. Effects of pre-reading training in auditory conceptualization on subsequent reading achievement. Ph.D. diss., Brigham Young University.

Hulme, C. 1981. *Reading Retardation and Multi-Sensory Teaching*. London: Routledge and Kegan Paul.

Hulme, C. 1988. The implausibility of low-level visual deficits as a cause of children's reading difficulties. *Cognitive Neuropsychology* 5:369–74.

Hulme, C., and Bradley, L. 1984. An experimental study of multisensory teaching with normal and retarded readers. In *Dyslexia: A Global Issue*, eds. R. Malatesha and H. Whitaker. The Hague: Martinus Nijhoff.

Hunt-Berg, M., Rankin, J. L., and Beukelman, D. R. 1994. Ponder the possibilities: Computer-supported writing for struggling writers. *Learning Disabilities Research and Practice* 9:169–78.

Hutcheson, L., Selig, H., and Young, N. 1990. A success story: A large urban district offers a working model for implementing multisensory teaching into the resource and regular classroom. *Annals of Dyslexia* 40:79–96.

Inhelder, B., and Piaget, J. 1958. *The Growth of Logical Thinking from Childhood to Adolescence*. New York: Basic Books.

Institute for Training and Research in Auditory Conceptualization (INTRAC). 1983. Santa Monica Preventive Study. San Luis Obispo, CA.

International Dyslexia Association. Winter 2002. What is dyslexia? *Perspectives* 52:9.

Iverson, S., and Tunmer, W. E. 1993. Phonological processing skills and the reading recovery program. *Journal of Educational Psychology* 85:112–26.

Jenkins, J. R., Johnson, E., and Hileman, J. 2004. When is reading also writing: Sources of individual differences on the new reading performance assessments. *Scientific Studies of Reading* 1:125–52.

Jenkins, J. R., Peyton, J. A., Sanders, E. A., and Vadasy, P. F. 2004. Effects of reading decodable texts in supplemental first-grade tutoring. *Scientific Studies of Reading* 8:53–85.

Jensen, A. R. 1980. *Bias in Mental Testing*. New York: Macmillan.

Jimerson, S. R., and Kaufman, A. M. 2003. Reading, writing, and retention: A primer on grade retention research. *The Reading Teacher* 56:622–35.

Johnson, D. J., and Carlisle, J. F. 1996. A study of handwriting in written stories of normal and learning disabled children. *Reading and Writing: An Interdisciplinary Journal* 8:45–59.

Johnson, W. T. 1977. *The Johnson Handwriting Program*. Cambridge, MA: Educators Publishing Service.

Jorm, A. F. 1983. Specific reading retardation and working memory: A review. *British Journal of Psychology* 74:311–42.

Juel, C., and Roper-Schneider, D. 1985. The influence of basal readers on first grade reading. *Reading Research Quarterly* 20:134–52.

Just, M. A., and Carpenter, P. A. 1980. Theory of reading: From eye fixations to comprehension. *Psychological Review* 87:3329–54.

Kame'enui, E. J., Simmons, D. C., Good, R. H., and Harn, B. A. 2001. The use of fluency-based measures in early identification and evaluation of intervention efficacy in schools. In *Dyslexia, Fluency, and the Brain*, ed. M. Wolf. Baltimore: York Press.

Kamil, M. L., Mosenthal, P. B., Pearson, P. D., and Barr, R. eds. 2000. *Handbook of Reading Research, Volume III*. Mahwah, NJ: Lawrence Erlbaum Associates, Publishers.

Kaminski, R. A., and Good, R. H., III. 1996. Toward a technology for assessing basic early literacy skills. *School Psychology Review* 25:215–27.

Karweit, N. L., Coleman, M. A., Waclawiw, I., and Petza, R, 1990. *Story Telling and Retelling (STaR): Teachers' Manual*. Baltimore, MD: Johns Hopkins University, Center for Research on Effective Schooling for Disadvantaged Students.

Kavanagh, J. F., and Truss, T. J. Eds. 1988. *Learning Disabilities: Proceedings of the National Conference*. Parkton, MD: York Press.

Keogh, B. D., and Pelland, M. 1985. Vision training revisited. *Journal of Learning Disabilities* 18:228–36.

Kibel, M., and Miles, T. R. 1994. Phonological errors in spelling of taught dyslexic children. In *Reading Development and Dyslexia*, eds. C. Hulme and M. Snowling. San Diego, CA: Singular Publishing Group.

King, D. H. 1985. *Writing Skills for the Adolescent*. Cambridge, MA: Educators Publishing Service.

King, D. H. 1986. *Keyboarding Skills*. Cambridge, MA: Educators Publishing Service.

Kinsbourne, M., and Hiscock, M. 1981. Cerebral lateralization and cognitive development: Conceptual and methodological issues. In *Neuropsychological Assessment of the School-Age Child*, eds. G. W. Hynd and J. E. Obrzut. New York: Grune and Stratton.

Kirk, U. 1981. The development and use of rules in the acquisition of perceptual motor skills. *Child Development* 52:299–305.

LaBerge, D., and Samuels, S. J. 1974. Toward a theory of automatic information processing in reading. *Cognitive Psychology* 6:293–323.

Leslie, L., and Caldwell, J. 2001. *Qualitative Reading Inventory*. New York: Longman.

Levin, J. R. 1985. Educational applications of mnemonic pictures: Possibilities beyond your wildest imagination. In *Imagery in Education: Imagery in the Educational Process*, eds. A. A. Sheikh and K. S Sheikh. Farmingdale, NY: Baywood.

Liberman, I. Y. 1973. Segmentation of the spoken word and reading acquisition. *Bulletin of The Orton Society* 23:65–77.

Liberman, I. Y. 1984. A language-directed view of reading and its disabilities. *Thalamus* 4:1–41.

Liberman, I. Y., Liberman, A. M., Mattingly, I., and Shankweiler, D. 1983. Orthography and the beginning reader. In *Orthography, Reading, and Dyslexia*, eds. J. P. Kavanagh and R. L. Venezky. Baltimore: University Park Press.

Liberman, I. Y., and Shankweiler, D. 1979. Speech, the alphabet, and teaching to read. In *Theory and Practice of Early Reading, Vol. 2*, eds. L. B. Resnick and P. A. Weaver. Hillsdale, NJ: Lawrence Erlbaum Associates.

Liberman, I. Y., and Shankweiler, D. 1985. Phonology and the problems of learning to read and write. *Remedial and Special Education* 6:8–17.

Liberman, I. Y., Shankweiler, D., Fischer, F. W., and Carter, B. 1974. Explicit syllable and phoneme segmentation in the young child. *Journal of Experimental Child Psychology* 18:201–12.

Liberman, I. Y., Shankweiler, D., Liberman, A. M., Fowler, C., and Fischer, F. W. 1977. Phonetic segmentation and recoding in the beginning reader. In *Toward a Psychology of Reading*, eds. A. S. Rober and D. L. Scarborough. Hillsdale, NJ: Lawrence Erlbaum Associates.

Lichter, J. H., and Roberge, L. P. 1979. First grade intervention for reading achievement of high risk children. *Bulletin of The Orton Society* 29:238–44.

Lindamood, C. H., and Lindamood, P. C. 1975. *The A.D.D. Program, Auditory Discrimination in Depth: Books 1 and 2.* Austin, TX: PRO-ED.

Lindamood, C. H., and Lindamood, P. C. 2004. *The LAC Test: Lindamood Auditory Conceptualization Test.* Austin, TX: PRO-ED.

Lindamood, P. C. 1994. Issues in researching the link between phonological awareness, learning disabilities, and spelling. In *Frames of Reference for the Assessment of Learning Disabilities*, ed. G. R. Lyon. Baltimore: Paul H. Brookes Publishing Co.

Lindamood, P. C., Bell, N., and Lindamood, P. 1992. Issues in phonological awareness assessment. *Annals of Dyslexia* 42:242–59.

Lindamood, P. C., and Lindamood, C. H. 1980. Diagnosing and remediating auditory conceptual dysfunction. *Proceedings of the 18th Congress of the International Association of Logopedics and Phoniatrics* 2:148–77.

Lindamood, P., and Lindamood, P. 1998. *The Lindamood Phoneme Sequencing Program for Reading, Spelling, and Speech (LiPS).* Austin, TX: PRO-ED.

Lindamood, P., and Lindamood, P. 2004. *Lindamood-Bell Auditory Conceptualization Test–Third Edition.* Austin, TX: PRO-ED.

Livingstone, M. 1993. Parallel processing in the visual system and the brain: Is one subsystem selectively affected in dyslexia? In *Dyslexia and Development: Neurobiological Aspects of Extra-Ordinary Brains*, ed. A. M. Galaburda. Cambridge, MA: Harvard University Press.

Lloyd, J., Epstein, M., and Cullinan, D. 1981. Direct teaching for learning disabilities. In *Developmental Theory and Research in Learning Disabilities*, eds. J. Gottlieb and S. S. Strichart. Baltimore: University Park Press.

Lovegrove, W. 1992. The visual deficit hypothesis. In *Learning Disabilities: Nature, Theory, and Treatment*, eds. N. Singh and I. Beale. New York: Springer-Verlag.

Lovegrove, W. J., and Williams, M. J. 1993. Visual temporal processing deficits in specific reading disability. In *Visual Processes in Reading and Reading Disabilities*, eds. D. M. Willows, R. S. Kruk, and E. Corcos. Hillsdale, NJ: Lawrence Erlbaum Associates.

Lovett, M., Lacerenza, L., Borden, S. L., Frijters, J. C., Steinbach, K. A., and De Palma, M. 2000. Components of effective remediation for developmental reading disabilities: Combining phonological and strategy-based instruction to improve outcomes. *Journal of Educational Psychology* 92:263–83.

Lovett, M., and Steinbach, K. 1997. The effectiveness of remedial programs for reading disabled children of different ages: Does the benefit decrease for older children? *Learning Disabilities Quarterly* 20:189–210.

Lovett, M., Warren-Chaplin, P. M., Ransby, M. J., and Borden, S. L. 1990. Training the word recognition skills of reading disabled children: Treatment and transfer effects. *Journal of Educational Psychology* 82:769–80.

Lovitt, T. C., and DeMier, D. M. 1984. An evaluation of the Slingerland method with LD youngsters. *Journal of Learning Disabilities* 17:267–72.

Lubs, H., Duara, R., Levin, B., Jallad, B., Lubs, M., Rabin, M., Kushch, A., and Gross-Glenn, K. 1991. Dyslexia subtypes: Genetics, behavior, and brain imaging. In *The Reading Brain: The Biological Basis of Dyslexia*, eds. D. D. Drake and D. B. Gray. Parkton, MD: York Press.

Lubs, H., Rabin, M., Feldman, E., Jallud, B. J., Kushch, A., and Gross-Glenn, K. 1993. Familial dyslexia and medical findings in eleven three-generation families. *Annals of Dyslexia* 43:44–60.

Lundberg, I., Frost, J., and Petersen, O. P. 1988. Effects of an extensive program for stimulating phonological awareness in preschool children. *Reading Research Quarterly* 23:263–84.

Lyon, G. R. 1994. Ed. *Frames of Reference for the Assessment of Learning Disabilities.* Baltimore: Paul H. Brookes Publishing Co.

Lyon, G. R. 1995. Research initiatives in learning disabilities: Contributions from scientists supported by the National Institute of Child Health and Human Development. *Journal of Child Neurology* 10:120–26.

Lyon, G. R., Shaywitz, S. E., and Shaywitz, B. A. 2003. A definition of dyslexia. *Annals of Dyslexia* 53:1–14.

Lyons, C. A., Pinnell, G. S., and DeFord, D. E. 1993. *Partners in Learning: Teachers and Children in Reading Recovery.* New York: Teachers College Press.

MacArthur, C. A., and Graham, S. 1988. Learning disabled students composing under three methods of text production: Handwriting, word processing, and dictation. *The Journal of Special Education* 21:22–42.

MacArthur, C. A., and Schneiderman, B. 1986. Learning disabled students' difficulties in learning to use a word processor: Implications for instruction and software evaluation. *Journal of Learning Disabilities* 19:248–53.

MacArthur, C. A., Schwartz, S. S., and Graham, S. 1991. A model for writing instruction: Integrating word processing and strategy instruction into a process approach to writing. *Learning Disabilities Research and Practice* 6:230–36.

Maclean, M., Bryant, P. E., and Bradley, L. 1987. Rhymes, nursery rhymes, and reading in early childhood. *Merrill-Palmer Quarterly* 33:255–81.

Madden, N. A. 1995. *Reading Roots: Teachers' Manual.* Baltimore: Johns Hopkins University, Center for Research on Effective Schooling for Disadvantaged Students.

Madden, N. A., Slavin, R. E., Farnish, A. M., Livingston, M. A., Calderon, M., and Stevens, R. J. 1996. *Reading Wings: Teachers' Manual.* Baltimore: Johns Hopkins University, Center for Research on the Education of Students Placed at Risk.

Madden, N. A., Slavin, R. E., Karweit, N. L., Dolan, L. J., and Wasik, B. A. 1993. Success for all: Longitudinal effects of a restructuring program for inner-city elementary schools. *American Educational Research Journal* 30:123–48.

Madden, N. A., Wasik, B. A., and Petza, R. 1989. *Writing from the Heart: A Writing Process Approach for First and Second Graders.* Baltimore: Johns Hopkins University, Center for Research on Effective Schooling for Disadvantaged Students.

Makar, B. W. 1995. *Mac and Tab Primary Phonics Series.* Cambridge, MA: Educators Publishing Service.

Mann, V. A., and Liberman, I. Y. 1984. Phonological awareness and verbal short-term memory. *Journal of Learning Disabilities* 17:592–99.

Mann, V. A., Liberman, I. Y., and Shankweiler, D. 1980. Children's memory for sentences and word strings in relation to reading ability. *Memory and Cognition* 8:329-35.

Mann, V. A., Shankweiler, D., and Smith, S. 1984. The association between comprehension of spoken sentences and early reading ability: The role of phonetic representation. *Journal of Child Language* 11:627–43.

Mann, V. A., Tobin, P., and Wilson, R. 1987. Measuring phonological awareness through the invented spellings of kindergarten children. *Merrill-Palmer Quarterly* 33:365-91.

Mannis, F. R., Seidenberg, M. S., and Doi, L. M. 1999. See Dick RAN: Rapid naming and the longitudinal prediction of reading subskills in first and second graders. *Scientific Study of Reading* 3:129–57.

Maria, K. 1987. A new look at comprehension instruction for disabled readers. *Annals of Dyslexia* 37:264–78.

Maria, K. 1990. *Reading Comprehension Instruction: Issues and Strategies.* Parkton, MD: York Press.

Markwardt, F. C. 1989. *Peabody Individualized Achievement Test–Revised.* Circle Pines, MN: American Guidance.

Marsh, G., Freidman, M., Welch, V., and Desberg, P. 1981. A cognitive-developmental theory of reading acquisition. In *Reading Research: Advances in Theory and Practice: Vol. 3*, eds. G. Mackinnon and T. G. Waller. New York: Academic Press.

Martin, J. H. 1985. The Writing to Read system and reading difficulties: Some preliminary observations. In *Understanding Learning Disabilities: International and Multidisciplinary Views*, eds. D. Duane and C. K. Leong. New York: Plenum Press.

Martin, J. H., and Friedberg, A. 1986. *Writing to Read*. New York: Warner Books.

Martinez, M., Roser, N., and Strecker, S. 1999. " I never thought I could be a star": A readers theatre ticket to fluency. *The Reading Teacher* 52:326–34.

Masonheimer, P. E., Drum, P. A., and Ehri, L. C. 1984. Does environmental print identification lead children into word reading? *Journal of Reading Behavior* 16:257–72.

McCulloch, C. 1985. The Slingerland approach: Is it effective in a specific language disability classroom? M.A. thesis, Seattle Pacific University, Seattle, WA.

McCully, E. A. 1988. *The Grandma Mix-up*. New York: Harper.

McMahon, S. I., and Goatley, V. J. 1995. Fifth graders helping peers discuss texts in student-led groups. *Journal of Educational Research* 89:23–35.

McMahon, S. I., Raphael, T. E. with Goatley, V. J., and Pardo, L. S. 1997. *The Book Club Connection: Literacy Learning and Classroom Talk*. New York: Teachers College Press.

Merzenich, M., Jenkins, W. M., Johnston, Schreiner, C., Miller, S. L., and Tallal, P. 1996. Temporal Processing deficits of language-learning impaired children ameliorated by training. *Science* 271:77–81.

Metzger, R. L., and Werner, D. B. 1984. Use of visual training for reading disabilities: A review. *Pediatrics* 73:824–29.

Meyer, L. A. 1984. Long-term academic effects of the direct instruction project Follow-Through. *Elementary School Journal* 84:380–94.

Meyer, L. A., Gersten, R. M., and Gutkin, J. 1983. Direct instruction: A project follow-through success story in an inner-city school. *Elementary School Journal* 84:241–52.

Moats, L. C. 1983. A comparison of the spelling errors of older dyslexic and second grade normal children. *Annals of Dyslexia* 33:121–39.

Moats, L. C. 1993. Spelling error interpretation: Beyond the phonetic/dysphonetic dichotomy. *Annals of Dyslexia* 43:174–85.

Moats, L. C. 1994a. Assessment of spelling. In *Frames of Reference for the Assessment of Learning Disabilities*, ed. G. R. Lyon. Baltimore: Paul H. Brookes Publishing Co.

Moats, L. C. 1994b. The missing foundation in teacher education: Knowledge of the structure of spoken and written language. *Annals of Dyslexia* 44:81–102.

Moats, L. C. 1995. *Spelling: Development, Disabilities, and Instruction*. Baltimore: York Press.

Moats, L. C. 2000. *Speech to Print: Language Essentials for Teachers*. Baltimore: Paul H. Brookes Publishing Company.

Montessori, M. 1915. *The Montessori Method*. London: Heinemann.

Montessori, M. 1964. *The Montessori Method*. New York: Shocken Books.

Morais, J. Cary, L., Alegria, J., and Bertelson, P. 1979. Does awareness of speech as a sequence of phones arise spontaneously? *Cognition* 7:323–31.

Morris, D. 1983. Concept of word and phoneme awareness in the beginning reader. *Research in the Teaching of English* 17:359–73.

Morris, D. 1993. The relationship between children's concept of word in text and phoneme awareness in learning to read: A longitudinal study. *Research in the Teaching of English* 27:133-53.

Morris, D. 1999. *Case Studies in Teaching Beginning Readers: The Howard Street Tutoring Manual*. New York: Guilford Press.

Morris, D., Bloodgood, J. W., Lomax, R. G., and Perney, J. 2003. Developmental steps in learning to read: A longitudinal study in kindergarten and first grade. *Reading Research Quarterly* 38:302-28.

Morris, D., and Perney, J. 1984. Developmental spelling as a predictor of first-grade reading achievement. *The Elementary School Journal* 84:441–57.

Morris, D., Shaw, B., and Perney, J. 1990. Helping low readers in grades 2 and 3: An after-school volunteer tutoring program. *Elementary School Journal* 91:133–50.

Nagy, W. E. 1988. *Teaching Vocabulary to Improve Reading Comprehension*. Urbana, IL: NCTE.

Nagy, W., and Herman, P. 1987. Breadth and depth of vocabulary knowledge: Implications for acquisition and instruction. In *The Nature of Vocabulary Acquisition*, eds. M. G. McKeown and M. E. Curtis. Hillsdale, NJ: Lawrence Erlbaum Associates.

Nagy, W., and Scott, J. 2000. Vocabulary processes. In *Handbook of Reading Research*, *Vol. III*, eds. M. Kamil, P. Mosenthal, P. D. Pearson, and R. Barr. Mahwah, NJ: Lawrence Erlbaum Associates.

National Reading Panel. 2000. *Report of the National Reading Panel: Teaching Children to Read: An Evidence-based Assessment of the Scientific Research Literature on Reading and its Implications for Reading Instruction*. Rockville, MD: NICHD Clearinghouse.

Nockleby, D. M., and Galbraith, G. G. 1984. Developmental dyslexia subtypes and the Boder Test of Reading-Spelling Patterns. *Journal of Psychoeducational Assessment* 2:91–100.

Notari-Syverson, A., O'Connor, R. E., and Vadasy, P. F. 1998. *Ladders to Literacy: A Preschool Activity Book*. Baltimore: Paul H. Brookes Publishing Company.

O'Connor, P. D., Sofo, F., Kendall, L., and Olsen, G. 1990. Reading disabilities and the effects of colored filters. *Journal of Learning Disabilities* 23:597–603.

O'Connor, R., Jenkins, J., and Slocum, T. 1995. Transfer among phonological tasks in kindergarten: Essential instructional content. *Journal of Educational Psychology* 87:202–17.

O'Connor, R., Notari-Syverson, A., and Vadasy, P. 1996. Ladders to literacy: The effects of teacher-led phonological activities for kindergarten children with and without disabilities. *Exceptional Children* 63:117–30.

O'Connor, R. E., Notari-Syverson, A., and Vadasy, P. F. 1998a. *Ladders to Literacy: A Kindergarten Activity Book*. Baltimore: Paul H. Brookes Publishing Company.

O'Connor, R., Notari-Syverson, A., and Vadasy, P. 1998b. First-grade effects of teacher-led phonological activities in kindergarten for children with mild disabilities: A follow-up study. *Learning Disabilities Research and Practice* 13:43–52.

Oakhill, J., and Garnham, A. 1988. *Becoming a Skilled Reader*. Oxford: Basil Blackwell.

Oakland, T., Black, J. L., Stanford, G., Nussbaum, N. L., and Balise, R. R. 1998. An evaluation of the Dyslexia Training Program: A multisensory method for promoting reading in students with reading disabilities. *Journal of Learning Disabilities* 31:140–47.

Obrzut, J. E., and Boliek, C. A. 1986. Lateralization characteristics in learning disabled children. *Journal of Learning Disabilities* 19:308–14.

Olson, R. K., Conners, F. A., and Rack, J. P. 1991. Eye movements in normal and dyslexic readers. In *Vision and Visual Dyslexia*, ed. J. F. Stein. London: Macmillan.

Olson, R. K., Kliegl, R., Davidson, B. J., and Folz, G. 1985. Individual and developmental differences in reading disability. In *Reading Research: Advances in Theory and Practice: Vol. 4*, eds. C. E. MacKinnon and T. G. Waller. New York: Academic Press.

Olson, R. K., Wise, B., Conners, F. A., and Rack, J. P. 1990. Organization, heritability, and remediation of component word recognition and language skills in disabled readers. In *Reading and its Development: Component Skills Approaches*, eds. T. H. Carr and B. A. Levy. New York: Academic Press.

Olson, R. K., Wise, B., Conners, F., Rack, J. P., and Fulker, D. 1989. Specific deficits in component reading and language skills: Genetic and environmental influences. *Journal of Learning Disabilities* 22:339–48.

Open Court Reading. 1995. *Collections for Young Scholars*. Chicago: SRA/McGraw-Hill.

Orton, J. 1964. *A Guide to Teaching Phonics*. Cambridge, MA: Educators Publishing Service.

Orton, S. T. 1928. Specific reading disability—strephosymbolia. *The Journal of the American Medical Association* 90:1095-99.

Orton, S. T. 1937. *Reading, Writing, and Speech Problems in Children*. New York: Norton.

Owens, R. E. 2001. *Language Development: An Introduction*. Boston: Allyn and Bacon.

Palincsar, A. S. 1986. The role of dialogue in providing scaffolded instruction. *Educational Psychologist* 21:73–98.

Palincsar, A., and Brown, A. 1983. Reciprocal teaching of comprehension-monitoring activities Technical Report No. 269. Urbana, IL: The University of Illinois, Center for the Study of Reading.

Palincsar, A., and Brown, A. 1984. Reciprocal teaching of comprehension-fostering and monitoring activities. *Cognition and Instruction* 1:117-75.

Palincsar, A., and Brown, A. 1985. Reciprocal teaching: A means to a meaningful end. In *Reading Education: Foundations for a Literate America*, eds., J. Osborn, P. T. Wilson, and R. C. Anderson. Lexington, MA: D. C. Heath.

Paris, S., Wasik, B. A., and Turner, J. C. 1991. The development of strategic readers. In *Handbook of Reading Research, Vol. II*, eds. R. Barr, M. L. Kamil, P. B. Mosenthal, and P. D. Pearson. Mahwah, NJ: Lawrence Erlbaum Associates.

Patterson, K. E., Marshall, J. C., and Coltheart, M. 1985. Eds. *Surface Dyslexia: Neuropsychological and Cognitive Studies of Phonological Reading*. Hillsdale, NJ: Lawrence Erlbaum Associates.

Pavlidis, G. T. 1985. Eye movements in dyslexia: Their diagnostic significance. *Journal of Learning Disabilities* 18:42–50.

Pearson, P. D., and Fielding, L. 1991. Comprehension instruction. In *Handbook of Reading Research, Vol. II*, eds. R. Barr, M. L. Kamil, P. B. Mosenthal, and P. D. Pearson. New York: Longman.

Peister, P., Fadiman, S., Pierce, K., and Fayne, H. 1978–1980. Integrative review of basic reading skills. *Integrative Reviews of Research: Vol. 1*. New York: Teachers College, Institute for the Study of Learning Disabilities.

Pennington, B. F. 1991. *Diagnosing Learning Disorders: A Neuropsychological Framework*. New York: Guilford Press.

Perfetti, C. A. 1984. Reading acquisition and beyond: Decoding includes cognition. *American Journal of Education* 93:40–60.

Perfetti, C. A. 1985a. Continuities in reading acquisition, reading skills, and reading disability. *Remedial and Special Education* 7:11–21.

Perfetti, C. A. 1985b. *Reading Ability*. New York: Oxford University Press.

Peters, E. E., and Levin, J. R. 1986. Effects of a mnemonic imagery strategy on good and poor readers' prose recall. *Reading Research Quarterly* 21:179–92.

Phelps, J., and Stempel, M. 1987. Handwriting: Evolution and evaluation. *Annals of Dyslexia* 37:228–39.

Piaget, J. 1970. *Structuralism*. New York: Basic Books.

Pilcher, H. 2004. Chinese dyslexics have problems of their own. *Nature News*. Retrieved September, 2004 from http://www.nature.com/news/2004/040830/full/0408305.html

Pinnell, G. S., Lyons, C. A., DeFord, D. E., Bryk, A. S., and Seltzer, M. 1994. Comparing instructional models for the literacy education of high-risk first graders. *Reading Research Quarterly* 29:8–39.

Pollatsek, A. 1993. Eye movements in reading. In *Visual Processes in Reading and Reading Disabilities*, eds. D. M. Willows, R. S. Kruk, and E. Corcos. Hillsdale, NJ: Lawrence Erlbaum Associates.

Polloway, E. A., and Epstein, M. H. 1986. The use of Corrective Reading (SRA) with mildly handicapped students. *Direct Instruction News* 2–3.

Poplin, M. 1983. Assessing developmental writing abilities. *Topics in Learning and Learning Disabilities* 3:63–75.

Poplin, M., Gray, R., Larsen, S., Banikowski, A., and Mehring, T. 1980. A comparison of components of written expression abilities in learning disabled and non-disabled students at three grade levels. *Learning Disability Quarterly* 3:46–59.

Pressley, M. 2003. *Reading Instruction that Works.* New York: The Guilford Press.

Pressley, M., Allington, R. L., Wharton-McDonald, R., Block, C. C., and Morrow, L. M. 2001. *Learning to Read: Lessons from Exemplary First-Grade Classrooms.* New York: The Guilford Press.

Pressley, M., El-Dinary, P. B., Gaskins, I., Schuder, T., Bergman, J. L., Almasi, J., and Brown, R. 1992. Beyond direct explanation: Transactional instruction of reading comprehension strategies. *The Elementary School Journal* 92:513–55.

Pressley, M., Gaskins, I. W., Cunicelli, E. A., Burdick, N. J., Schaub-Matt, M., Lee, D. S., and Powell, N. 1991. Strategy instruction at Benchmark School: A faculty interview study. *Learning Disability Quarterly* 14:19–48.

Pressley, M., Hogan, K., Wharton-McDonald, R., Mistretta, J., and Ettenberger, S. 1996. The challenges of instructional scaffolding: The challenges of instruction that supports student thinking. *Learning Disabilities Research and Practice* 11:138–46.

Pressley, M., Levin, J. R., and McDaniel, M. A. 1987. Remembering versus inferring what a word means: Mnemonic and contextual approaches. In *The Nature of Vocabulary Acquisition*, eds. M. G. McKeown and M. E. Curtis. Hillsdale, NJ: Lawrence Erlbaum Associates.

Pugh, K. R., Mencl, W. E., Jenner, A. R., Katz, L., Frost, S. J., Lee, J. R., Shaywitz, S. E., and Shaywitz, B. A. 2001. Neurobiological studies of reading and reading disability. *Journal of Communication Disorders* 34:479–92.

Pugh, K. R., Mencl, W., Shaywitz, B., Shaywitz, S., Fulbright, R., Constable, R., Skudlarski, P., Marchione, K., Jenner, A., Fletcher, J., Liberman, A., Shankweiler, D., Katz, L., Lacadie, C., and Gore, J. 2000. The angular gyrus in developmental dyslexia: Task specific differences in functional connectivity within posterior cortex. *Psychological Science* 11:51–56.

Punnet, A. F., and Steinhauer, G. D. 1984. Relationship between reinforcement and eye-movements during ocular motor training with learning disabled children. *Journal of Learning Disabilities* 17:16–20.

Rack, J. P., Snowling, M. J., and Olson, R. K. 1992. The nonword reading deficit in developmental dyslexia: A review. *Reading Research Quarterly* 27:28–53.

Raphael, T. E., and Englert, C. S. 1990. Reading and writing: Partners in constructing meaning. *The Reading Teacher* 43:388–400.

Raphael, T. E., and McMahon, S. I. 1994. Book club: An alternative framework for reading instruction. *The Reading Teacher* 48:102–16.

Rashotte, C. A. 1983. Repeated reading and reading fluency in learning disabled children. Pd.D. diss., The Florida State University, Tallahassee, Fl.

Rashotte, C. A., and Torgesen, J. K. 1985. Repeated reading and reading fluency in learning disabled children. *Reading Research Quarterly* 20:180–88.

Rasinski, T. V. 1995. Commentary on the effects of Reading Recovery: A response to Pinnell, Lyons, DeFord, Bryk, and Seltzer. *Reading Research Quarterly* 30:264–70.

Rasinski, T. V. 2000. Speed does matter in reading. *The Reading Teacher* 54:145–51.

Rasmussen, D. E., and Goldberg, L. 1976. *SRA Basic Reading.* Chicago, IL: Science Research Associates.

Rayner, K. 1985. The role of eye movements in learning to read and reading disability. *Remedial and Special Education* 6:53-60.

Rayner, K. 1992. Ed. *Eye Movements and Visual Cognition: Scene Perception and Reading.* New York: Springer-Verlag.

Rayner, K. 1993. Directions for research and theory. In *Visual Processes in Reading and Reading Disabilities*, eds. D. M. Willows, R. S. Kruk, and E. Corcos. Hillsdale, NJ: Lawrence Erlbaum Associates.

Rayner, K., and Pollatsek, A. 1987. Eye movements in reading: A tutorial review. In *Attention and Performance XII: The Psychology of Reading*, ed. M. Coltheart. London: Lawrence Erlbaum Associates Ltd.

Read, C. 1970. Children's perceptions of the sounds of English phonology from three to six. Ph.D. diss., Harvard Graduate School of Education, Cambridge, MA.

Read, C. 1971. Preschool children's knowledge of English phonology. *Harvard Educational Review* 41:1–34.

Read, C. 1975. Lessons to be learned from the preschool orthographer. In *Foundations of Language Development: Vol. 2*, eds. E. H. Lennenberg and E. Lennenberg. New York: Academic Press.

Read, C. 1986. *Children's Creative Spellings*. London: Routledge and Kegan Paul.

Read, C., and Ruyter, L. 1985. Reading and spelling skills in adults of low literacy. *Remedial and Special Education* 6:43–52.

Richardson, E., and DiBenedetto, B. 1985. *Decoding Skills Test*. Parkton, MD: York Press.

Richardson, E., DiBenedetto, B., and Adler, A. 1982. Use of the Decoding Skills Test to study the differences between good and poor readers. In *Advances in Learning and Behavioral Disabilities*, eds. K. D. Gadow and I. Bialer. Greenwich, CT: JAI Press.

Robbins, C., and Ehri, L. C. 1994. Reading storybooks to kindergartners helps them learn new vocabulary words. *Journal of Educational Psychology* 86:54–64.

Robinson, G. L. W., and Conway, R. N. F. 1990. The effects of Irlen colored lenses on students' specific reading skills and their perception of ability: A 12-month validity study. *Journal of Learning Disabilities* 23:588–96.

Rosenblatt, L. M. 1978. *The Reader, the Text, and the Poem: The Transactional Theory of the Literary Work*. Carbondale, IL: Southern Illinois University Press.

Rosenblatt, L. M. 1989. Writing and reading: The transactional theory. In *Reading and Writing Connections*, ed. J. M. Mason. Boston: Allyn and Bacon.

Rosenshine, B. 1983. Teaching functions in instructional programs. *Elementary School Journal* 83:335–40.

Rosenshine, B., and Stevens, R. 1984. Classroom instruction in reading. In *Handbook of Reading Research*, ed. P. D. Pearson. New York: Longman.

Rosner, J. 1974. Auditory analysis training with prereaders. *The Reading Teacher* 27:379–81.

Rosner, J. 1975. Test of auditory analysis skills. In *Helping Children Overcome Learning Difficulties*, ed. J. Rosner. New York: Walker and Co.

Rosner, J. 1999. *Phonological Awareness Skills Program*. Austin, TX: PRO-ED.

Ross, S. M., Smith, L. J., Casey, J., and Slavin, R. E. In press. Increasing the academic success of disadvantaged children: An examination of alternative early intervention programs. *American Educational Research Journal*.

Roswell, F. G., and Chall, J. S. 1997. *Roswell-Chall Auditory Blending Test*. Cambridge, MA: Educators Publishing Service.

Roswell, F. G., and Chall, J. S. 1992. *Diagnostic Assessment of Reading*. Chicago, Riverside Publishing Co.

Roy, B. J. January 1986. A cooperative teacher education and language retraining program for dyslexics in west Texas. Paper presented at the Action in Research V, Conference, Lubbock, TX.

Rubin, H., and Eberhardt, N. C. 1996. Facilitating invented spelling through language analysis instruction: An integrated model. *Reading and Writing: An Interdisciplinary Journal* 8:27–43.

Rumelhart, D. E. 1977. Toward an interactive model of reading. In *Attention and Performance VI*, ed. S. Dornic. Hillsdale, NJ: Lawrence Erlbaum Associates.

Rumelhart, D. E. 1980. Schemata: The building blocks of cognition. In *Theoretical Issues in Reading Comprehension*, eds. R. J. Spiro, B. C. Bruce, and W. F. Brewer. Hillsdale, NJ: Lawrence Erlbaum Associates.

Rutter, M. 1978. The prevalence and types of dyslexia. In *Dyslexia: An Appraisal of Current Knowledge*, eds. A. L. Benton and D. Pearl. New York: Oxford University Press.

Ryan, M. C., Miller, C. E., and Witt, J. C. 1984. A comparison of the use of orthographic structure in word discrimination by learning disabled and normal children. *Journal of Learning Disabilities* 17:38–40.

Sadoski, M., and Paivio, A. 2001. *Imagery and Text: A Dual Coding Theory of Reading and Writing*. Mahwah, NJ: Lawrence Erlbaum Associates.

Samuels, S. J. 1974/1997. The method of repeated readings. *The Reading Teacher* 50:376–81.

Samuels, S. J. 1986. Automaticity and repeated readings. In *Reading Education: Foundations for a Literate America*, eds. J. Osborn, P. T. Wilson, and R. C. Anderson. Lexington, MA: D. C. Heath.

Santa, C. M. 1998. *Early Steps: Learning from a Reader*. Kalispell, MT: Scott.

Santa, C. M., and Høien, T. 1999. An assessment of Early Steps: A program for early intervention of reading problems. *Reading Research Quarterly* 34:54–75.

Satz, P., Saslow, E., and Henry, R. 1985. The pathological left-handedness syndrome. *Brain and Cognition* 4:27–46.

Schatschneider, C., Francis, D., Foorman, B., Fletcher, J., and Mehta, P. 1999. The dimensionality of phonological awareness: An application of item response theory. *Journal of Educational Psychology* 91:439–49.

Sears, S., and Keogh, B. 1993. Predicting reading performance using the Slingerland procedures. *Annals of Dyslexia* 43:78–89.

Seidenberg, M. S., and McClelland, J. L. 1989. A distributed, developmental model of word recognition and naming. *Psychological Review* 96:523–68.

Shaywitz, B. A. April 1993. Medical symposium of the New York Orton Dyslexia Society Annual Meeting.

Shaywitz, B. A., Pugh, K. G., Jenner, A. R., Fulbright, R. K., Fletcher, J. M., Gore, J. C., and Shaywitz, S. E. 2000. The neurobiology of reading and reading disability dyslexia. In *The Handbook of Reading Research, Vol. III*, eds. M. L. Kamil, P. B. Mosenthal, P. D. Pearson, and R. Barr. Mahwah, NJ: Lawrence Erlbaum Associates.

Shaywitz, B. A., Shaywitz, S. E., Blachman, B. A., Pugh, K. R., Fullbright, R. K., Skudlarski, P., Mencl, W. E., Constable, R. T., Holahan, J. M., Marchione, K. E., Fletcher, J. M., Lyon, G. R., and Gore, J. C. 2004. Development of left occipitotemporal systems for skilled reading in children after a phonologically-based intervention. *Biological Psychiatry* 55:926–33.

Shaywitz, S. E. 2003. *Overcoming Dyslexia*. New York: Alfred A. Knopf.

Shaywitz, S. E., and Shaywitz, B. A. Eds. 1991. Introduction to the special issue on attention deficit disorder. *Journal of Learning Disabilities* 24:68–71.

Shaywitz, S. E., Escobar, M. D., Shaywitz, B. A., Fletcher, J. M., and Makuch, R. 1992. Evidence that dyslexia may represent the lower tail of a normal distribution of reading disability. *The New England Journal of Medicine* 326:145–50.

Shaywitz, S. E., and Shaywitz, B. A. Eds. 1992. *Attention Deficit Disorder Comes of Age: Towards the Twenty-First Century*. Austin, TX: PRO-ED.

Shaywitz, S. E., Shaywitz, B. A., Fletcher, J. M., and Escobar, M. D. 1990. Prevalence of reading disability in boys and girls. *Journal of the American Medical Association* 264:998–1002.

Shaywitz, S. E., Shaywitz, B. A., Pugh, K. G., Fulbright, R. K., Constable, R. T., Mencl, W. E., Shankweiler, D. P., Liberman, A. M., Skudlarski, P., Fletcher, J. M., Katz, L., Marchione, K. E., Lacadie, C., Gatenby, C., and Gore, J. C. 1998. Functional disruption in the organization of the brain for reading in dyslexia. *Proceedings of the National Academy of Sciences* 95:2636–41.

Shaywitz, S. E., Shaywitz, B. A., Schnell, C., and Towle, V. R. 1988. Concurrent and predictive validity of the Yale Children's Inventory: An instrument to assess children with attentional deficits and learning disabilities. *Pediatrics* 81:562–71.

Sheikh, A. A., and Sheikh, K. S. 1985. *Imagery in Education.* Farmingdale, NY: Baywood Publishing Company.

Shepherd, M. J., and Uhry, J. K. April 1993. Phonological awareness training: Case studies of children at-risk for dyslexia. Paper presented at the annual meeting of the American Educational Research Association in Atlanta.

Siegel, L. S. 1985. Psycholinguistic aspects of reading disabilities. In *Cognitive Development of Atypical Children,* eds. L. S. Siegel and F. J. Morrison. New York: Springer Verlag.

Siegel, L. S. 1989. IQ is irrelevant to the definition of learning disabilities. *Journal of Learning Disabilities* 22:469–78.

Silver, L. A. 1987. The "magic cure:" A review of the current controversial approaches for treating learning disabilities. *Journal of Learning Disabilities* 20:498–512.

Silverman, R., Zigmond, N., Zimmerman, J. M., and Vallescorsa, B. 1981. Improving written expression in learning disabled adolescents. *Journal of Learning Disabilities* 16:478-82.

Siok, W. T., Perfetti, C. A., Jin, Z., and Tan, L. H. September 2, 2004. Biological abnormality of impaired reading is constrained by culture. *Nature* 431:71–76.

Slavin, R. E., and Madden, N. A. December 1999. *Success for All/Roots and Wings: Summary of Research on Achievement Outcomes.* Baltimore, MD: Johns Hopkins University and Howard University, Center for Research on the Education of Students Placed at Risk, Report #41.

Slavin, R. E., Madden, N. A., Dolan, L. J., and Wasik, B. A. 1996. *Every Child, Every School: Success for All.* Thousand Oaks, CA: Corwin Press.

Slavin, R. E., Madden, N. A., Karweit, N. L., Dolan, L., and Wasik, B. A. 1992. *Success for All: A Relentless Approach to Prevention and Early Intervention in Elementary Schools.* Arlington, VA: Educational Research Service.

Slepian, J., and Seidler, A. 1967. *The Hungry Thing.* New York: Scholastic.

Slingerland, B. H. 1971. *A Multi-Sensory Approach to Language Arts for Specific Language Disability Children: A Guide for Primary Teachers, Books 1–3.* Cambridge, MA: Educators Publishing Service.

Slingerland, B. H. 1976. *Basics in Scope and Sequence of a Multi-Sensory Approach to Language Arts for SLD Children.* Cambridge, MA: Educators Publishing Service.

Smith, F. 1979. Conflicting approaches to reading research and instruction. In *Theory and Practice of Early Reading: Vol. 2,* eds. L. B. Resnick and P. A. Weaver. Hillsdale, NJ: Lawrence Erlbaum Associates.

Smith, F. 2004. *Understanding Reading.* Mahwah, NJ: Lawrence Erlbaum Associates.

Smith, L., and Stayton, B. 1998. *Poppin Auditory Discrimination Reading Series.* Austin, TX: PRO-ED.

Smith, S. D., Kimberling, W. J., and Pennington, B. F. 1991. Screening for multiple genes influencing dyslexia. In *Neuropsychology and Cognition, Vol. 4: Reading Disabilities: Genetic and Neurological Influences,* ed. B. F. Pennington. Dordrecht, Netherlands: Kluwer Academic Publishing.

Snow, C. E., Burns, M. S., and Griffin, P. 1998. Eds. *Preventing Reading Difficulties in Young Children.* Washington, DC: National Academy Press.

Snowling, M. J. 1980. The development of grapheme-phoneme correspondences in normal and dyslexic readers. *Journal of Experimental Child Psychology* 29:294–305.

Snowling, M., Goulandris, N., and Stackhouse, J. 1994. Phonological constraints on learning to read: Evidence from single case studies of reading difficulty. In *Reading Development and Dyslexia,* eds. C. Hulme and M. Snowling. San Diego, CA: Singular Publishing Group.

Snowling, M. J., and Hulme, C. 1989. A longitudinal case study of developmental phonological dyslexia. *Cognitive Neuropsychology* 6:379–401.

Solan, H. 1990. An appraisal of the Irlen technique of correcting reading disorders using tinted overlays and tinted lenses. *Journal of Learning Disabilities* 23:621–23.

Spalding, R. B., and Spalding, W. T. 1986. *The Writing Road to Reading*. New York: Quill/William Morrow.

Stahl, S. 1998. *Vocabulary Development*. Cambridge, MA: Brookline Press.

Stahl, S. A. 2004. Scaly? Audacious? Debris? Salubrious? Vocabulary learning and the child with learning disabilities. *Perspectives* 30:5–12.

Stahl, S., and Fairbanks, M. 1986. The effects of vocabulary instruction: A model-based meta-analysis. *Review of Education Research* 56:72–110.

Stahl, S. A., and Murray, B. A. 1994. Defining phonological awareness and its relationship to early reading. *Journal of Educational Psychology* 86:221–34.

Stanback, M., and Hansen, M. 1980. Integrative review of spelling. In *Integrative Reviews of Research: Vol. 1*. New York: Teachers College, Institute for the Study of Learning Disabilities.

Stanovich, K. E. 1980. Toward an interactive-compensatory model of individual differences in the development of reading fluency. *Reading Research Quarterly* 1:32–37.

Stanovich, K. E. 1981. Relationships between word decoding speed, general name-retrieval ability, and reading progress in first-grade children. *Journal of Educational Psychology* 73:809–15.

Stanovich, K. E. 1984. The interactive-compensatory model of reading: A confluence of developmental, experimental, and educational psychology. *Remedial and Special Education* 5:11–19.

Stanovich, K. E. 1986a. Cognitive processes and the reading problems of learning disabled children: Evaluating the assumption of specificity. In *Psychological and Educational Perspectives on Learning Disabilities*, eds. J. K. Torgesen and B. Y. L. Wong. New York: Academic Press.

Stanovich, K. E. 1986b. Matthew effects in reading: Some consequences of individual differences in the acquisition of literacy. *Reading Research Quarterly* 21:360–407.

Stanovich, K. E. 1988a. The right and wrong places to look for the cognitive locus of reading disability. *Annals of Dyslexia* 38:154–77.

Stanovich, K. E. 1988b. Explaining the differences between the dyslexic and the garden-variety poor reader: The phonological-core variable-difference model. *Journal of Learning Disabilities* 21:590–604.

Stanovich, K. E. 1991. Discrepancy definitions of reading disability: Has intelligence led us astray? *Reading Research Quarterly* 26:7–29.

Stanovich, K. E., Cunningham, A. E., and Cramer, B. 1984. Assessing phonological awareness in kindergarten children: Issues of task comparability. *Journal of Experimental Child Psychology* 38:175–90.

Stanovich, K. E., Cunningham, A. E., and Feeman, D. J., 1984. Intelligence, cognitive skills, and early reading progress. *Reading Research Quarterly* 19:278–303.

Stark, R. E., Bernstein, L. E., Condino, R., Bender, M., Tallal, P., and Catts, H. 1984. Four-year follow-up study of language impaired children. *Annals of Dyslexia* 34:49–68.

Stevens, R. J., Madden, N. A., Slavin, R. E., and Farnish, A. M. 1987. Cooperative integrated reading and composition: Two field experiments. *Reading Research Quarterly* 22:433–54.

Stevenson, J. 1991. Which aspects of processing text mediate genetic effects? In *Neuropsychology and Cognition, Vol. 4: Reading Disabilities: Genetic and Neurological Influences*, ed. B. F. Pennington. Dordrecht, Netherlands: Kluwer Academic Publishing.

Stothard, S. 1994. The nature and treatment of reading comprehension difficulties in children. In *Reading Development and Dyslexia*, eds. C. Hulme and M. Snowling. San Diego, CA: Singular Publishing Group.

Strominger, A. Z., and Bashir, A. S. 1977. Longitudinal study of language-delayed children. Paper presented at the Annual Convention of the American Speech and Hearing Association.

Tallal, P. 1980. Language and reading: Some perceptual prerequisites. *Bulletin of the Orton Society* 30:170–78.

Tallal, P., Miller, S. L., Bedl, G., Byma, G., Wang, X., Nagarajan, S. S., Schreiner, C., Jenkins, W. M., and Merzenich, M. M. 1996. Language comprehension in language-learning impaired children improved with acoustically modified speech. *Science* 271:81–84.

Tallal, P., Miller, S. L., Jenkins, W. M., and Merzenich, M. M. 1997. The role of temporal processing in developmental language-based learning disorders: Research and clinical implications. In *Foundations of Reading Acquisition and Dyslexia: Implications for Early Intervention*, ed. B. Blachman. Mahwah, NJ: Lawrence Erlbaum Associates.

Tallal, P., and Stark, R. E. 1982. Perceptual/motor profiles of reading impaired children with or without concomitant oral language deficits. *Annals of Dyslexia* 32:163–76.

Tan, A., and Nicholson, T. 1997. Flashcards revisited: Training poor readers to read words faster improves their comprehension of text. *Journal of Educational Psychology* 89:276–88.

Tangel, D. M., and Blachman, B. A. 1992. Effect of phoneme awareness on instruction on kindergarten children's invented spelling. *Journal of Reading Behavior* 24:233–61.

Tangel, D. M., and Blachman, B. A. 1995. Effect of phoneme awareness instruction on the invented spelling of first-grade children: A one-year follow-up. *Journal of Reading Behavior* 27:153–83.

Templeton, S., and Morris, D. 2000. Spelling. In *Handbook of Reading Research, Vol. III*, eds. M. Kamil, P. Mosenthal, P. D. Pearson, and R. Barr. Mahwah, NJ: Lawrence Erlbaum Associates.

Terman, L. M. 1916. *The Measurement of Intelligence*. Boston: Houghton-Mifflin.

Tierney, R. J., and Cunningham, J. W. 1984. Research on teaching reading comprehension. In *Handbook of Reading Research*, ed. P. D. Pearson. New York: Longman.

Torgesen, J. K. April 1995. Modeling growth in early reading skills: Individual and group differences. Paper presented at the annual meeting of the American Educational Research Association in San Francisco.

Torgesen, J. K. 2000. Individual differences in response to early interventions in reading: The lingering problem of treatment resisters. *Learning Disabilities Research and Practice* 15:55–64.

Torgesen, J. K. 2002. The prevention of reading difficulties. *Journal of School Psychology* 40:7–26.

Torgesen, J. K., and Barker, T. A. 1995. Computers as aids in the prevention and remediation of reading disabilities. *Learning Disabilities Quarterly* 18:76–87.

Torgesen, J. K., and Bryant, B. R. 1994a. *Phonological Awareness Training for Reading*. Austin, TX: PRO-ED.

Torgesen, J. K., and Bryant, B. R. 1994b. *Test of Phonological Awareness*. Austin, TX: PRO-ED.

Torgesen, J. K., and Davis, C. April 1993. Individual difference variables that predict response to training in phonological awareness. In *Does Phonological Awareness Training Enhance Children's Acquisition of Written Language Skills?* ed. R. Wagner. Symposium conducted at the annual meeting of the American Educational Research Association in Atlanta.

Torgesen, J. K., Morgan, S., and Davis, C. 1992. The effects of two types of phonological awareness training on word learning in kindergarten children. *Journal of Educational Psychology* 84:364–70.

Torgesen, J. K., Rashotte, C. A., and Alexander, A. W. 2001. Principles of fluency instruction in reading: Relationships with established empirical outcomes. In *Dyslexia, Fluency, and the Brain,* ed. M. Wolf. Baltimore: York Press.

Torgesen, J. K., and Wagner, R. K. 1998. Alternative diagnostic approaches for specific developmental reading disabilities. *Learning Disabilities Research and Practice* 13:220–32.

Torgesen, J. K., Wagner, R., and Rashotte, C. 1997. Prevention and remediation of severe reading disabilities: Keeping the end in mind. *Scientific Studies of Reading* 1:217–34.

Torgesen, J. K., Wagner, R., and Rashotte, C. 1999. *Test of Word Reading Efficiency.* Austin, TX: PRO-ED.

Torgesen, J. K., Wagner, R., Rashotte, C. A., Alexander, A. W., and Conway, T. 1997. Preventive and remedial interventions for children with severe reading disabilities. *Learning Disabilities: A Multi-Disciplinary Journal* 8:51–61.

Torgesen, J., Wagner, R., Rashotte, C., Rose, E., Lindamood, P., Conway, T., and Garvan, C. 1999. Preventing reading failure in young children with phonological processing disabilities: Group and individual responses to instruction. *Journal of Educational Psychology* 91:579–93.

Traub, N. 1982. Reading, spelling, handwriting: Traub Systematic Holistic Method. *Annals of Dyslexia* 32:135–45.

Traub, N., and Bloom, F. 2000. *Recipe for Reading.* Cambridge, MA: Educators Publishing Service.

Treiman, R. 1985. Onsets and rimes as units of spoken syllables: Evidence from children. *Journal of Experimental Child Psychiatry* 39:161–81.

Treiman, R. 1993. *Beginning to Spell.* Oxford: Oxford University Press.

Treiman, R. 1994. Use of consonant letter names in beginning spelling. *Developmental Psychology* 30:567–80.

Treiman, R., and Baron, J. 1983. Individual differences in spelling: The Phoenician-Chinese distinction. *Topics in Learning Disabilities* 3:33–40.

Troia, G. A., and Graham, S. 2002. The effectiveness of a highly explicit, teacher-directed strategy instruction route: Changing the writing performance of students with learning disabilities. *Journal of Learning Disabilities* 35:290–305.

Uhry, J. K. 1993a. Predicting reading from print awareness and phonological awareness skills: An early reading screening. *Educational Assessment* 1:349–68.

Uhry, J. K. 1993b. The spelling/reading connection and dyslexia: Can spelling be used to teach the alphabetic strategy? In *Reading Disabilities: Diagnosis and Component Processes,* eds. R. M. Joshi and C. K. Leong. Dordrecht, The Netherlands: Kluwer Publishers.

Uhry, J. K. 1997. Case studies of dyslexia: Young readers with rapid serial naming deficits. In *Cross-language Studies of Learning to Read and Spell: Phonological and Orthographic Processing,* eds. M. Joshi and C. K. Leong. Dordrecht, The Netherlands: Kluwer Academic Publishers.

Uhry, J. K. 1999. Invented spelling in kindergarten: The relationship with finger-point reading. *Reading and Writing: An Interdisciplinary Journal* 11:441–64.

Uhry, J. K. 2001. Rapid serial letter naming: The role of orthography. Paper presented at the annual conference of the American Educational Researach Association in Seattle.

Uhry, J. K. 2002a. Finger-point reading in kindergarten: The role of phonemic awareness, one-to-one correspondence, and rapid serial naming. *Scientific Studies of Reading* 6:319–42.

Uhry, J. K. 2002b. Phonological awareness and rapid serial naming as predictors of reading and spelling: Longitudinal evidence. In *Basic Mechanisms of Language and Language Disorders,* eds. E. Witruk, A. D. Friederici, and T. Lachman. Dordrecht, The Netherlands: Kluwer Academic Publishers.

Uhry, J. K. 2003. Teachers' phonemic knowledge and skills and first graders' reading outcomes. Paper presented at the June meeting of the Society for the Scientific Study of Reading in Boulder.

Uhry, J. K., and Ehri, L. C. 1999. Ease of segmenting two- and three-phoneme words in kindergarten: Rime cohesion or vowel salience? *Journal of Educational Psychology* 91:594–603.

Uhry, J. K., and Shepherd, M. J. 1993a. Segmentation/spelling instruction as part of a first grade reading program: Effects on several measures of reading. *Reading Research Quarterly* 28:218–33.

Uhry, J. K., and Shepherd, M. J. 1993b. Writing disorder. In *Child and Adolescent Psychiatry Clinics of North America*, ed. L. B. Silver. 2:209–19.

Uhry, J. K., and Shepherd, M. J. 1997. Teaching phonological recoding to young children with dyslexia: The effect on sight vocabulary acquisition. *Learning Disabilities Quarterly* 20:104–125.

Vaughn, S., Schumm, J. S., and Gordon, J. 1993. Which motoric condition is most effective for teaching spelling to students with and without learning disabilities? *Journal of Learning Disabilities* 26:191–98.

Vellutino, F. 1978. Toward an understanding of dyslexia: Psychological factors in specific reading disability. In *Dyslexia: An Appraisal of Current Knowledge,* eds. A. L. Benton and D. Pearl. New York: Oxford University Press.

Vellutino, F. 1979. *Dyslexia: Theory and Research.* Cambridge, MA: The MIT Press.

Vellutino, F. 1983. Dyslexia: Perceptual deficiency of perceptual inefficiency. In *Orthography, Reading, and Dyslexia*, eds. J. P. Kavanagh and R. L. Venezky. Baltimore: University Park Press.

Vellutino, F. 1987. Dyslexia. *Scientific American* 256(3):34–41.

Vellutino, F., Steger, J. A., Kaman, M., and DeSetto, L. 1975. Visual form perception in deficient and normal readers as a function of age and orthographic linguistic familiarity. *Cortex* 11:22–30.

Vellutino, F., Steger, J. A., and Kandel, G. 1972. Reading disability: An investigation of the perceptual deficit hypothesis. *Cortex* 8:106–18.

Vellutino, F., Steger, J. A., and Pruzek, R. 1973. Inter- vs. intrasensory deficit in paired associate learning in poor and normal readers. *Canadian Journal of Behavioral Science* 5:111–23.

Venezky, R. L. 1970. *The Structure of English Orthography*. The Hague, Holland: Moulton.

Venezky, R. L. 1999. *The American Way of Spelling: The Structure and Origins of American English Orthography.* New York: Guilford Press.

Vickery, K. S., Reynolds, V. A., and Cochran, S. W. 1987. Multisensory teaching for reading, spelling, and handwriting, Orton-Gillingham based, in a public school setting. *Annals of Dyslexia* 37:189–202.

Vogel, S. A. 1990. Gender differences in intelligence, language, visual-motor abilities, and academic achievement in students with learning disabilities: A review of the literature. *Journal of Learning Disabilities* 23:44–52.

Vygotsky, L. S. 1978. *Mind in Society*. Eds. and trans. M. Cole, V. John-Steiner, S. Scribner, and E. Souberman. Cambridge, MA: Harvard University Press.

Wagner, R. K., Muse, A. E., Stein, T. L., Cukrowicz, K. C., Harrell, E. R., Rashotte, C. A., and Samwel, C. S. 2003. How to assess reading-related phonological abilities. In *Preventing and Remediating Reading Difficulties*, ed. B. R. Foorman. Baltimore: York Press.

Wagner, R. K., and Torgesen, J. K. 1987. The nature of phonological processing and its causal role in the acquisition of reading skills. *Psychological Bulletin* 101:192–212.

Wagner, R. K., Torgesen, J. K., Laughon, P., Simmons, K., and Rashotte, C. A. 1993. Development of young readers' phonological processing abilities. *Journal of Educational Psychology* 85:83–103.

Wagner, R. K., Torgesen, J. K., and Rashotte, C. A. 1999 *Comprehensive Test of Phonological Processing*. Austin, TX: PRO-ED.

Wasik, B. A. 1998. Volunteer tutoring programs in reading: A review. *Reading Research Quarterly* 33:266–92.

Wasik, B. A., and Slavin, R. E. 1993. Preventing early reading failure with one-to-one tutoring: A review of five programs. *Reading Research Quarterly* 28:179–200.

Wechsler, D. 1989. *Wechsler Preschool and Primary Scale of Intelligence–Revised*. San Antonio, TX: The Psychological Corporation.

Wechsler, D. 1991. *Wechsler Intelligence Scale for Children–III*. San Antonio, TX: The Psychological Corporation.

Wechsler, D. 1992. *Wechsler Individual Achievement Test*. San Antonio, TX: The Psychological Corporation.

Wechsler, D. 2002. *Wechsler Intelligence Scale for Children–IV*. San Antonio, TX: The Psychological Corporation.

Weintraub, N., and Graham, S. 1998. Writing legibly and quickly: A study of children's ability to adjust their handwriting to meet classroom demands. *Learning Disabilities Research and Practice* 13:146–52.

Werner, H., and Strauss, A. A. 1940. Causal factors in low performance. *American Journal of Mental Deficiency* 45:213–18.

White, E. B. 1952. *Charlotte's Web*. New York: Harper Collins Publishers.

Wiederbolt, J. L., and Bryant, B. R. 2001. *Gray Oral Reading Test–4*. Austin, TX: PRO-ED.

Willcutt, E. G., and Pennington, B. F. 2000. Comorbidity of reading disability and attention-deficit/hyperactivity disorder: Differences by gender and subtype. *Journal of Learning Disabilities* 33:179–91.

Williams, J. P. 1975. Training children to copy and discriminate letter like forms. *Journal of Educational Psychology* 67:790–95.

Williams, J. P. 1980. Teaching decoding with an emphasis on phoneme analysis and phoneme blending. *Journal of Educational Psychology* 72:1–15.

Williams, J. P. 1986. Teaching children to identify the main idea of expository texts. *Exceptional Children* 53:163–68.

Williams, J. P. 1993. Comprehension of students with and without learning disabilities: Identification of narrative themes and idiosyncratic text representations. *Journal of Educational Psychology* 85:631–41.

Willows, D. M., and Jackson, G. April 1992. Differential diagnosis of reading disability subtypes based on the Boder reading spelling test: Issues of reliability and validity. Paper presented at the annual conference of the American Educational Research Association.

Willows, D. M., and Terepocki, M. 1993. The relation of reversal errors to reading disabilities. In *Visual Processes in Reading and Reading Disabilities*, eds. D. M. Willows, R. S. Kruk, and E. Corcos. Hillsdale, NJ: Lawrence Erlbaum Associates.

Wilson, B. A. 1988a. *Instructor Manual*. Millbury, MA: Wilson Language Training.

Wilson, B. A. 1988b. *Wilson Reading System Program Overview*. Millbury, MA: Wilson Language Training.

Wilson, B. A. 1995. Wilson reading system: MSLE research report. Unpublished report from Wilson Language Training, 162 West Main Street, Millbury, MA 01527.

Wilson, B. A. 2002. *Fundations Teacher's Manual, Levels K-1*. Millbury, MA: Wilson Language Training Corporation.

Wilson, B. A. 2004. *Fundations Teacher's Manual, Level 2*. Millbury, MA: Wilson Language Training Corporation.

Wilson, B. A., and O'Connor, J.. 1995. Effectiveness of the Wilson Reading System used in public school training. In *Clinical Studies of Multisensory Structured Language*

Education, eds. C. McIntyre and J. Pickering. Salem, OR: International Multisensory Structured Language Education Council.

Wise, B. W. April 1995. Orthographic and phonological influences in computerized remedial reading. Paper presented at the annual meeting of the American Educational Research Association in San Francisco.

Wise, B. W., Olson, R. K., Anstett, M., Andrews, L., Terjak, M., Schneider, V., and Kostuch, J. 1989. Implementing a long term computerized remedial reading program with synthetic speech feedback: Hardware, software, and real world issues. *Behavior Research Methods, Instruments, and Computers* 21:173–80.

Wise, B., Olson, R., Anstett, M., Andrews, L., Terjak, M., Schneider, V., Kostuch, J., and Driho, L. 1989. Implementing a long-term computerized remedial reading program with synthetic speech feedback: Hardware, software, and real-world issues. *Behavior Research Methods, Instruments, and Computers* 21(2):173–80.

Wise, M. 1924. *On the Techniques of Manuscript Writing.* New York: Scribner's and Sons.

Wolf, B. J. 1985. The effect of Slingerland instruction on the reading and language of second grade children. Ph.D. diss., Seattle Pacific University, Seattle, WA.

Wolf, M. 1991. Naming speed and reading: The contribution of the cognitive neurosciences. *Reading Research Quarterly* 26:123–41.

Wolf, M. 1999. What time may tell: Towards a new conceptualization of developmental dyslexia. *Annals of Dyslexia* 49:3–28.

Wolf, M. 2001. Ed. *Dyslexia, Fluency, and the Brain.* Baltimore: York Press.

Wolf, M., and Bowers, P. 1999. The "double deficit" hypothesis for the developmental dyslexias. *Journal of Educational Psychology* 91:1–24.

Wolf, M., Miller, L., and Donnelly, K. 2000. Retrieval, Automaticity, Vocabulary Elaboration, Orthography (RAVE-O): A comprehensive, fluency-based reading intervention program. *Journal of Learning Disabilities* 33:375–86.

Wolff, P. H., Michel, G. F., and Ovrut, M. 1990a. Rate variables and automatized naming in developmental dyslexia. *Brain and Language* 39:556–75.

Wolff, P. H., Michel, G. F., and Ovrut, M. 1990b. The timing of syllable repetitions in developmental dyslexia. *Journal of Speech and Hearing Research* 33:281–89.

Wood, F. B. April 1993. Mrs. Orton's now adult dyslexics. Paper presented at the New York Orton Dyslexia Society's annual meeting in New York City.

Wood, F. 2002. Data analysis of the Wilson Reading System. Published in *Wilson Literacy Solutions: Evidence of Effectiveness.*

Wood, F. B., and Felton, R. H. 1994. Separate linguistic and attentional factors in the development of reading. *Topics in Language Disorders* 14:42–57.

Wood, F., Felton, R., Flowers, L., and Naylor, C. 1991. Neurobehavioral definition of dyslexia. In *The Reading Brain: The Biological Basis of Dyslexia*, eds. D. D. Duane and D. B. Gray. Parkton, MD: York Press.

Woodcock, R. 1987. *Woodcock Reading Mastery Tests–Revised.* Circle Pines, MN: American Guidance.

Woodcock, R., and Mather, N. 1989a. *Woodcock-Johnson Tests of Cognitive Ability.* Allen, TX: DLM.

Woodcock, R., and Mather, N. 1989b. *Woodcock-Johnson Tests of Achievement.* Allen, TX: DLM.

Woods, M. L., and Moe, A. J. 2002. *Analytical Reading Inventory.* New York: Macmillan Publishing.

Yee, A H. 1966. The generalization controversy on spelling instruction. *Elementary English* 43:154–63.

Yopp, H. 1992. Developing phonological awareness in young children. *The Reading Teacher* 45:696–703.

Yopp, H. K. 1988. The validity and reliability of phonemic awareness tests. *Reading Research Quarterly* 23:159–77.

Yopp, H. K. 1995. Read-aloud books for developing phonemic awareness: An annotated bibliography. *The Reading Teacher* 48:538–42.

Yopp, H. K., and Yopp, R. H. (2000). Supporting phonemic awareness development in the classroom: Playful and appealing activities that focus on the sound structure of language. *The Reading Teacher* 54:130–43.

Zigmond, N. 1966. *Intrasensory and intersensory processes in normal and dyslexic children.* Ph.D. diss., Northwestern University, Chicago. IL.

Zigmond, N., and Miller, S. E. 1986. Assessment for instructional planning. *Exceptional Children* 52:501–9.

Resource and Teacher Training Guide

International Dyslexia Association
Chester Building, Suite 382
8600 LaSalle Road
Baltimore, Maryland 21286
(410) 296-0232

> Once named the Orton Dyslexia Society, the International Dyslexia
> Association (IDA) is an extremely useful resource for parents as well as teachers
> of students with dyslexia. This organization has branches in many areas of the
> United States, and in Canada, Israel, Brazil, Czechoslovakia, and The
> Philippines. Often, the local branches can provide referrals to tutors trained in
> multisensory techniques or schools specializing in services for children with
> dyslexia. Some branches also provide training in multisensory techniques or
> information about local resources for this.

TEACHER TRAINING CENTERS

Association for Direct Instruction
P.O. Box 10252
Eugene, OR 97440
Tel: (541) 485-1293
Fax: (541) 683-7543
www.adihome.org

Carroll School
25 Baker Bridge Road
Lincoln, MA 01773
(781) 259-8342

Centers for Youth and Families—Dyslexia Training Center
Stacey L. Mahurin, Director
6601 West 12th Street
Little Rock, AR 72204
(501) 666-8686 or (501) 660-6886 ext. 1129
E-mail: smahurin@aristotle.net
www.iser.com/dyslexiactr-AR.html

Dyslexia Training Program (Training plus videotapes for classroom use)
Martha Sibley, Dyslexia Coordinator
Texas Scottish Rite Hospital for Children
2222 Welborn St.
Dallas, TX 75219-3993
(214) 559-7800

Edmar Educational Services (MTA training)
Margaret Smith & Edith Hogan, Directors
P.O. Box 2
Forney, TX 75126
(214) 552-1500 or (214) 542-2323

The Greenwood Institute
14 Greenwood Lane
Putney, VT 05346
(802) 387-4545
greenwood@sover.net
www.greenwood.org

Institute in Multisensory Teaching of Basic Language Skills
Mary Rowe, Director
Box 223, Department of Special Education
Teachers College, Columbia University
525 West 120th Street
New York, NY 10027
(212) 678-3080

James Phillips Williams Memorial Foundation
2133 Office Park Drive
San Angelo, TX 76904
(325) 655-2331

Katheryne B. Payne Education Center
Ann Richardson, Director
3240 W. Britton Road, Suite 104
Oklahoma City, OK 73120
(405) 755-4205
Email: payneedu@accessacg.net
www.payneeducationcenter.org

Katheryne B. Payne Education Center
Ginny Little, Director
P.O. Box 1807
Ardmore, OK 73402
(405) 226-2341

Lindamood-Bell Learning Process
416 Higuera Street
San Luis Obispo, CA 93401
(805) 541-3836

Multisensory Structured Language Training of the
University of New Mexico
Sandra Dillon, Director
6344 Buenos Aires, N.W.
Albuquerque, NM 87120
(505) 898-7500

Neuhaus Education Center
Kay Allen, Director
4433 Bissonnet
Bellaire, TX 77401
(713) 664-7676
www.neuhaus.com

Project Read: Enfield and Greene
The Language Circle
P.O. Box 20631
Bloomington, MN 55420
Tel: (800) 450-0343
Fax: (952) 884-6787
Email: projread@gwest.net
www.projectread.com

Reading Disabilities Unit of the Language Disorders Unit
A.C.C.—Room 737
Massachusetts General Hospital
Boston, MA 02114
(617) 726-2764

Recipe for Reading
Mrs. Connie Russo
323 Concord Street
Dix Hills, NY 11746
(516) 242-8943

Reading Reform Foundation of New York
333 West 57th Street
New York, NY 10019
(212) 307-7320

Scottish Rite Learning Center of West Texas
Dorris Haney, Director of Teacher Training
602 Avenue Q
P.O. Box 10135
Lubbock, TX 79401
(806) 765-9150

The Slingerland Institute
Sue Heinz, Dean
1 Bellevue Center
411 108th Avenue, N.E.
Bellevue, WA 98004
Tel: (425) 453-1190
Fax: (425) 635-7762
Email: mail@slingerland.org
www.slingerland.org

Southern Methodist University, Learning Therapy Program
SMU Box 750384
Dallas, TX 75275-0384
(214) 768-7323

Southwest Multisensory Training Center
Beverly Dooley, Director
600 S. Jupiter
Allen, TX 75002-4065
Tel: (972) 359-6646
Fax: (972) 359-8291
Email: BevDool@aol.com
www.southwestacademy.org

Texas Scottish Rite Hospital for Children
Gladys Kolenovsky, Director
Connie Burkhalter, Education Coordinator & Coordinator of Teacher
Training
2222 Welborn Street, Room 425
Dallas, TX 75219-3993
(214) 559-7800

TSRH Literacy Program (Videotapes for adolescents and adults)
Elizabeth Cantrell, Outreach Director
Texas Scottish Rite Hospital for Children
2222 Welborn Street
Dallas, TX 75219-3993
(214) 559-7800

Wilson Language Training Corporation
Barbara A. Wilson
175 West Main Street
Millbury, MA 01527-1943
Tel: (800) 899-8454 or (508) 865-5699
Fax: (508) 865-9644
Email: info@wilsonlanguage.com
www.wilsonlanguage.com

ACCREDITATION

Academic Language Therapy Association (ALTA)
4020 McEwen, Suite #105
Dallas, TX 75244
(972) 907-3924

Academy of Orton-Gillingham Practitioners and Educators
East Main Street
Post Office Box # 234
Amenia, NY 12501
(914) 373-8919

International Multisensory Structured Language Education Council
(IMSLEC)
The June Shelton School
15720 Hillcrest Road
Dallas, TX 75248
(972) 774-1772

MATERIALS FOR TESTING AND INSTRUCTION

Addresses for publishers for the following materials are included at the end of this section (see the key).

ALPHABETIC PHONICS	EPS
Blocks and tokens for phoneme segmenting	Delta

Delta's math catalog lists two wonderful materials that can be used for phoneme segmentation and blending: (1) 2 cm colored wooden blocks and (2) rubber tokens with yellow on one side and blue on the other for consonants and vowels.

CLEAR AND LIVELY WRITING	Walker

(Priscilla Vail's book of ideas for teaching writing)

DIRECT INSTRUCTION READING	Merrill

Carnine, Silbert, and Kame'enui's book about the methods used in the DISTAR and Corrective Reading programs

DYSLEXIA TRAINING PROGRAM
DTP print materials	EPS
DTP tapes	Scottish Rite Hospital

FUNDATIONS
Wilson for K–2	Wilson

Puppets, Sound Cards, Word Cards, Student Readers, Instructor Manual, etc.

THE HOWARD STREET TUTORING MANUAL: TEACHING AT-RISK READERS IN THE PRIMARY GRADES	Guilford

(Darrell Morris's book with his developmental spelling test)

INSTA-LEARN MATERIALS	Step
J&J LANGUAGE READERS	Sopris
LADDERS TO LITERACY	Brookes

Teachers' manuals for Pre-K and K

LET'S READ	EPS

Readers by Bloomfield, Barnhart, and Barnhart used in Alphabetic Phonics

LINDAMOOD MATERIALS   PRO-ED
LiPs is the remedial program.
Lindamood Auditory Conceptualization Test (LAC)
is the test.

MERRILL LINGUISTIC READERS   Merrill

MULTISENSORY TEACHING APPROACH (MTA)   EPS

PREVENTING ACADEMIC FAILURE   EPS
Orton–Gillingham program by Phyllis Bertin
and Eileen Perlman which can be used with
the Merrill readers.

PHONOLOGICAL AWARENESS SKILLS PROGRAM   PRO-ED
AND PASP Test by Jerome Rosner

PRIMARY PHONICS   EPS

RECIPE FOR READING   EPS

SPELLMASTER   PRO-ED
Curriculum-based spelling tests

SLINGERLAND   EPS
Testing and remedial materials

STORY BOX BOOKS   Wright
A series of picture books (both big books and
little books) with predictable text used in
Reading Recovery and in many grade K-1 classrooms.

WILSON READING SYSTEM FUNDATIONS   Wilson or
(Wilson for K-2)   PRO-ED
Sound Cards, Word Cards, Student Readers,
Student Workbooks, Supplemental Readers,
Instructor Manual, etc.

WINSTON GRAMMAR PROGRAM   Hewitt
Parts-of-speech cards by Paul Irwin

WORDS   PRO-ED
Marcia Henry's Integrated Decoding and Spelling
Instruction Based on Word Origin and Word Structure.

WRITING SKILLS FOR ADOLESCENTS by Diana King   EPS
Teacher's guide and two workbooks for Grades 4 to adult

ADDRESSES FOR PUBLISHERS LISTED ABOVE

Academic Therapy Publishers   Academic
20 Commerical Boulevard
Novato, CA 94949
(415) 883-3314 or (800) 422-7249

Paul H. Brookes Publishing Company   Brookes
P.O. Box 10624
Baltimore, MD 21285-0624
www.brookespublishing.com

Delta Education, Inc.   Delta
P.O. Box 3000
Nashua, NH 03061
(800) 260-9577 or (603) 579-3494
Fax: (603) 579-3499
www.delta-education.com

Educators Publishing Service   EPS
P.O. Box 9031
Cambridge, MA 02139-9031
Tel: (800) 225-5750
Fax: (888) 440-2665
www.epsbooks.com

The Guilford Press   Guilford
72 Spring Street
New York, NY 10012

Hewitt Educational Resources   Hewitt
P.O. Box 9
Washougal, WA 98671-0009
(800) 348-1750 or (360) 835-8708

Lex Press   Lex
P.O. Box 859
Los Gatos, CA 95031

Merrill/Prentice Hall   Merrill
Professional Development for the Professional Educator
E-mail: csweb@pearsoned.com.

PRO-ED   PRO-ED
8700 Shoal Creek Boulevard
Austin, TX 78757
Tel: (800) 897-3202
Fax: (800) 397-7633
www.proedinc.com

Riverside Publishing Company   Riverside
425 Spring Lake Drive
Itasca, IL 60143-2079
Tel: (800) 323-9540 or (312) 693-0040
Fax: (630) 467-7162
www.riverpub.com

Sopris West, Inc.   Sopris
4093 Specialty Place
Longmont, CO 80504
(303) 651-2829 or (800) 547-6747
Fax: (888) 819-7767
Email: customerservice@sopriswest.com
www.sopriswest.com

Step, Inc.   Step
P.O. Box 887
Mukilteo, WA 98275-0887
(800) 225-7837

Wilson Language Training Corporation   Wilson
175 West Main Street
Millbury, MA 01527-1956
Catalog inquiries at: (508) 865-5699
Fax: (800) 218-9367
www.wilsonlanguage.com

Wright Group   Wright
19201 120th Avenue, N.E.
Bothell, WA 98011-9512
(800) 523-2371

Glossary of Terms

Affix — a letter or group of letters attached to the beginning or ending of a base word that changes the meaning of that word.

Alphabetic principle — the understanding or awareness that a temporal sequence of phonemes in spoken words (e.g., the sounds /b/-/u/-/g/) map onto a left-to-right sequence of letters in written words (e.g., bug). The alphabetic principle requires phoneme awareness as well as letter-sound knowledge.

C-V-C — a word composed of letters with the consonant-vowel-consonant pattern. These short vowel words are a common starting point for reading phonetically regular words.

Digraph — two successive letters in the same syllable representing a single speech sound. A consonant digraph is made up of two successive letters representing a single consonant sound, e.g., *sh, th, ph*. A vowel digraph involves two successive letters representing a single vowel sound, e.g., *oa, ai*.

Diphthong — two adjacent vowels in the same syllable whose sounds slide as they blend together. Cox lists four English dipthongs: *ou* as in *out*, *ow* as in *cow*, *oi* as in *oil*, and *oy* as in *boy* (1984, p.15).

Dysgraphia — severe handwriting disorder due to poor eye-hand coordination.

Etymology — the study of the origins and derivations of words.

Gestalt — a pattern or configuration that constitutes, and is conceived as, a unit or whole.

Grapheme — a single letter or letter cluster representing a single speech sound, e.g., *i*, *igh* (Cox, 1984, p. 17).

Inflectual ending — a morpheme added to the end of a word that changes its meaning in terms of grammatical case, number, gender, or tense, e.g., *ing* in *ending*, *ed* in *ended*.

Laterality — the choice of hand, eye, or foot in performing everyday activities.

Lateralization — dominance of one or the other cerebral hemispheres for any form of brain functioning.

Lexicon — a body of word knowledge, either spoken or written.

Morpheme — a meaningful unit of speech. A morpheme may be a whole word, e.g., *child*; a base word, e.g., *child* in *childhood*; a suffix, e.g., *hood* in *childhood*; or a prefix, e.g., *un* in *untie*. A single morpheme may have many forms, as for example, the morpheme for plurality: *s* in *dogs*, *es* in *foxes*, *a* in *data*. Each of these forms is an allomorph of the morpheme for plurality.

Morphograph — written form of a word part that has meaning such as the ending -tion.

Morphological — in linguistic terms, an adjective referring to meaningful units of speech; a suffix, for example, is a morphological (or inflectional) ending.

Multisensory — involving three or more senses, usually visual, auditory, kinesthetic (awareness of muscle movement), or tactile.

Neuron — a nerve cell.

Onset — the initial portion of a word, spoken or written, which, when segmented, leaves the rime, e.g., *c* in *cat* and *str* in *stretch*.

Orthography — the spelling of written language.

Orthographic — pertaining to the spelling of written language.

Phoneme — an individual sound unit in spoken words. The "smallest unit of speech that distinguishes one utterance from another . . . in the speech of a particular person or particular dialect . . ." (Webster's third edition).

Phonics — 1. "The science of sound" (Webster's third edition). 2. "The central use of letter-sound connections in the teaching of reading and spelling" (Cox, 1984, p. 25).

Phonogram — "A symbol or symbols used to represent a single speech sound" (Cox, 1984, p.25).

Phonological — pertaining to the speech sounds in words.

Phonology — the science of speech sounds, including the development of speech sounds in one language or comparison of speech sound development in different languages (Webster's third edition).

Prefix — a morpheme (unit of meaning) involving a letter or combination of letters attached to the beginning of a base word that changes the meaning of that word, e.g., *tri* in *tricycle*.

Rime — the vowel and final consonant(s) portion of a word, in contrast with the onset or initial consonant(s), e.g., *at* in *cat*, and *itch* in *switch*. The term is sometimes used to indicate printed words alone and sometimes oral rhyme as well.

Scheme or schema — in psychological terms, a theoretical framework of knowledge. Plural form: schemata.

Schwa — an unaccented vowel whose pronunciation approximates the short/u/sound, as the first and last *a* in *banana* or the *o* in *carrot*.

Suffix — a morpheme (unit of meaning) involving a letter or combination of letters attached to the end of a word that changes the meaning of that word, e.g., *s* in *cats*.

Syntax — sentence structure. "That part of grammar which treats the relation of words, according to established usage" (Cox., 1984, p. 31).

Index